The Roots of Cognitive Neuroscience

The Roots of Cognitive Neuroscience

Behavioral Neurology and Neuropsychology

EDITED BY ANJAN CHATTERJEE

and

H. BRANCH COSLETT

OXFORD
UNIVERSITY PRESS

OXFORD
UNIVERSITY PRESS

Oxford University Press is a department of the University of Oxford.
It furthers the University's objective of excellence in research, scholarship,
and education by publishing worldwide.

Oxford New York
Auckland Cape Town Dar es Salaam Hong Kong Karachi
Kuala Lumpur Madrid Melbourne Mexico City Nairobi
New Delhi Shanghai Taipei Toronto

With offices in
Argentina Austria Brazil Chile Czech Republic France Greece
Guatemala Hungary Italy Japan Poland Portugal Singapore
South Korea Switzerland Thailand Turkey Ukraine Vietnam

Published in the United States of America by
Oxford University Press
198 Madison Avenue, New York, NY 10016

Library of Congress Cataloging-in-Publication Data
The roots of cognitive neuroscience : behavioral neurology and neuropsychology / edited by
Anjan Chatterjee, H. Branch Coslett.
pages cm
Includes bibliographical references and index.
ISBN 978-0-19-539554-9
1. Cognitive neuroscience. 2. Clinical neuropsychology. 3. Neuropsychiatry.
I. Chatterjee, Anjan, editor of compilation. II. Coslett, H. Branch, editor of compilation.
QP360.5.R66 2014
612.8′233—dc23
2013012874

9 8 7 6 5 4 3 2 1
Printed in the United States of America
on acid-free paper

CONTENTS

PREFACE

Cognitive neuroscience is in high fashion. Images with colored patches showing brain regions that are active when we think, perceive, feel, and make decisions grace the covers of the most prestigious scientific journals. Every month, neuroscientists seem to be making new discoveries about why we are the way we are. Even the general public has an inexhaustible appetite for neural explanations for our behavior. Advanced technologies promise to demystify the mind as they reveal detailed workings of the brain. Most research universities now have imaging centers in which scientists can picture brains functioning in vivo. Many use novel electrical recording techniques and non-invasive stimulation methods to understand how the brain works. In this climate of progress, driven by technology that was inconceivable only a generation ago, why publish a book focused on an old approach to the brain? The answer is simple. As the chapters in this volume demonstrate, behavioral neurology and neuropsychology remain just as relevant to advancing our understanding of the biology of cognitive and affective systems as they were 150 years ago.

Examining the behavior of individuals with neurologic disease, sometimes referred to as "the lesion method," informs our understanding of cognitive and affective systems in several ways. Firstly, as has been noted in the past, patients reveal how large-scale systems can be "carved at their joints." Understanding the nature of these joints and the way that different components articulate reveals the nature of the system under consideration. Secondly, the lesion method allows us to test hypotheses about the role of neural structures in a way not possible by other methods. Whether or not a particular region of the brain is necessary for a mental operation is tested directly by assessing the consequences of damage to that part of the brain. Finally, the striking phenomenology in patients, behaviors that most of us would not have imagined possible, allows us to generate hypotheses about the organization of the mind. How is it possible for someone to know facts about the world and not facts about their own life? Why does someone speak, but not understand? What does it mean for a person to recognize some, but not other parts of their body? How can an intelligent and articulate person behave as if one side of the universe has vanished? These and many other deeply counterintuitive phenomena reveal something about the structure of the mind as implemented in the brain. They generate hypotheses to be tested, and, as occurred with the most celebrated case in all of behavioral neurology and neuropsychology, Henry Molaison (better known as H. M.), they can radically change the basic understanding of how our minds are organized.

Beyond making the case for the central importance of behavioral neurology and neuropsychology today, we have another aim in publishing this book. We wish to acknowledge the contributions and influence of our mentor, Dr. Kenneth M. Heilman. We both have been deeply affected by Dr. Heilman, whom we met at critical times in our peculiarly similar academic paths. We were both medical students at the University of Pennsylvania (separated by several years) at a time when a career of studying cognition as a neurologist was at best regarded with bewilderment, and, more typically, with condescension. After our neurology residencies, we both did post-doctoral fellowships at the University of Florida under Dr. Heilman's guidance. Branch went on to work at Temple University for several years. Anjan started his academic career at the University of Alabama in Birmingham. In the late 1990s, we both returned to the University of Pennsylvania to join the neurology department and to work at the Penn Center for Cognitive Neuroscience. The rise of neuroimaging had made behavioral neurology attractive even in a place like Penn that had long been a bastion of neuromuscular research.

Over the last 45 years, Dr. Heilman has been and remains one of the most productive and creative thinkers in this field. The chapters in this book, in addition to showing the relevance of patient studies, reveal Dr. Heilman's influence, which extends beyond his own research into his impact on subsequent generations of neurologists, neuropsychologists, and speech pathologists. These chapters, written by his students, represent but a small sample of those whose thinking has been touched by his agile mind.

The book begins with a chapter by Dr. Heilman. He reminds us of the importance of single case studies. This contribution is followed by a chapter that shows that the questions asked in the Golden Age of neurology, from the 1860s to the beginning of the First World War, were prescient in identifying concerns that we still face when theorizing about how mind arises from brain. The other chapters cover diverse areas such as language and semantics, emotion, attention, praxis, body representations, the nature of self, pharmacology, plasticity, and even art and creativity. Dr. Heilman has made his own mark in each of these fields. However, the chapters are not reviews of his contribution. Rather, they reflect the current understanding of these fundamental areas of cognitive neuroscience as informed by the study of people with neurological disease.

This is a book for cognitive neuroscientists, neurologists, psychiatrists, psychologists, physiatrists, and scholars in general interested in the biology of the human mind. Importantly, the book is also aimed at medical, neuroscience, and psychology students who are still forming their views of cognitive neuroscience. We hope the book will disabuse readers of two (in our view) wrong-headed notions. The first notion is that cognitive neuroscience is synonymous with functional neuroimaging. This misconception confuses a domain of scientific inquiry with a method. While functional neuroimaging has certainly invigorated cognitive neuroscience, the field has deep roots tracing back at least to the second half of the 19th century. The second notion is that while patient studies might be of historical interest, the real way forward is through new technologies such as functional neuroimaging. This view is misguided because the interpretation of imaging data is now relatively unconstrained. The widespread use of reverse inferences (inferring a mental operation based on neural locations of activation patterns) begs to be corralled. Lesion studies offer the perfect foil for functional neuroimaging studies as a method for confirming or rejecting hypotheses generated by activation patterns. The tremendous growth of functional imaging research makes lesion studies more important than they have ever been, if we are to ground our cognitive theorizing.

Finally, we should mention that this book would not have been possible without the help and patience of the staff at Oxford University Press. Joan Bossert, our editor, who also edited Dr. Heilman and Dr. Valenstein's classic *Clinical Neuropsychology,* was unfailingly supportive of our efforts

Anjan Chatterjee
H. Branch Coslett

CONTRIBUTORS

A.M. Barrett
Kessler Institute of Rehabilitation
West Orange, NJ

David Q. Beversdorf
University of Missouri
Columbia, MO

Lee X. Blonder
University of Kentucky
Lexington, KY

Anjan Chatterjee
University of Pennsylvania
Philadelphia, PA

H. Branch Coslett
University of Pennsylvania
Philadelphia, PA

Valeria Drago
IRCCS Fatebenefratelli, Laboratorio LENITEM
Brescia, Itlay

Todd Feinberg
Albert Einstein College of Medicine
Bronx, NY

Glen R. Finney
University of Florida
Gainesville, FL

Anne Foundas
Louisiana State University
New Orleans, LA

Kenneth M. Heilman
University of Florida
Gainesville, FL

Margaret M. Keane
Wellesley College
Wellesley, MA

Elizabeth Lacey
Johns Hopkins University
Baltimore, MD

Victor W. Mark
University of Alabama in Birmingham
Birmingham, AL

Kimford J. Meador
Emory University
Atlanta, GA

Mark Mennemeier
University of Arkansas for Medical Sciences
Little Rock, AR

Steven E. Nadeau
University of Florida
Gainesville, FL

Steven Rapscak
University of Arizona
Tucson, AZ

Anastasia M. Raymer
Old Dominion University
Norfolk, VA

David Roeltgen
Cape Regional Medical Center
Cape May Court House, NJ

Heidi Roth
University of North Carolina
Chapel Hill, NC

Leslie J. Gonzalez Rothi
University of Florida
Gainesville, FL

Edward Valenstein
University of Florida
Gainesville, FL

MiekeVerfaellie
Boston University
Boston, MA

Robert T. Watson
Florida State University
Tallahassee, FL

CHAPTER 1

The Case for Case Reports

Kenneth M. Heilman

In the motion picture *Flash of Genius*, the engineer who invented the intermittent windshield wiper sued Ford Motor Company for stealing his idea. A witness for Ford explained that this engineer did not invent the transistors, condensers, or other major elements of this wiper system, and that all of this had already been invented. The engineer who invented this intermittent wiper held up a book, *A Tale of Two Cities*, and started reading. He read the first word, "It" and then asked this witness if Dickens invented the word *it*? The witness said, "No." The engineer then asked if Dickens invented the word *was*, or the next words, "the best...," or any of the words in this book, and the witness said, "No." He then asked the witness, "If Dickens did not invent these words, why should he get credit for writing this book?" The engineer won the suit against Ford because it was the *means* by which he put these components together to develop a system that he created that was significant, and creating systems is as important as creating components.

Many basic science researchers do not consider the research performed in cognitive neuroscience, neuropsychology, and behavioral neurology as sciences because cognitive systems neuroscientists, unlike basic scientists, do not discover new proteins, neurotransmitters and neuromodulators, genes, or new structures. Cognitive systems neuroscientists do, however, discover how complex systems in the brain perform their functions, and also learn how failures in these systems adversely influence behavior. Perhaps these same basic scientists would argue that, since Dickens did not invent words, he should not be given credit for his great novel.

One of the aspects of behavioral neurology-neuropsychology that is most despised by many basic as well as clinical scientists is the case study. Recently, there has been a movement to severely limit these reports because many people do not consider them scientific. Several journals have also decided not to publish case studies. For example, Johnston and Hauser (2007), editors of the *Annals of*

Neurology, define case reports as "descriptions of fewer than 10 cases." They state that "one must always be concerned about reliability of inference based on an n of one. No statistics are possible in case reports. Inference is entirely dependent, then, on subjective judgment." These editors also noted that, of the various articles published, reviews were the most highly quoted, and that case reports were the least quoted. Those case reports published in the *Annals* received 60 percent fewer citations than "research articles." Since case reports do receive fewer citations, these editors believe the research community acknowledges the limited quality of these reports. Based on this reasoning, the editors state that they will continue to consider case reports. "However, we expect that the vast majority will be rejected without review."

The editors of the *Annals* are not alone in their de-evaluation of case reports. In an editorial in *Brain,* John Newsome-David and John Rothwell noted *Brain*'s high impact factor and also felt that limiting case reports will help further improve that impact factor. Recently, we (Torres, Heilman and Poizner, in press) contrasted the reaching movements, in the dark, of patients with Parkinson's disease (PD) who have basal-ganglia network dysfunction with those of a patient with a discrete injury to his posterior parietal cortex (PPCL) under three different sensory-guidance conditions: (1) brief and temporary viewing of the allocentric spatial target location and no viewing of the moving forelimb; (2) continuous viewing of the spatial target location (allocentric guidance) with no viewing for the forelimb; and (3) brief and temporary viewing of the target with continuous viewing of the moving finger (egocentric guidance). While the patient with the PPCL was helped most with continuous allocentric-based guidance, the patients with PD were helped most with continuous egocentric based guidance. These results suggest that for the programming and planning of reaching movements, the basal-ganglia-frontal circuits and the posterior-parietal cortex default to complementary sources of sensory (egocentric versus allocentric) information. We thought that this finding was novel and important and sent this paper to *Brain.* The paper was never reviewed, and we received the following response from the editors, "Thank you for submitting the above manuscript which we have considered carefully, but regret to inform you will not be considered further as a submission to *Brain.* Our current policy is very rarely to publish single case studies..."

Hospital and medical schools often consider surgeons more important than neurologists because surgeons make much more money than do neurologists, unless the neurologist brings in large sums of research funding. Recently, I was told by the director of our Gainesville VAMC Geriatric Research and Educational Clinical Center (GRECC) that he had to do his yearly report, and he needed to know about our research activities. When I told him that I would get him a list of the papers we published this past year, he apologetically told me that, while he was interested in these papers, the VA director and chief of staff were not interested in papers; they wanted to know the amount of research funds we brought in.

There are several serious errors in the Johnston's and Hauser editorial published in the *Annals of Neurology*. For example, they state, "No statistics are possible in case reports." There are many means of performing statistical analyses in case reports. These statistics can allow the investigator to know whether whatever is being measured in the case is different from a demographically matched normal population. There are statistical methods that can also inform the investigators about the reliability of the findings. Johnston and Hauser also state "Inference is entirely dependent, then, on subjective judgment." In single-subject studies, there are even statistical means of testing possible causation. For example, a patient can be repeatedly tested until they form a stable baseline, and after a stable baseline is established, a treatment can be instituted. If this treatment is either beneficial or harmful, the patient's performance will be altered from this baseline, and this alteration can be tested for significance.

Some critics of case reports are of the opinion that many case reports are nothing more than a serendipitous event. It is possible that a person might have a genetic defect or some other unique event that caused a disease, and that the mutation or event that led to this disease is unique to that person; however, while some case reports of previously unreported diseases do turn out to be rare diseases, the vast majority of case reports are subsequently demonstrated not to be unique. The knowledge that a clinician has discovered a new and unreported finding is also not serendipitous. No matter how many patients a clinician sees in their practice, it is the prepared mind that discovers the new findings that make a case reportable. To know that an observation is novel and that this novel observation is important, the clinician has to know that which is known, that which is not known, and that which may be important for others to know. Louis Pasteur stated that, "In the fields of observation, chance favors only the prepared mind."

Compared with population studies that may examine diagnostic tests or treatments (i.e., "evidence-based medicine"), case reports intensely investigate and describe the individual with the disease-disorder in the context of comorbidities and individual characteristics. It is often the individual differences that produce variability, and thus, population studies require statistical analyses to learn whether whatever result they observe is just a random event or unlikely to be a random event. It is exceedingly rare with a group or population study to have no variability. Learning the factors that caused this variation may be very important. However, to learn what caused this variability, the investigators would have to perform a series of case studies. Unless all subjects in a population study show the same effect, shouldn't a clinician and investigator still be concerned about reliability and making inferences based on these population studies?

Many people will state that case reports, case studies, or case series are uncontrolled, and since they are uncontrolled, are likely to be incorrect. When people prepare to write up case reports or n = 1 studies to submit to a journal, they attempt to learn if there have been other similar reports. Now with Internet tools such as PubMed, this task has become relatively easy. If the clinician-investigator learns that his or her observation has not been previously reported, and that he or she might have a new observation, this observation should be shared with others who might see the same phenomenon or who might want to do further research. However, it is important for this novel contribution to be confirmed by future studies and reports. If the clinician investigator does find prior reports of patients with the same finding, he or she might want to perform some type of meta-analysis that might allow them to find a thread that unites the findings, and thus leads to them to a new level of understanding.

These anti-case report messages from editors may be a very serious sign of a deeper sociological disorder, and it is possible that this disorder may seriously retard medical progress. The editorials mentioned above suggest that the "bean counters" have even taken control of our journals. And, unfortunately, the bean-counter mentality appears to be infectious, and is even corrupting the minds of brilliant scientists who make decisions about the type of papers that should be accepted for publication. Journals are ranked by "impact factors," and the impact factor is highly dependent on citations of the articles published in that journal. The editors of the *Annals of Neurology* as well as of *Brain* boast about their high impact factor. Thus, editors can increase the prestige of their journal by accepting papers that are likely to be frequently cited, and rejecting those that are cited less frequently, such as case reports. Review papers rarely present information that stimulates what Kuhn (1996) termed a "paradigmatic shift." These papers are often highly quoted because they summarize advances in a domain of research, and when people write papers, a reference to a review paper will often reduce the number of references required. But are citations really a valid means of measuring an article's importance? The real measure of the importance of an article is the novelty of the information, and how this information will affect clinical care as well as future research.

Jenicek (1999) states that case reports may be the "weakest" level of evidence, but they often remain the first line of evidence, and it is with the publication of a case report that discovery and education about a disease often begins. Anyone who is familiar with the history of neurology knows that most paradigmatic shifts in neurology have been initiated by case reports. It is difficult to think of a neurological disease that was not originally a case report, or a small series of case reports. Thus case reports or case studies have been a critical element in advancing neurology, and especially the sub-specialty of behavioral and cognitive neurology (Heilman, 2004).

In the clinic, the clinician-scientist has the opportunity to observe anomalies. By an anomaly, we mean a novel observation (i.e., an observation which has not been previously reported). The observation of an anomaly suggests that the scientific theory that attempted to explain the order in a system is inadequate, and a new theory that can accounts for this anomaly must be developed. The development of a major new theory based on the awareness of anomaly would be a paradigmatic shift.

There are many definitions of creativity. In a prior publication, I defined creativity as "the ability to understand, develop, and express in a systematic fashion novel orderly relationships" (Heilman et al., 2003). In this definition, novelty is a critical element of creativity, and novel ideas are a product of disengagement and divergent thinking. Thomas Kuhn (1996) in his book, *The Structure of Scientific Revolutions,* also stated that, "Discovery commences with the awareness of an anomaly." Awareness of an anomaly is a whisper of nature, and the people who hear this whisper are able to recognize that our knowledge is incomplete or that current theories might be either inadequate or incorrect. When some investigators hear this whisper of nature, they can develop and test new theories that will help account for these anomalies. These new theories and research that are performed to test these new theories often lead to a paradigmatic shift.

Traditionally, psychiatrists have studied disorders of the mind, and neurologists have studied disorders of the brain; however, it was with the development of behavioral and cognitive neurology that physicians started to study how disorders-diseases of the brain caused disorders of the mind. Modern behavioral and cognitive neurology began with four critical papers. The first, was the report of Phineas Gage by Harlow (1848). Gage, who had a severe frontal injury from an iron bar that was propelled into his brain, had a profound change in his personality, and Gage's story is still quoted in many reports about frontal lobe function and dysfunction. The interest in Gage has remained so strong that a reconstruction of Gage's skull and brain, after his injury, was reported by Damasio et al in 1994.

The second important paper was that of Paul Broca (1861), who reported a patient who sustained a left anterior hemispheric stroke that resulted in a loss of speech fluency. The patient, Leborgne, made few meaningful utterances, but frequently repeated the word "tan." This patient had relatively intact comprehension, but also impaired naming and ability to repeat. The third report, by Karl Wernicke (1874), described a patient who, unlike Lebourgne, spoke fluently, but spoke in jargon, and could not understand or repeat speech. Wernicke not only reported this patient with what is now known as Wernicke's aphasia, but also based his case as well as upon knowing about the patient reported by Broca Wernicke developed a speech-language information processing model, and based on this model, he was able to predict the observation of patients with conduction aphasia. Lichtheim (1885) described two patients with different forms of aphasia. One, like Wernicke's patient, could not comprehend, but unlike Wernicke's patient, could repeat. The other, like Broca's patient, was non-fluent, but unlike Broca's patient, Lichtheim's patient could repeat. Based on these cases, Lichtheim modified and enhanced Wernicke's speech information processing model that helped to explain several new types of aphasia.

Important case reports which produced paradigmatic shifts are neither limited to speech disorders-aphasia, nor were they just reported at the founding of behavioral and cognitive neurology in the 19th century. For example, the world famous patient H. M. recently died. H. M. had epilepsy that could not be controlled by medications. Since he had seizures emanating from both his left and right anterior-medial temporal lobes, both anterior temporal lobes were surgically removed. When H. M. recovered from surgery, he had a profound deficit of his episodic memory. H. M. was subsequently studied by more than 100 different investigators, and there have been several hundred papers and reports written about different aspects of H. M.'s memory. These case studies of H. M. produced a paradigmatic shift in our understanding of memory. Before the initial report by Scoville and Milner (1957), it was not known that removal of both hippocampi would induce this devastating amnesic disorder. Papez posited that a circuit comprised of the hippocampus, fornix, mammillary bodies, thalamus, cingulate gyrus, and retrosplenial cortex was important for mediating emotions; however, the studies initiated by the novel observation that H. M. had impaired episodic memory, but not impaired semantic or procedural memory after ablation of a portion of this "Papez" circuit (i.e., hippocampus) revolutionized our understanding of the neural basis of episodic memory.

Temporal lobectomy remains an important treatment of poorly medically controlled epilepsy, but now, the neurologists, psychologists, and neurosurgeons who take care of these patients attempt to protect the normal hippocampus in one hemisphere as well as other portions of the Papez circuit in this hemisphere. If Scoville and Milner submitted the report of H. M. to *Annals of Neurology* or *Brain,* there is a high probability that it would have been rejected without a review because it was just a case report.

Since Broca's and Wernicke's initial reports, studies of behavioral-anatomic fractionation have provided cognitive neuroscientists and clinicians with important information as to the modular organization of the brain and how local brain dysfunction might lead to specific forms of aberrant behavior. Many of the cognitive behaviors performed by humans, such as speech, sensory recognition, and memory (episodic, semantic, and procedural) are complex functions that are mediated by systems that have many components, and many of these component functions are mediated by anatomically distinct areas of the brain.

Caramazza (1986) noted that the experimental method used in a study is heavily dependent on the type of question that this research is attempting to answer. According to Caramazza, when cognitive scientists are attempting to understand brain function in normal subjects, as well as how brain function is altered with injury, the case study methods are highly valuable. Although Caramazza notes that studies that use large sample of participants do provide information about this group's average performance there is the assumption with group data that if there are individual differences, these differences are random and irrelevant. In certain studies this irrelevant assumption might be acceptable; however, if group data is used to understand the cognitive changes induced by injury, the group study of patients with brain damage would only be valid if each patient is identical in "all theoretically relevant respects...." When studying patients with brain damage, such as stroke, it is rare for any two subjects to have exactly the same anatomic lesion, and even when studying patients with degenerative diseases, it is rare that all participants will have the same severity and loci of degeneration. According to Caramazza, since these homogeneity criteria can rarely be met, grouped observations cannot be validly used to draw inferences about normal cognitive systems. Caramazza also notes that since group studies do not contain homogeneous participants, these studies have to use statistical analyses, and any conclusions drawn from such studies must contain probabilistic statements. In most group studies, there are no detailed analyses of the exceptions, and as discussed above, it is the exceptions or anomalies that often will provide important insights that lead to paradigmatic shifts in understanding.

Unfortunately, there is no single perfect method of studying the brain, and the lesion-case study method, even with double dissociations, also has its limitations. Hughlings Jackson (1932) recognized that with brain injuries, there are changes in behavior, and that injuries alter behaviors by two major mechanisms. The injury to a specific area of the brain causes a loss of the functions mediated by this portion of the brain; however, in addition to mediating specific functions, the injured area might have been inhibiting another more phylogenetic "primitive" area that performs a more stereotypical form of behavior, and this injury "releases" these more stereotypical primitive behaviors. In addition, as Monakow (Finger et al., 2004) noted, brain injury causes diaschisis, in which areas of the brain that have not been directly damaged, but are connected with the damaged area, malfunction; malfunction of an area not directly injured can also produce behavioral changes. Lastly, although a specific portion of the brain might be mediating a function, there might be other areas of the brain that can also perform this function (functional plasticity), and, with damage to an area, other areas can compensate for the damaged area. Thus, even damage to an area that mediates a specific function might not lead to permanent changes in that function.

There are several other theoretical problems-limitations of case reports. When a report appears in a journal, the authors, editors, and readers want to know whether that which has been reported is valid (sound and cogent). Validity in medicine and science requires that the findings -observations be replicable-reliable, and that conclusions drawn from this case report be demonstrated to be correct. Since case studies are based on individual patients, these observations have not been replicated, and thus, might not be valid. When reporting a case, the authors should invite others to replicate the findings of this case to help establish reliability. However, people have to be aware of the disorder before they can attempt to replicate the prior observations. Validity also depends on further testing of the hypotheses that are raised by the case report, which might include gaining a better understanding of pathophysiology.

For the reasons mentioned above, cognitive-systems neuroscientists have to be cautious when deducing the function of a specific brain area based on injury to or degeneration of that area. It is important to obtain converging evidence. In regard to behavioral neurology, neuropsychology, and speech pathology, in addition to behavioral analyses designed to determine the functional systems that are impaired and, by inference, the systems that normally mediate specific behaviors, there are now many powerful tools that will allow us to provide converging evidence and help understand pathophysiology, including: electroencephalography and evoked potentials, fMRI, positron emission tomography (PET), magneto-encephalography, electrical stimulation, magnetic stimulation, and neurochemical-neurotransmitter analyses.

Case studies can also have an important influence on the training of clinical investigators. A part of my career that has been very rewarding is introducing new neurobehavioral fellows into research. Many of the former fellows had never done research, and were concerned as to whether or not they had the ability to perform research. One of the things I do is to remind them that, during their training, they have already learned to perform research. In their practice, neurologists see patients who are often referred from other physicians. Typically, based on the history they obtain and their findings on examination, they use convergent thinking to decide where in the brain-spinal cord-neuromuscular system these patients are having their dysfunction. Then, based on this localization, they may use divergent thinking to come up with a list of possible causes, and based on these possibilities, they may then order tests that will help confirm or disconfirm each of the possibilities. In many respects, almost all new patients seen by clinical neuroscientists are research projects in which the clinician, based on her or his observations, develops a-priori hypotheses, and then tests these hypotheses. Thus, case studies come closest to the type of clinical functions that the fellows have performed. There are times when seeing patients, and asking "where, why and how" questions, that there is a surprise finding. This unexpected or novel finding may be an opportunity to learn something new about the nervous system, and share it with others who will find this novel finding to be important in their understanding of the nervous system and the diseases that might affect it.

In summary, although there is little doubt that controlled studies and evidence-based medicine are crucial to the advancement of medicine, these advancements are often initiated by case reports. One of the fundamental components of creativity is novelty, and novelty in the medical, speech, and psychological sciences is often the product of a careful clinical evaluation. In medicine, and especially in neurology, we are continuing to discover new diseases. Clinicians and scientists need to know about new diseases so that patients can be diagnosed, mechanisms can be determined, and treatments developed. The only means of reporting the observation of new diseases are case reports and case series. Case reports and studies also may allow us to uncover the mechanisms of certain diseases. Many medicines currently in use to treat diseases were not developed for the purpose that they are currently being used, and these beneficial, as well as adverse, effects were often initially observed and reported as case reports. Just as hospitals' administrative "bean counters" are attempting to reduce the time a physician spends with each patient, several journal editors are trying to reduce the number of case reports, case studies, and case series reported in journals. By implementing this policy, these editors may be increasing their journal's citations and ranking; however, just as seeing patients more rapidly might make more money for departments, clinics and health centers, this reduction of time spent with patients reduces the quality of care. Not publishing case studies will no doubt retard the advancement of medicine. As mentioned by Jenicek (1999), case reports may be the "weakest" level of evidence, but they often remain the first line of evidence, and it is in the publication of case reports that discovery and education about a disease often begins.

We have had a neurobehavioral fellowship program at the University of Florida for almost 40 years. One of the greatest gifts in my life has been the privilege of helping to train these fellows, many of whom are now leaders in behavioral and cognitive neurology, neuropsychology, speech therapy and even anthropology. When many of these fellows started their fellowship, they were concerned about their ability to perform research, and often it was a case study that introduced them to research. In this book, several of our most prominent former neurobehavioral fellows write about some of their important research contributions, including case studies. It will be apparent to people who read these chapters that case studies have done much to advance our science, and hopefully they will continue to help.

References

Broca, P. Remarques sur le siege de la faculté de la parole articulée, suives d'une observation d'aphemie (perte de parole). *Bulletins de la Société Anatomique de Paris.* 1861; 36: 330–357.

Caramazza, A. The logic of neuropsychological research and the problem of patient classification in aphasia. *Brain and Language.* 1984; 21:9–20.

Damasio, H., Grabowski, T., Frank, R., Galaburda, A. M., Damasio, A.R. The return of Phineas Gage: clues about the brain from the skull of a famous patient. *Science.* May 20; 1994; 264(5162): 1102–5.

Finger, S., Koehler, P.J., Jagella, C. The Monakow concept of diaschisis: origins and perspectives. *Archives of Neurology.* 2004;61: 283–288.

Harlow, J.M. Passage of an iron rod through the head. *The Boston Medical and Surgical Journal.* 1848; 39:389–393.

Heilman, K. M., Nadeau, S. E., Beversdorf, D. O. Creative innovation: Possible brain mechanisms. *Neurocase.* 2003; 9: 369–379.

Heilman, K.M. Case reports and case studies: An endangered species. *Cognitive and Behavioral Neurology.* 2004; 17: 121.

Jackson, J.H. *Selected Writing of John Hughlings Jackson.* Taylor, I., ed. London: Hodder and Stoughton, 1932.
Jenicek, M. Clinical Case Reporting. In *Evidence Based Medicine,* Oxford, U.K, Butterworth-Heinemann, 1999.
Johnston, C. and Hauser, S. L. Message from the Editor: The Value of a Case Report. *Annals of Neurology.* 2007; 62(2):A11–A12.
Kuhn, T.S. *The Structure of Scientific Revolutions,* 3rd ed. Chicago: University Chicago Press, 1996.
Lichtheim, L. On aphasia. *Brain.* 1885; 7:433–485.
Scoville, W.B. and Milner, B. Loss of recent memory after bilateral hippocampal lesions. *Journal of Neurology, Neurosurgery, & Psychiatry.* 1957; 20:11–21.
Wernicke, C. *Der aphasische Symptomencomplex.* Breslau: Frank und Weigert, 1874.

CHAPTER 2

We Stand on the Shoulders of Giants: The Golden Era of Behavioral Neurology 1860–1950 and Its Relevance to Cognitive Neuroscience Today

Heidi L. Roth

The golden era of behavioral neurology from 1860 to the mid-20th century generated an enormous literature filled with careful clinical observations and comprehensive models of cognitive function. The extent of this literature can easily be underappreciated, but a review of publications by leading scientists and physicians of the time reveals its vastness and depth.

Among other topics, this period is filled with active debates and thoughtful consideration of the neurological organization of language, action, and perception. The models derived from this period have in some cases directly shaped, and in others, strongly influenced modern models in these areas.

Here, we will examine important models from this period and highlight how they remain relevant to our current understanding of cognition. We will also highlight some of the challenges faced by the researchers from the past which are not unlike those faced by scientists today. Much of this work was based on the examination of patients with brain lesions. We begin with a review of the challenges faced at the beginning of the 1860s when the concept of modularity of higher functions was first established by Paul Broca in his reports on his cases of aphasia in France. After that, we will consider Carl Wernicke's contribution to the understanding of language and aphasia and his use of diagrams and connectionist flow models of higher cognitive function. Finally, we will consider subsequent studies of apraxia and visual agnosia that were influenced by Wernicke's approach. Throughout, we will try to elucidate how and why the early contributions were accepted, the criticisms to which they were vulnerable, and how our current models of function are indebted to them.

Language and Aphasia

BROCA: MODULARITY OF HIGHER-LEVEL FUNCTIONS AND THE USE OF THE CLINICAL-PATHOLOGICAL METHOD

Language is one of the "highest" cognitive functions, closely associated with a person's identity and intelligence. In the early 19th century, there were both scientific and ideological arguments opposing the view that language might be localized in the brain, but the paper entitled "Remarks on the Seat of the Faculty of Articulate Speech, Followed by a Case of Aphemia (Loss of Speech)," published in 1861, by Pierre Paul Broca (1824–1880) in represented an important turning point (Broca 1861/1977). Broca's report and the debates that followed began to convince people, at least in France, that higher-level cortical functions might be associated with injury in a particular area of the brain.

Broca's description of aphasia was certainly not the first, and there were fairly detailed reports of the characteristics of aphasic language that had been previously recorded. The fact that language dysfunction could occur from a head injury was even mentioned in the Egyptian Surgical Papyrus from 2300 B.C.E. (Breasted, 1930). In the early 19th century, not long before Broca, the phrenological program introduced by Franz Joseph Gall (1758–1828) and popularized by Johann Spurzheim, posited that psychological/cognitive functions were localized in circumscribed areas of the cortex. They even proposed that language ability or verbal memory was located in the front part of the brain. They also suggested that the size of the cortical regions should correlate with the degree of development of that function, and that differences between people could be assessed by feeling bumps on the skull, which would reflect the underlying topography of the brain (Gall & Spurzheim, 1810–1819, 1835).

By the time Broca was active, the phrenological ideas of Gall had been strongly discredited, and the enthusiasm for searching for the brain basis for higher-level cognitive functions had lost momentum. Gall failed to provide scientific evidence for his theories. At the same time, experimental physiologists failed to find evidence for regional specialization in the cortex of higher-level behavior in their studies of animals. The most prominent experimental physiologist in France, Pierre Flourens (1794–1867), ablated parts of the cerebral hemispheres of pigeons and observed that specific functions in the higher-level domain (excluding respiration and vital functions, which were controlled by the brain stem, and motor functions, which were controlled by the cerebellum) were not affected by where the ablation took place (Flourens, 1824). He found only that overall loss of function occurred with cortical lesions, irrespective of where they were placed, and the final impairment seemed to depend only on the total amount of brain removed. This supported a view of the brain organization called the "law of mass action." According to the law of mass action, all tissue in the brain could contribute to the performance of any specific task of higher behavior, and performance of any specific kind would degrade depending on the amount, not on the specific area of tissue removed. Flourens's conclusion and opinions, especially in the context of the political and religious milieu at the time, which favored more anti-materialistic views of mind, were quite influential. A physician named Francois Bouillaud was a lonely crusader during this time for the view that language abilities were located in the anterior part of the brain, and he collected over 100 clinical-pathological cases to support this view (Bouillaud, 1847–1848).

Paul Broca was a surgeon interested in brain and skull morphometry, who also served as president of the Anthropological Society. He entered the debate on language localization when the Anthropological Society was discussing whether intelligence could be related to brain volume and skull size. Bouillaud's son-in-law, Ernst Aubertin, suggested that, instead, they should turn their attention to the localization of brain functions. He thought that language localization and the localization thesis in general could be tested, and challenged the group to find a case of language disturbance in which there was not a lesion affecting the anterior part of the brain. Only a week later, Broca encountered a patient who had been transferred to his hospital service with cellulitis of the leg and a language problem. The patient, a man named Lelong, had suffered from epilepsy since childhood and had developed severe loss of the ability to speak at the age of 30, followed 10 years later by a slowly progressive right hemiparesis. Lelong died six days after being on Broca's service, and Broca had the opportunity to analyze his brain. Lelong became known as "Tan" since that was the only word he uttered, other than a swear word when exasperated. In the next several months, Broca saw a second patient with an aphasic disturbance who died and whose brain he was able to evaluate pathologically.

Broca (1861/1977) described speech function affected in these cases very carefully. He emphasized that what was affected was not intelligence, nor the concept of the word, nor the understanding of words, but rather the ability to *produce* words. This ability was not related simply to motor function of the tongue or vocal apparatus, since the tongue and mouth movement worked well when producing complex non-word sounds, but rather was related to the patients having lost the power to "execute the series of systematic and coordinated movements" that correspond to the syllable they are looking for. Broca wrote, "What has vanished is not the language faculty, nor word memory, neither is it the action of the nerves or muscles of phonation and articulation; it is something else, a particular faculty, considered by M. Bouillaud to be *the faculty of coordinating the movements necessary for spoken language....*" (Broca 1861/ 1994, 44). Broca explained that the ability to produce speech is clearly distinct from the ability to understand language, as is demonstrated by childhood language acquisition. Children acquiring language learn to understand many words before they learn to use these words in speech. Broca argued, "The gradual perfecting of the spoken language among children is due to the development of a particular kind of memory, which is not the memory of words, but the memory of the movement necessary to articulate words. And this particular memory has no relation whatsoever to other memory, nor to the rest of intelligence" (Broca 1861/1994, 44). Broca called the loss of this ability to produce speech, in the absence of any difficulty understanding speech or loss of intelligence, "aphemia," a term later replaced by "aphasia," by a physician named Armand Trousseau (1864).

When Broca examined Tan's brain, he found an oblong lesion "about the size of a hen's egg" in the anterior left hemisphere. It was fairly extensive, including the inferior portions of the frontal lobe, as well as portions of the insula, corpus striatum, and the anterior superior temporal lobe (Broca 1861/1977, 142–143). In spite of its extent, Broca argued that the critical area for speech was likely to be the area of the third frontal convolution, since that area appeared to be the first involved pathologically, and Tan's speech problem was the first symptom he had developed. The second patient who came to Broca's attention had a smaller lesion that mostly affected the third inferior frontal convolution. Based on these two cases, Broca argued that this particular "convolution" in the cortex might be in some way responsible for this specific language symptom. He admitted that the evidence was by no means definitive and further cases needed to be examined.

Broca's paper reportedly "galvanized" the scientific community in France (Harrington 1987, 44), but was by no means fully accepted initially. Heated debate about language localization continued for years afterwards. Why was the report so influential and what barriers prevented others from accepting it? As briefly described above, localization of mental function had been discredited in the first half of the 19th century in France, despite evidence of clinical-pathological correlations supporting language localization presented by observers like Bouillaud. But Broca's report distinguished itself from others. His discussion of cerebral convolutions and sulcal anatomy was new. Rather than simply talking about an anterior lesion in the brain, he referred more precisely to a specific part of the anterior lobe. Also, his discussion of the language deficit, was advanced, by the standards of the day, specifying the most prominent aspect of language that was affected—the production of speech—and contrasting it with other aspects of language that were spared, including comprehension. He also noted that in contrast to speech production, other aspects of communication including that of using gestures and emotional melodic intonation were intact.

Broca's reception was also helped by his explicit refutation of Gall's thesis that skull topography provided information about localization. Broca stated, with obvious reference to Gall, that the anatomy of the convolutions was not correlated with "any system of bumps" on the skull. Furthermore, because there was a variable relationship between brain convolutions and skull topography, any negative conclusions that went against language localization using Gall's method were invalid. Another positive factor for Broca's reception was the cautious tone of his conclusion. Broca's scientific style of arguing from facts, and not theories, was becoming ascendant in his time, and contrasted sharply with the dogmatic scientific styles of Bouillaud and Gall. Finally, the conservative religious and cultural ideologies, which had presented major obstacles for the idea of localization of mental function in the earlier part of the century, were no longer as strong.

Broca's personality may have facilitated his success. The topic of language localization had been associated with lively debates, and localizationists had been largely discredited. Broca was willing to voice controversial opinions that represented progressive scientific thinking. Attesting to this, in 1859, the year that Darwin published *The Origin of the Species*, Broca endorsed the idea that species might be transmuted from one another (see Harrington, 1987). Broca was also able to frame his presentation sensitively in the context of the history of the debate, so as to recognize allies and offer credit to others to whom it was due. While clearly rejecting the failed program of Gall, he graciously acknowledged continuity with Bouillaud, who had pursued the language localization effort in the absence of much interest from the intellectual community for decades.

While Broca's initial report represents a landmark in the history of behavioral neurology and neuropsychology, one could ask whether his contribution is sophisticated by today's standards. Over the years there have been a variety of criticisms of Broca's work.

A number of studies have shown that the area identified by Broca does not necessarily alone produce Broca's aphasia. Often, the full syndrome requires additional regions beyond those which Broca initially identified. But, it should be borne in mind that whether or not a little more brain territory is necessary, or whether a closely associated territory is sufficient in some cases, the fundamental finding established by Broca is not negated. His fundamental point was that a constellation of language deficits are associated with a disrupted area in a particular region of the cortex, and that this area was located near the anterior region that he identified.

Pierre Marie (1853–1940) was one of those who famously attacked Broca's findings in a paper entitled "The Third left frontal convolution plays no special role in the function of language" (Marie, 1906). He cited cases in which lesions in that area did not produce Broca's aphasia as well as cases of aphasia like those presented by Broca which did not have a lesion in that area. Marie also argued that all cases of aphasia were associated with some degree of dementia or loss of general intellectual function. We know now that although modularity of function may be apparent for a specific function based on lesions studies, the precision may not be apparent in every case because of the dynamic and variable nature of brain structure. We also know that, in some cases, language impairment can be associated with dementia (e.g., in vascular dementia or Alzheimer's disease), but that does not necessarily mean that these abilities cannot be dissociated.

Linguists, both then and now, have argued that Broca's description of his patients' language deficits lacked sophistication. In particular, there have been accusations that grammatical features of language, word formation, and sentence level structural impairments were not adequately addressed. One scholarly psycholinguist recently found Broca's papers to show "severe shortcomings" and to lack "originality." He concluded that Broca failed to characterize sufficiently the process of language production, and that his inferences with regard to neuroanatomical localization were deficient and would be "unacceptable to any scientifically oriented medical doctor." (Eling 1994, 38). But, it is important to keep in perspective Broca's achievement in the context of his own time. Although Broca did not address grammar or other linguistic phenomena, he did address the essential question of his time, whether functions of language could be dissociated and related to specific brain lesions. Also, with regard to neuroanatomy, Broca's work was uniformly regarded as exceptional. Even Wernicke, who had trained with the great neuroanatomist, Theodor von Meynert, complimented Broca on his anatomical precision. The test of time has also supported Broca's conclusions. No one today would argue that the ability to articulate language is not located in the anterior region of the brain close to Broca's area (possibly in the anterior insula region or in regions affecting the underlying white matter as well). Broca's great achievement was to give a clear example of regional specialization of a distinct brain function rooted in neuroscience and anatomy.

LANGUAGE LATERALIZATION AND THE BIRTH OF HEMISPHERIC SPECIALIZATION

Another watershed development in the history of cognitive neuroscience was the recognition that language function could be lateralized in the left hemisphere of the brain. Two years after his original report, in 1863, Broca reported a case series of eight patients with language disorders, all of whom had lesions on the left side of the brain. In 1865, he speculated about how left hemisphere specialization of language might occur (Broca, 1865). Prior to the 1860s, there had been very little consideration that language might be lateralized in the brain.

In order to more fully appreciate the significance of this development, it is important to understand that the idea of asymmetry of localization did not naturally follow from the idea of localization. Throughout the 1700s and 1800s the entrenched view was that the cerebral hemispheres should be symmetric in all functions (Harrington, 1987). The original defenders of localization of functions in the brain had never spoken of lateralization. Even Broca, when he was arguing for localization of the capacity for articulate speech in the third frontal convolution of the brain in his original paper had not suggested that this was on the left side of the brain. From the perspective of the time, the idea of asymmetric specialization of function in the hemispheres might have seemed even more heretical than the localization of functions per se.

To understand why the idea of the functional asymmetry of the hemispheres was so revolutionary, it is worth reviewing the fundamental principles in biology taught at the time. After the success of Newtonian mechanics and its predictive laws, biologists sought to discover similar laws in biology. Much of this work focused on attempting to discover laws that explained structural anatomy in biology. Influential theories postulated that the cerebral hemispheres were duplicate and symmetric, because as organs that interact with the environment in space, they have to be able to have spatially balanced interactions (Bichat 1805/1978). Biological organs had been divided into two categories, those that did not need to interact with the environment, which could be more variable in structure and did not need to occur in pairs (e.g., digestive organs), and those which do interact with the both sides of the environment, and need to be in pairs to have balanced interactions with the world (e.g., arms, legs, eyes). The cerebral hemispheres, operating at the highest level of processing and perception and interaction with the environment, were entrusted with the most delicate and complex processing of the external environment, and it was thought that it was especially important that they have this balanced processing in the two hemispheres.

The pervasiveness of the belief that the hemispheres were symmetric organs is seen even in the work of Gall. Despite his localizationist agenda, he never questioned the brain hemisphere symmetry thesis. He was likely influenced by Johann Gottfried Herder, a leader of the *Naturphilosophie* school, which sought laws governing the structure of biology. While Gall's model made detailed claims about the localization of functional modules in the hemispheres, according to Gall, each functional module had a corresponding module in the other hemisphere, which allowed the module on one side to substitute for the corresponding one on the other in the case of damage.

As a corollary to the entrenched belief about the natural state of cerebral symmetry, some physicians explained pathological conditions, including mental illness, as resulting from a loss of symmetry of function and a failure of the coordination of the two "minds" located in the two hemispheres. They suggested that patients with asymmetric functioning in the hemispheres failed to process signals in the two hemispheres in a balanced way that allowed integration. Some writers went so far as to suggest that one of the purposes of education and schooling was to promote better cooperation and balance between the two minds represented in the two hemispheres (See Harrington, 1987, pp. 19–26, for discussion of Wigan (1844) and other theories of Benjamin Rush, Jean Esquirol, Hewett Watson, Sir Henry Holland, and Karl Friedrich Burdach for variations on the theme that the hemispheres need to be balanced and have integrated capacities, and that pathology that results when they do not). Although some anatomists had noted structural asymmetries between the two hemispheres, or a "lack of correspondence of the convolutions on the hemispheres," these were not interpreted as a reflection of differences in functions, specialization, or capacities.

With the systematic collection of further cases of aphasia, asymmetry could no longer be ignored. Broca was the first to comment on this officially from Paris, when he reported his "surprise" at finding that the eight cases of language disturbance he had collected by 1863 all had lesions in the left hemisphere. But Broca avoided making strong conclusions, indicating how uncomfortable he felt about the finding. He described how "if it were necessary to admit that the two symmetrical halves of the encephalon have different attributes... (it would be) a veritable subversion of our knowledge of cerebral physiology...." (Broca 1877, p. 509, quoted in Harrington 1987, 52). He added that this finding might be due to a small sample size, and hoped that "others more fortunate" than he would "find an example of aphemia caused by a lesion of the right hemisphere."

That same year, in 1863, Gustav Dax brought to the attention of the Paris medical societies that 27 years earlier his father, Marc Dax, who had practiced as a country doctor, had collected 40 cases of language disturbances, all of which were associated with left-sided brain pathology. Marc Dax had presented the findings to medical colleagues in 1836 (Dax 1836/1974), but the prominent contributors to the language localization debate in the1860s had been unaware of them.

In discussing Dax's observations, the anti-localizationist physician Paul Briquet ridiculed the idea of asymmetry, asking "Is it possible that the right eye would see only blue, black, and red, whereas the left eye would be constructed for seeing only green, yellow, and blue? Could the right ear hear in music only *do, re, mi, fa*? And the left ear *so, la, ti*? (Briquet, Discussion sur la faculté (1864–5, 714; quoted in Harrington 1987, p. 56). Another anti-localizationist physician, Louis Francisque Lélut, commented: "We could suppose that "there is only one eye, the left, for example, which sees, (while) the right was used for some wholly different thing. But as is well known, and speaking seriously, matters are the same for the hemispheres as for the two eyes; they serve the same functions...." (Lélut, Discussion sur la faculté 1864–1865, 174, quoted in Harrington, p. 54). But other commentators were willing to defend the possibility of asymmetric localization. Bouillaud argued that asymmetry was not so unprecedented and absurd as others were making it out to be, and drew on the analogy with handedness. Trousseau commented upon how other diseases derived from brain function disorders can affect the body asymmetrically, including hysterical symptoms, which more often affect the left side of the body. Trousseau also pointed out that the weight of evidence favored the Dax position, and that there must be differences in localization in the brain for language on the left side. He offered the hypothesis that this might be due to differences in cerebral blood flow to the left and right hemispheres. In June of 1865, Jules Baillarger introduced the idea of a degree of specialization rather than full asymmetry of function, such that the left hemisphere could be more adept at certain functions than the right. He discussed how with writing, if one loses function of the right hand with which one usually writes, it may be difficult to develop the ability to write with the left hand, though it is not impossible. Furthermore, Baillarger suggested that structural asymmetry in the development of the hemispheres might lead to specialization. He reminded everyone of the findings of the anatomist and anthropologist, Louis Pierre Gratiolet, who had posited that the left frontal area developed faster in fetal life than the right. Baillarger discussed how faster development in the left side of the brain might be the basis for the tendency to develop greater use of the right hand than the left, and similarly to account for preferential development of speech abilities in the left hemisphere.

In June, 1865, just weeks after Baillarger's comments at the Society of Medicine, Broca read his famous treatise on the asymmetry of language localization to the Anthropological Society. To explain the language function asymmetry, he relied on some of the same arguments as did Baillarger (although precedence cannot be established for certain, it is likely that Broca conceived of his ideas independently, since he had long been aware of Gratiolet's work and claimed that he had shared his ideas with students the preceding year (Harrington 1987, p. 58)). Broca's explanation posited that the brain starts out functionally symmetric, but differential structural growth of the left hemisphere, as described by Gratiolet, causes the left hemisphere to learn things sooner. This results in humans utilizing and relying on this side "to the exclusion of the other" as they develop skilled tasks such as the ability to produce language. Broca summarizes: "... the two halves of the encephalon, being perfectly identical from an anatomical point of view, cannot have different characteristics: but the more precocious development of the left hemisphere predisposes us, during our first groping activities, to execute with that side of the brain, the most complicated physical and intellectual acts; among these it being certainly necessary to include the expression of ideas by means of language, and more particularly by articulate language... But this specialization of functions does not imply the existence of a functional disparity between the two halves of the encephalon (Broca 1865, 393; quoted in Harrington 1987, p. 59).

Broca's thesis about lateralization has been dubbed "the maturational hypothesis for asymmetric specialization." Broca seems to try to avoid endorsing anything too radical when he refers to the asymmetry in development. He makes it clear that the specialization is an artifact of learning, so as not to undermine the idea that the hemispheres were designed fundamentally to be equal. In his 1865 paper, however, he also famously stated that most of us are "left brained." In his words: "It comes down to the fact that, for language as well as for the much less complicated and refined actions about which I will speak later, we are left-brained. In the same way that we direct our movements in writing, drawing, embroidering, etc., with our left hemisphere, we talk with our left hemisphere. It is a habit we have had since our earliest infancy" (Broca 1865/1977, 57).

Broca made two further points in his treatise of 1865. First, he discussed left handers. He explained that exceptional cases in which the right brain may have developed slightly faster than the left might explain left-handedness. Similarly, he noted that, with differences in maturational rates, some people might be right-brained for language. Interestingly, Broca cautioned people from believing that all left handers should also be right-brained for language, since these might not necessarily always be linked together. Second, he discussed what became known as the doctrine of substitution. Since Broca's hypothesis for specialization of language function rests on a slight difference in maturational rates of the hemisphere, it does not posit that either hemisphere is theoretically restricted in its abilities. This means that if there were damage in one hemisphere at birth, the other hemisphere could take over the functions of the originally favored hemisphere (similar to what Gall had suggested). Thus, if one were to have damage in one hemisphere in a particular area important for motor function, then the other hemisphere would be perfectly able to develop skilled functions in these capacities. Broca explains: "From the preceding, it follows that a subject whose third convolution of the left frontal lobe, normally the seat of spoken language, had been atrophied since birth would learn to speak and would indeed speak with the third convolution of the right frontal lobe, as a child born without a right hand becomes as skillful with its left hand as one normally is with the right." (Broca 1865/1977, 58). This doctrine of substitution was invoked by Broca to explain recovery following language impairment from injury to one side. The opposite hemisphere could take over some of the injured hemisphere's capacities.

By the late 1860s, left-sided language lateralization was generally accepted. New theories proposed that a variety of cognitive abilities were asymmetrically localized. Some of these theories were fueled by prejudices of the day, that the left side of the brain is the seat of more lofty and highly cultured abilities, and the right side, the seat of more primitive or basic sensory or nutritional functions, and of irrational thinking. John Hughlings Jackson had a more complex and balanced view of specialization. In his model, "voluntary functions" were often localized laterally in one specific hemisphere, whereas more "automatic functions" were distributed bilaterally (and thus less resistant to damage by specific lesions). Both the right and left sides of the brain participated in the highest forms of symbolic thinking. The left anterior side was specialized for what he called propositional language (which was contrasted with emotional utterances that might be preserved after unilateral left hemisphere damage). The posterior right side of the brain was specialized for the highest level of perceptual integration of thinking and visual ideation, something that British philosophers at the time, as well as Hughlings Jackson, thought was the critical foundation of our concepts and knowledge.

WERNICKE AND LICHTHEIM: FURTHER APPLICATION OF THE CLINICAL-PATHOLOGICAL METHOD TO THE STUDY OF HIGHER COGNITIVE FUNCTION AND THE USE OF THE "DIAGRAM" HEURISTIC

The general impact of Broca's work in Germany was not as great as in France. In part, this was because of the differences in approach taken by the French scientists as compared to the Germans. French scientists were more likely to think of psychological functions as separate and unified distinct entities or faculties, which might be mapped onto brain regions. Accordingly, Broca had described the function of articulating words as a distinct "faculty," and defined a location for it in the brain on the basis of the clinical-pathological correlation. In Germany, physiology was the dominant science partly because of the influence of Hermann Helmholtz and his mentor Johannes Mueller. Physiological models emphasized the mapping of smaller subcomponents of functions onto physiological processes, and uncovering principles of biological function through experimentation and fine-scaled measurement. With the standard of science based on physiological measurement, findings based on clinical correlation and large psychological entities did not seem as reliable and did not translate well into physiological terms. It was not immediately clear, however, how the physiological perspective applied to the study of aphasia, and even less so to faculty psychology. In Germany, there were also other challenges to the acceptance of Broca's findings. A preeminent psycholinguist in Germany, Heymann Steinthal, argued that clinicians' descriptions of aphasic language deficits were sorely lacking and uninformed about concepts well established in linguistics. Carl Westphal, a prominent Berlin physician, personally reviewed cases of aphasia himself, and reported back to Steinthal that, in his opinion, aphasic language disturbances also did not seem to be explained very well by current linguistics concepts. An exciting physiological discovery related to higher cortical function reported in Germany in 1870, was Gustav Fritsch and Eduard Hitzig's demonstration of specialization of motor function in the cortex. Fritsch and Hitzig demonstrated how physiological stimulation in the cortex of dogs, and later, monkeys, could produce movements in the forelegs and hindlegs. That cortical regions could be specialized for motor function was a surprise at the time. It was considered a well established fact "that the cerebral convolutions are not motor organs" because physiologists had never been able to obtain movement from cortical stimulation previously. This new physiological finding might have helped paved the way for acceptance of language localization, or at least the motor component of speech, but Hitzig was not initially able to provide any satisfactory explanation for how speech could be related to cortical specialization of movement control (Hagner, 1997).

Carl Wernicke's watershed paper: "The Aphasia Symptom Complex: A Psychological Study on an Anatomical Basis" was published in 1874 when he was only 26 years old. It satisfied many of the concerns raised about language localization in the German scientific community. Wernicke presented a new model of speech production that was based on motor and sensory components and connections between them. The emphasis on the motor and sensory dichotomy and their connections (which he discussed in terms of a reflex arc) used terminology that was different from that of faculty psychology and seemed more physiological in nature. Wernicke's paper also represented a new approach to thinking about higher cognitive functions in which a cognitive function could be supported by a variety of component centers in the brain and the connections between them. This approach was stimulated by the Austrian neuroanatomist Theodor Meynert, with whom he trained.

According to Wernicke, Broca's aphasia results from destruction of the motor component for speech located in the frontal operculum or at the posterior part of the third frontal gyrus. This motor center (or Broca's area) contains the memory for the motor image of words, or the knowledge of how to produce words. A second type of aphasia, called sensory aphasia, results from the destruction of the sensory component for speech, located in the posterior portion of the superior temporal gyrus. The sensory center for speech (subsequently called Wernicke's area) contains the memory for the acoustic image of words, how words sound, or what some might now call the acoustic phonological lexicon or phonological input lexicon. When Broca's area is damaged, the familiar symptomatology of Broca's aphasia results, namely non-fluent speech with reduced vocabulary, along with spared ability to comprehend speech. When the sensory language area is damaged, patients have more fluent speech and larger vocabularies because Broca's area is spared, but they have difficulty comprehending speech because they cannot identify the acoustic images of words or recognize them. Wernicke also explained that the speech of patients with sensory aphasia, while having well-formed utterances and relatively fluent phrasing, is marked by word confusion and transpositions and neologisms (including semantic and phonemic paraphasic errors) because patients are faulty at monitoring their speech output due to the acoustic difficulties. He explained that when the sensory center is damaged, Broca's area (the output lexicon) is no longer constrained by information about acoustic knowledge from the sensory center (Wernicke's area) which could affect speech output accuracy. Compared to patients with Broca's aphasia, patients with sensory aphasia are less aware of their speech problems, since they are not able to acoustically recognize words accurately even as they utter them. Patients with sensory aphasia still identify non-speech sounds without difficulty (keys jingling, or door bell ringing), since it is only the acoustic level of speech recognition that is affected. To summarize, disruption of the sensory center, and the new sensory aphasia described by Wernicke, is characterized by relatively fluent speech output, word and sound confusions, impaired comprehension, and lack of full awareness of speech deficits.

Wernicke's model, which identified the two main speech centers, also led him to predict that, in addition to the motor and sensory types of aphasia, there might be a third type of aphasia in which the centers themselves would be spared, but the connection between them disrupted. He initially thought the connections between the two might run through the insula region, though when Constantin von Monakow later identified the arcuate fasciculus, Wernicke thought this might be the basis for the connection. This third type of aphasia has been called *Leitungsaphasie* or conduction aphasia. In this aphasia, damage in the connection between the sensory and motor word centers produce failures in repetition, because of loss of fidelity in transferring information from the word that is heard to the word that is spoken. In this aphasia, word production in spontaneous speech, was expected to be characterized by paraphasic errors because motor output would fail to be constrained properly by phoneme selection from the sensory center. Wernicke described this aphasia as likely to be characterized by very hesitant speech, with long pauses "in which the patient gropes for correct expression." In contrast to patients with sensory aphasia, the patients with this type of aphasia would still be able to comprehend speech because their acoustic word memories in the sensory center were still intact. They would also be aware of their errors and be able to monitor their speech acoustically, since the sensory center was intact. This theoretically hypothesized aphasia was subsequently recognized clinically and is now classically associated with the findings of relatively spared comprehension and relatively fluent output, but with markedly impaired repetition and paraphasic errors of which the patient is aware and tries to correct. Since these patients are able to monitor their speech, they have been noted to exhibit a phenomenon that has been called *conduit d'approche* in which they keep correcting themselves when they make paraphasic errors, gradually coming closer and closer to the correct target.

To understand the basic components of Wernicke's model, it is useful to think of a reflex arc, an analogy used by Wernicke. The concept of the reflex arc brings together the understanding of the sensory and motor components of speech while providing a model to explain how they are intimately related. Many physiological processes can be divided into sensory and motor components, but in the case of speech, these are particularly interdependent. With respect to the reflex arc, Wernicke argued that children first learn to speak in great part by repeating what they hear, and the process of mimicry allows them to associate the sensory impressions of words they hear with the motor programs for uttering those words. These associations form the basis for sensori-motor associations in the speech apparatus. In later papers, Ludwig Lichtheim and others emphasized how disruption of Wernicke's arc can be specifically detected by failures of repetition, since all elements of Wernicke's arc, including both the sensory and motor center and the connections between them must remain intact in order for people to repeat spoken words that they hear. Wernicke, like most investigators at the time, maintained that higher thought, i.e., ideas and concepts, were unlikely be localized in any particular brain area. Thus, his model is limited to elements of speech input and speech output and the sensory and motor correlates of speech.

Interestingly, in the schematic drawing of the language components in his original paper Wernicke depicted the components of language on the right side of the brain since it was not yet known that language was primarily localized on the left. In Wernicke's diagram, which is depicted in Figure 2.1, "M" represents the "Motor" area for speech which contains the motor memories for speech production. "A" represents the "Auditory area" for speech that contains the auditory memories of how words sound. When a person listens to speech, the sound is first heard in the external acoustic apparatus (ear), depicted as "a," these sounds then travel to the center for recognition of how words sound, "A," located in the posterior superior temporal lobe. In order to produce speech, the center "M" in Broca's area near the premotor oral area must be activated, which contains the memories for the motor production of words. "M" in turn sends impulses that direct oral facial speech motor neurons in the medulla depicted as "m," which direct the activation of musculature to execute speech sounds. The arc a → A → M→ m forms the core sensorimotor substrate for speech and language in the brain. The relationships between sensory and motor speech components develop in childhood when children mimic what they hear. During the course of mimicry or repetition, signals must be transferred from the sensory word center "A" through the pathway

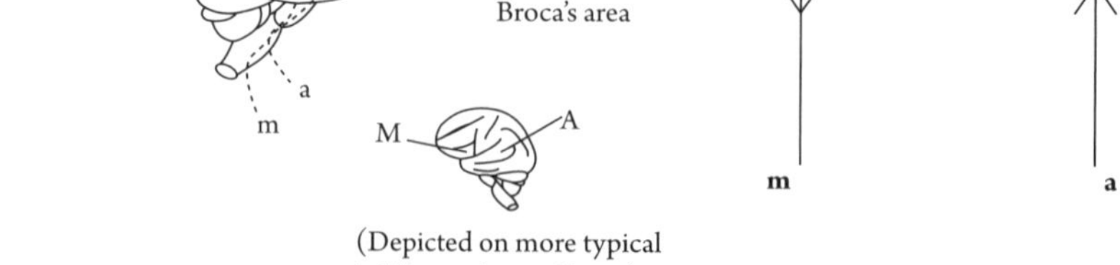

Figure 2.1 Wernicke's Arc: Schematic of Wernicke's model adapted from the figure in his original paper.

A–M to reach "M," which can direct the production of speech. Sensory aphasia results from a lesion in A; Broca's aphasia from a lesion in M; conduction aphasia from a lesion in the connection between A and M (A–M). Language impairments resulting from any lesion in the components of Wernicke's arc have disrupted repetition ability.

Wernicke's approach to explaining aphasia was very different from that of Broca and became the starting place for conceptualizing the brain as consisting of centers, connections, and distributed systems. Wernicke went beyond correlating a single function with a specific location in the brain and provided a more differentiated view of possible symptoms and types of language disorders. Many had previously felt that patients were not adequately described by the description in Broca's aphasia, and Wernicke provided a "theory of aphasia . . . (that permitted) . . . a consolidation of the diversified picture of the disorder" (Wernicke 1874/1977, 143). To further satisfy the physiologists and other experimental scientists of his day, he had even mentioned how changes in the nerve pathways in the brain might come about from changes in the quanta of energy required to activate them after training and exposure, similar to that later proposed by the principles of Hebbian learning that came much later. Wernicke also satisfied linguists of his day to some extent. He was informed of distinctions made by linguists and attempted in his paper to address differences between his observations of aphasics and the linguistic concepts. Wernicke's paper, like Broca's, maintained a positivistic scientific tone, modestly acknowledging that his model did not explain all the interesting features of abnormal language in aphasia. He conceded that "many of the oddities in the province of aphasia must remain unresolved, such as the isolated loss of substantives or verbs, etc." (Wernicke 1874/1977. 143). Wernicke noted that "An interpretation of such unexplained symptoms on the basis of our primary anatomic elements was deliberately avoided, and it must be clearly stated here that whole areas of brain physiology and the odd symptoms observed therein . . . are not accessible (in the medical sense) to scientific treatment" (Wernicke 1874/1977, 143)

Wernicke's paper was well received when it appeared. The approach that Wernicke took has subsequently been referred to as a "connectionistic" approach. Those who used this approach were also referred to as "diagram makers" because they often illustrated their models with diagrams which mapped centers onto different regions in the brain and showed the connections between them that could also be lesioned to produce different symptoms. The diagram makers provided a method both for explaining the effects of lesions, and for distilling theories of brain behavior relationships that allowed for the generation of new hypotheses about brain and behavior relationships.

FURTHER CONTRIBUTIONS TO THE DIAGRAM MODELS OF LANGUAGE: THE WERNICKE-LICHTHEIM MODEL AND THE EXPLANATION OF OTHER APHASIC SYNDROMES

Wernicke's model was expanded in 1885 by Ludwig Lichtheim (1845–1928), a student of Wernicke. Lichtheim's paper was a high water mark of sophistication in diagram models. His main addition to Wernicke's model was to add a concept center or a semantic field (*Begriffe*)(See Schematic of Lichtheim's Model, Figure 2.2). This component was not meant to be an anatomic center like that of the sensory repository for word images (Wernicke's area), or the motor repository for word images (Broca and its surrounding area), but, rather, it designated a distributed knowledge network of associations that contain the concepts to which words refer. With this addition to the model, Lichtheim described two new types of aphasia based on disruption of the connection of Broca's and Wernicke's areas to the center for concepts. In both these aphasias, because Wernicke's arc is intact, repetition is normal. In one case, however, the acoustic images or perception of speech sounds coming from Wernicke's center cannot be passed on to concepts for recognition, and thus comprehension is impaired (depicted in Lichtheim's model as a lesion 1 in the pathway A–C). In the other case, concepts, which are activated in preparation for generating spontaneous speech are not able to activate Broca's area for speech output, and thus, speech is not produced fluently (lesion 2 in the pathway C–M). These two aphasias have subsequently come to be known as transcortical sensory aphasia and transcortical motor aphasia.

Lichtheim's model can also explain the characteristics of other aphasic syndromes. Adolf Kussmaul (1822–1902), described "word deafness," in which patients have disruption in the connections between the primary auditory areas and Wernicke's acoustic-phonological center (Kussmaul, 1877). Since hearing occurs bilaterally, connections theoretically have to be disrupted from both

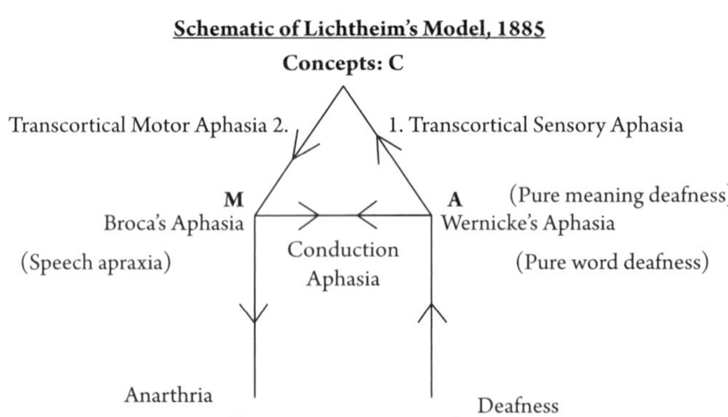

Figure 2.2 A schematic diagram of Lichtheim's influential model of the language system and aphasias.

primary auditory areas of the brain where they connect to Wernicke's area. In such cases, which disrupt the pathway a-A on the figure, sounds not related to speech are perceived well and understood, but speech sounds cannot be recognized because they cannot access the sensory-acoustic phonological input lexicon for speech sounds in Wernicke's area. Because this lesion occurs independently of any destruction of Wernicke's area or Broca's area or internal connections in the brain between these areas and between concepts, speech output is entirely normal, as is writing, reading, and naming. Only capacities which rely on processing auditory perception of speech are affected, including comprehension, the ability to repeat what is heard, and the ability to write to dictation. Speech output is normal because the ability to monitor speech internally is still intact due to the preservation of Wernicke's area.

Another type of aphasia which can be explained using Lichtheim's model and is mentioned in his paper is a condition that has subsequently been called "pure meaning deafness." (reported also by Bramwell and reviewed in Ellis, 1984). In this type of aphasia, acoustic information is processed in Wernicke's area in such a way that the phonological forms are recognized and can be repeated, but the information is blocked from activating concepts, which impairs comprehension. Unlike in Wernicke's aphasia or transcortical sensory aphasia, spontaneous speech is not affected by paraphasic errors because top-down connections to Wernicke's area remain intact, and the phonological word form recognition can monitor speech production. Since phonological word knowledge is intact, these patients can also make phonological-to-orthographic translations and write down words based on the phonological information, even when they cannot understand the words that they hear. After writing down the words that are incomprehensible to them, they can then read these and understand them. In short, these patients can repeat what they hear, but do not understand words they hear until they write them down.

Finally, disruption of the outflow tract from Broca's area to the musculature and innervation of the motor neurons to produce speech can explain another type of speech difficulty. This results in the loss of the ability to produce normal speech sounds even though knowledge of the words' phonology is preserved. There is isolated impairment of the execution of speech sounds, despite preservation of knowledge of word features. In Lichtheim's time, this type of speech difficulty was called either ataxic speech or aphemia. Today, it might be called apraxia of speech, or when impairment is more complete, aphemia. Impairment of production of speech in this disorder is different from that found in Broca's aphasia. In Broca's aphasia, there is also loss of knowledge of the sequence of phonemes that are part of the word form to be produced, whereas in apraxia of speech, the word phonemes are known, but the production of the word is distorted due to problems in the execution and programming of the phoneme sequences, i.e., motor activation of the appropriate motor neurons. This causes the distortion of vowels and phonemes and syllable sounds, particularly when words are longer or require more coordination from the execution standpoint. Despite distorted production, fluency can be relatively preserved, reading and writing are intact, and knowledge about the characteristics of the word components are also preserved. Kussmaul described these patients as having "freedom of intellect and of movement of the tongue" and they also write words without difficulty, but "when asked to articulate... (the signs)... as sounds or words, they cannot, even when they are shown how to shape their tongue and lips." The failure of these patients to produce the sounds despite the intact knowledge of acoustic features or phonological knowledge of the identity of the sequence of sounds can be understood in Lichtheim's model to arise from the disruption of the final pathway emanating from Broca's area to the musculature designated as (M–m) in the figure. This type of disruption would be expected to cause purely motor difficulty in production of speech while all other language functions including repetition, comprehension, writing, and reading could be completely intact.

LICHTHEIM'S MODEL: CRITICISMS, CONTROVERSIES, PREDICTIONS OF COMPETING MODELS, AND OTHER APHASIC SYNDROMES

In 1891 Sigmund Freud (1856–1939) criticized Lichtheim's model for failing to explain why patients should have disrupted repetition in conduction aphasia. He pointed out that in Lichtheim's model, patients with conduction aphasia should still be able to repeat words by accessing the word meaning and by taking the "detour" (A–C–M), which would allow them to bypass the disrupted direct connection between Wernicke's and Broca's area (A–M). An interesting consequence of this observation is that patients repeating by this route should only be able to repeat "real" words, but not non-words or unknown foreign words, because only known real words could activate specific meanings or concepts. As Freud explains: "If this detour is really available, patients with conduction aphasia would have to be characterized as a condition in which... repetition of comprehensible words... (is intact)..., but in which repetition of incomprehensible words, such as those of a foreign language, is abolished"(Freud 1891/1953, 14). This exact dissociation, as predicted by the Lichtheim's model and pointed out by Freud, was subsequently described (Katz & Goodglass, 1990). Patients with this condition have what has been called deep dysphasia. They are able to repeat *only* words that are real, and are unable to repeat non-words like "FLIG" or "BLUB." One interesting aspect of deep dysphasia is that repetition errors are almost always semantic because all repetition proceeds via the concepts or semantic route, thus they do not make phonological errors.

Lichtheim argued for bi-directionality in the information flow between Broca's and Wernicke's area. Lichtheim explained that this was necessary to support internal speech, in which one might generate ideas that would be translated directly into word output programs, but would then be transferred into acoustic form in Wernicke's area. Lichtheim argued that much of speech is supported by "internal speech," which we might today call phonological working memory. This allows us to review what we might say or what might have just said. In addition to using this bi-directionality to explain internal speech, Lichtheim relied on this bi-directionality to explain why speech output is still altered with paraphasic errors when people only have lesions of the acoustic recognition center and Wernicke's area. He argued that speech production, even when we generate our production spontaneously from ideas, always also activates the acoustic forms in Wernicke's area, and Wernicke's area is always involved internally in monitoring and constraining speech production.

Lichtheim tried to show that patients with lesions only in Broca's area and/or its surroundings have deficits of acoustic knowledge of speech. He thought that Broca's area was the only conduit for accessing acoustic information internally. Lichtheim famously suggested that this could be tested by asking patients with Broca's lesions to indicate the number of syllables in a word by squeezing their hand the appropriate numbers of times, even when they were unable to speak. If they still had access to the acoustic knowledge, or Wernicke's area, they should be able to indicate the number of syllables by squeezing, using their acoustic knowledge of these words. Lichtheim showed that his patients with Broca's- like aphasia were unable to indicate the number of syllables in words by squeezing, which supported his view that internal speech and knowledge of acoustic information have to pass through Broca's area first (this claim has subsequently been tested further, see Heilman, Tucker, & Valentein, 1976; Feinberg, Rothi, & Heilman, 1986).

Kussmaul's model (1877) contrasted with Lichtheim's because it emphasized a bi-directional connection from concepts to the acoustic center, but it had no direct connection from concepts to the motor production of words. Thus, all speech output in Kussmaul's model had to first be routed through the acoustic knowledge center, and there was no direct access to speech output that did not first utilize acoustic knowledge. Wernicke, in his later writings, also seemed to side with Kussmaul, and suggested that concepts might first activate the acoustic word form before the motor form (Wernicke, 1885–1886). Wernicke explained how this might make more sense based on speech development, since in speech development words are first heard, and speech develops from mimicry in which acoustic knowledge becomes intimately linked with motor speech knowledge. This link is so strong that it might be hard for one to proceed without the other. Thus, Wernicke suggested that all speech production relies to some degree on acoustic knowledge. Spontaneous speech might proceed by the pathway C–A–M instead of directly from C→M. This entire discussion was aimed at explaining why patients who only have lesions affecting the acoustic center still have problems with motor production. That is why patients with conduction or Wernicke's aphasia still make paraphasic errors (something that Freud also brought up as a concern in his critical analysis of the aphasia models). Kussmaul and Wernicke could explain the abnormal speech output very directly, because in their models, acoustic knowledge affects speech output because concepts often (Wernicke) or always (Kussmaul) first activate acoustic knowledge before proceeding to speech output production. Lichtheim, in contrast, argued that Broca's area is automatically influenced by Wernicke's area by its backward connections.

With both bottom-up and top-down directions for connections between concepts and acoustic word knowledge (Figure 2.3), Kussmaul's model more easily accounts for an isolated naming disorder or "anomia." *Anomia* is a residual sign of many different forms of aphasia, but it can also occur as a discrete lesion. Patients with lesions of the conceptual field, Broca's area, and Wernickes' area all have deficits in naming; but they also have deficits in repetition, speech production, or comprehension. An isolated deficit in naming occurs in Kussmaul's model when only the top-down connecting pathway between the concept/ semantic field to Wernicke's area is disrupted, leaving comprehension intact, as well as repetition and speech production. Kussmaul's model also predicts the opposite condition, in which only the bottom-up pathway is affected, such that the semantic field can access the phonological lexicon, but the phonological lexicon cannot access the semantic field. In this case, the patient can name, but have difficulty understanding, the name of the object that they are able to name. This would be expected to produce intact naming, repetition, and spontaneous speech, despite deficits in comprehension, a constellation of symptoms reminiscent of word-meaning deafness. (See Heilman, Rothi, McFarling, & Rottman, 1981).

Although language was the starting point for the golden era of behavioral neurology, after Broca and Wernicke's influential publications, the literature in higher-level cognition expanded greatly. In order to expand the consideration of the seminal models beyond the topic of language, we will highlight a few of the more influential contributions in relation to the study of apraxia and visual agnosia from this time.

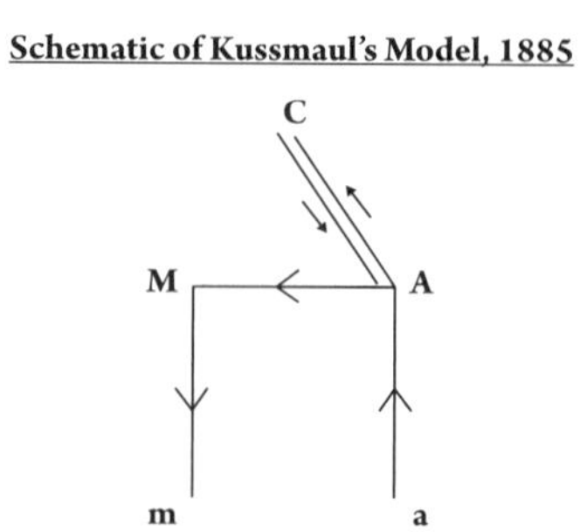

Figure 2.3 A schematic diagram of Kussmaul's model of the language system.

Apraxia and Praxis

Hugo Karl Liepmann (1863–1925) was the first to establish a systematic account of the motor planning and execution disorder known as apraxia. He was a student of Wernicke's and worked as Wernicke's assistant from 1895 to 1899. His approach was similar to that of other diagram makers, and involved the identification of underlying functional modules that supported the cognitive function in question and identification of the anatomical organization of the modules based on observations of patients with lesions. Liepmann very precisely discussed his use of the term *apraxia*, and clearly contrasted it with others from the time, which helped clarify the disorder and its features, and how it was distinct from other cognitive issues.

In general, *apraxia* refers to a deficiency in the ability to perform complex and learned motor acts in the absence of primary motor and sensory deficits that might affect execution of the learned motor activity. Although during spontaneous activities a person may demonstrate that the motor ability is possible, when the apraxic individual intentionally tries to perform these activities, the motor activity is incorrectly executed and characterized by a variety of deficiencies. The patient with apraxia might have difficulty using tools correctly or making hand gestures to indicate needs. While the deficiency might not at first seem particularly debilitating in milder forms, in severe cases it can render a patient strikingly disabled (e.g., in advanced corticobasal degeneration or in selected cases of severe apraxia after stroke). Apraxia can affect a variety of motor activities selectively, including writing, oral buccal movements, limb movements, and speech. The study of apraxia provides a window into the organization of complex motor programming in the brain.

THE CASE OF MR. T.

Liepmann's interest in apraxia, and much of the basis for his formulation of the deficit, was based on the extraordinary case of a 48-year-old, right-handed German government official (*Regieurungsrat*), referred to as Mr. T (Liepmann, 1900/1977). Mr. T. suffered a stroke that resulted in poor speech output and apparent lack of speech comprehension. His speech output initially was limited to fewer than 15 words, and he was unable to point reliably to designated objects, or select designated objects from an array. Mr. T. sometimes responded to requests with completely unrelated activities, or employed objects inappropriately. Liepmann's first impression was that Mr. T failed "almost everything" he was asked to do. Specifically when asked to do things with objects, he would handle the "objects quite absurdly" and overall "it appeared as if the patient did not understand—that he was cerebrally deaf, possibly also cerebrally blind." In part because of the bizarreness of his use of objects, he was thought to have a dementia, along with his aphasia affecting both speech production and comprehension.

But after working with Mr. T. over the course of several days, Liepmann noticed some of his abilities to do things and his comprehension were preserved. Mr. T. responded to whole body commands to get up and walk to the window and others quite readily. Liepmann also noticed that Mr. T. responded to almost every request with his right arm, and began to wonder what would happen if Mr. T were required to use the left. When required to use the left arm, Liepmann made the startling discovery, that "...all of a sudden, the picture changed" (Liepmann 1900/1977, 159). With the left arm, Mr. T. showed that he understood commands and was able to respond much more accurately. With the left arm, he could select tools from an array, point to specified objects in the room, and gesture accurate responses to *yes* and *no* questions. The preservation of responses when Mr. T. used his left arm meant that Mr. T. did not have a generalized comprehension disorder or confusional disorder. Instead, he had to have a problem specifically with motor execution affecting the right arm selectively. By requiring Mr. T to use the left arm, Liepmann discovered that Mr. T. was capable of performing the tasks, and understood what was being asked of him; he was just not able to do so volitionally with the right arm.

Liepmann concluded that Mr. T. had a specific problem with implementing intentional actions using the right side (arm and leg), but not the left. Rather than having a general comprehension disorder, Liepmann concluded, he had a severe motor execution disorder. Liepmann determined Mr. T.'s inability to implement actions with the right side occurred in many different circumstances with different modes of input or instruction. For example, using the right side, Mr. T. could neither imitate nor copy motor gestures, nor could he select an object correctly when the name of the object was given to him written on a piece of paper in written form. When given a hairbrush in his right hand, he used it like a spoon bringing it to his mouth. When given a comb, he used it as a pencil. He could not accurately scratch his right ear when tickled, or point to a bell that was ringing with his right side. He could do these tasks with the left hand.

Mr T. did not have visuospatial neglect or hemianopsia. However, in addition to the motor action errors affecting the right side, Mr. T. had some sensory problems on the right side, with decreased capacity to respond to touch and pinprick, poor ability to localize tactile stimuli, and poor ability to perceive the position of his right arm without seeing it (measured by the inability of the of left arm to produce the same posture as the right).

With respect to Mr. T's action deficiencies, Liepmann argued that Mr. T.'s problem was not a pure motor output disorder, but a deficiency of higher-level computation of how to produce purposeful movements. Liepmann emphasized that Mr. T. could perform some activities with good dexterity and capacity spontaneously, such as when buttoning buttons, but was not able to do the same activity when asked to do it intentionally. Thus, it was not the basic ability to do the task that was affected, but the inability to do it intentionally. Furthermore, the ability to execute the task depended on the specific circumstances. For example, Mr. T's ability to reach for targets was better when he was asked to pick up a single target object, compared to when he was asked to pick up a target object from among an array of objects. Right-hand movements were also sometimes in conflict with left-hand movements, such that when he poured water with the left hand, he simultaneously raised the glass to his lips with the right, and would get the sequence of events out of order. Thus, it was not simply a problem with motor output, but one that depended on the need or intention to perform more complex motor actions.

REDEFINING APRAXIA: LIEPMANN'S PROCESSING MODEL

Liepmann's case helped highlight some essential features of the disorder of apraxia that had not previously been as clearly differentiated. Prior investigators had noted that after developing aphasia, patients could have specific difficulty using objects in their environment (trying to use a spoon as a pencil for example) or could have a problem performing tasks when asked that involved tools. The linguist Steinthal is credited with first using the term *apraxia* when in the context of the misuse of objects in patients with aphasia in 1871. Steinthal suggested that apraxia could be a failure of connecting the purpose and mechanisms of tool use to the execution of the movements themselves. Steinthal noted that this deficiency was similar to the general loss of the connection between ideas and movements that was also evident in aphasia. He did not necessarily think that apraxia was secondary to aphasia, but noted the similarities in this underlying deficient cognitive component. Other explanations for apraxia included the following: Apraxia might be due to loss of knowledge for how objects or tools were to be used (what we might call the loss of knowledge for the semantics of tools); loss of the ability to perceive and recognize an object fully (agnosia) (Pick, Kussmaul, Flechsig, Starr); or the product of a general symbolic disorder, similar to that affecting language, such that it was due to an overall failure of giving symbols motor expression (Finkelnberg). Some saw the deficit as a disturbance in the central primary motor abilities, but had not explained well how there could be spared ability to move on the elemental level of dexterity and capacity for coordinated movement, despite an inability to elicit the program for complex movement or movement under more intentional circumstances (Nothnagel, Meynert).

Mr. T.'s case allowed Liepmann to define apraxia more systematically than had been done previously. This was aided to a great degree by the unilateral nature of Mr. T's deficit. Because Mr. T could demonstrate intact responses in the left hand, Liepmann was able to conclude that apraxia (1) was not due to a problem with perceiving the object (2) was not a problem with not having knowledge of an object, and (3) was not due to a general problem of expression of symbols.

Instead, Liepmann proposed that apraxia be understood as a deficiency that affects *higher-level execution of learned movement*, including the ability to initiate learned movements upon command, in imitation, or when the object is absent. It was importantly *not* a deficit of elemental motor ability or basic ability to execute or coordinate motor activity.

After publishing the case of Mr. T. in 1900, Liepmann continued to write and publish on apraxia for the remainder of his career. In 1905, his first extensive theoretical formulation of apraxia appeared. His model included three components that underlie motor execution. First, there was "the movement formula," the representation in the brain of the sensory image or pattern that contains knowledge of the features of a specific movement. Second, there was "the innervatory apparatus" of the motor system. This is where the motor neurons are able to produce innervatory patterns when guided by the movement formula to execute the movement action. Third, there was "kinetic memories." These could be stored in the innervatory apparatus for simple and overlearned movements and could be activated independently of any guidance by movement formulae.

In this theoretical formulation, the first step in performing an action is the activation of the memory or representation containing a spatial temporal map that defines that movement, called the "movement formula." This formula would, in most cases, be represented in a form like that of a visual image of the action (in some type of spatiotemporal map). That image would define information about the known spatiotemporal relationships of the action as they should appear. After the movement formula was identified, it would need to be connected to a "central" region that executed an innervatory pattern. The central region could stimulate motor output neurons required for execution of the movement, but had to be guided by the movement formula to produce the accurate pattern of activation. Some movements that were highly overlearned or elemental (such as finger tapping) could be represented directly in the innervatory machinery, without needing to be guided by a movement formula. These overlearned representations were called kinetic memories.

With this model, Liepmann defined different subtypes of apraxia. For example, Mr. T. had a problem related to disruption in the connection of the movement formula to the innervatory apparatus. He had the capacity to produce complex movements (thus the innervatory apparatus was intact), and the capacity to recognize them and implement them (thus the movement formula was intact). He lacked the connection between the two, so when he willfully wanted to produce the movement, the movement formula was not able to connect to or guide the innervatory machinery responsible for the action in the right hand. When Mr. T. was provided with visual examples of how to perform these movements (as in imitation), it did not help, since these still could not be connected to the innervatory machinery. Mr T.'s type of case, in which praxis is especially poor for the generation of purposeful movements upon command, but is also present at least to some degree when provided with the opportunity to copy the movement, Liepmann called "idio-kinetic" apraxia. The hyphen was used to emphasize that it is a defect in the *connection* between the knowledge of the movement form (in the movement formula) and the innervatory apparatus that executes the movement.

Unlike Mr. T., there are other cases in which a movement cannot be performed to command, but demonstrating the movement to the patient fully corrects the problem. These patients, in whom mimicry is profoundly better, Liepmann suggested, might have a problem with the activation or integrity of the movement formula. In these cases, when the movement formula is demonstrated in the form of the visual demonstration, it activates that spatiotemporal map better, which has an intact connection to the executor apparatus, which results in restored performance. In these cases, the visuo spatiotemporal movement image can still be applied to the innervatory apparatus if it is made available. Liepmann called these cases "ideational apraxia." Patients with this disorder might substitute the wrong whole movement for another, or make errors in the sequence of movements, but these errors were reduced by mimicry.

The final major form of apraxia Liepmann described was called limb-kinetic apraxia. This was a disturbance that affected the basic overlearned sequences contained in the primary motor-strip regions which he had called kinetic memories. Limb-kinetic apraxia affects basic elements of movements, such as precision, dexterity, and simple overlearned activities such as finger tapping. In some respects, it is unlike other kinds of apraxia, and in some publications, he described and included it only under an "extended concept of apraxia." Patients with limb kinetic apraxia have difficulties in manipulating any tool or object, since dexterity affects all movement. Liepmann emphasized that an individual apraxic patient might have more than one deficit of the apraxis spectrum. For example, patients with ideo-kinetic apraxia often have limb kinetic apraxia.

Liepmann described how different apraxic error types could be distinctive of different types of apraxia. When lesions are more posterior, and located nearer the occipito-temporal junction, he suggested there would be more ideational errors characterized by substitution and content mistakes (seen in ideational apraxia or ideo-kinetic apraxia), whereas the more anterior a lesion was, the more the errors could be morphological in nature, related to the faulty execution of the details of the movement sequence (seen in limb-kinetic or ideo-kinetic apraxia). In modern terminology, *ideo-kinetic apraxia* is most readily translated as ideo-motor apraxia. The term *ideational apraxia* has been differentiated into conceptual and ideational apraxia subtypes. Dissociation apraxias, which Liepmann did not address specifically, refer to apraxias that occur only in response to a single input modality (only to verbal instruction, but not to visual cues).

CONNECTING APRAXIA TO UNDERLYING NEUROANATOMICAL SUBSTRATES

Liepmann's legacy for the field of apraxia also lies in how he connected praxis to brain anatomy. He established unequivocally that the left hemisphere is dominant for praxis in right handers. He dramatically highlighted that the right hemisphere, which directs actions of the left hand, actually does not possess full control over the left hand, but is dependent on the left hemisphere. Essentially, the right hemisphere has to "borrow" knowledge from the left to complete left-hand movements. He summarizes: "A part of what the left hand 'can do' is not a possession of the right hemisphere which directs its mobility, but is a possession which is borrowed from the left hemisphere. The right hand centre... (may remain)... during the whole of life in a certain dependency on the left hemisphere (Liepmann 1908, pg. 34). He describes how the dependency on praxis with respect to the left hemisphere might vary between patients, but it was never the case that the left hemisphere was dependent on the right (page 220, Mr. T. Autopsy part II; 19: 1905; also in Section 2 of the *Drei Aufsaetze*).

His anatomical model was based on his careful examination of a large series of 83 right-handed patients with strokes causing hemiparesis (Liepmann, 1908, Essay 2). Patients were tested on their nonparetic hand with a battery of praxis tests, including: 1) Intransitive and transitive gestures to command (e.g., intransitive = scolding gesture, saluting gestures, snapping fingers vs. transitive = hammering, knocking on a door, catching a fly, counting out money, playing the piano), 2) intransitive and transitive gestures to imitation, and 3) transitive gestures with tools or props present.

Of the 83 patients, the syndrome of apraxia never occurred in the non-paretic right hand of any of the 42 patients with right hemisphere strokes, but occurred in the non-paretic left hand of about 50 percent (20/41) of patients with left hemispheric strokes. All those with apraxia had difficulty with gesture upon command; usually difficulties were not corrected by imitation. Twenty-five percent had problems with using tools. The finding that no patients with right-hemisphere stroke had apraxia in the right hand, but that 50 percent of patients with left hemisphere strokes had apraxia in the left hand, showed that the left hemisphere was particularly specialized as the repository of the movement formula or images important for directing movements, even when movement was facilitated by the right hemisphere.

Based on a number of cases, Liepmann also showed that lesions of the corpus callosum, particularly the anterior portion, but not the splenium, prevented critical information from the left hemisphere from reaching the right hemisphere, and produced similar apraxia (Liepmann &Maas 1907). In these cases, the apraxia was due to a pure disconnection problem (*Leitungsunterbrechung*), and apraxia would affect only the left hand. In one case, Liepmann also explained how left-sided agraphia could be a pure apraxic deficit caused by a colossal lesion.

Liepmann, Vertical Schema of Apraxia, 1908

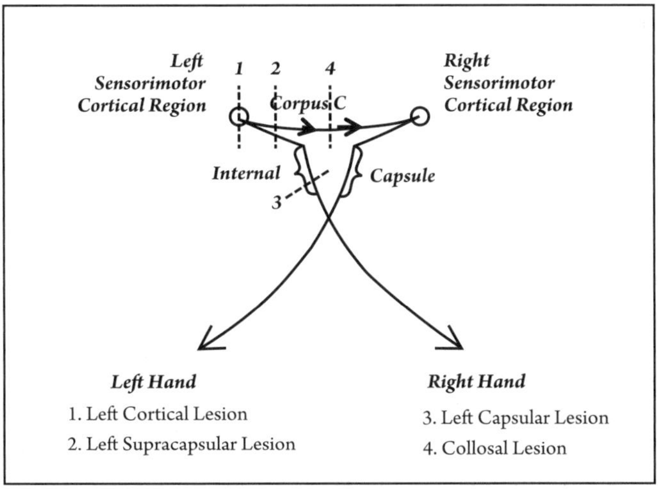

Figure 2.4 Liepmann's vertical schema of apraxia: This is a translation and adaptation of Liepmann's vertical schema of apraxia from his 1908 paper which shows how different types of lesions produce left-sided apraxia. The left sensorimotor cortex dominates the right for learned movements. Thus, the right cortex depends on input from the left, which is carried in the corpus callosum to produce skilled movements of the left hand. Lesions at 1, 2, and 4 which interrupt the corpus callosum pathway from left to right result in apraxia of the left hand. Lesions at 3, in contrast, do not affect apraxia of the left hand, since the left sensorimotor cortex and corpus callosum pathway remain intact. Lesions of 1, 2, and 3 all cause right-sided paralysis. A lesion of 4 causes only left-sided apraxia without right sided paralysis; the lesion at 3 causes only right-sided paralysis without left-sided apraxia.

Liepmann eventually proposed a model to predict when one would encounter a patient with left-hand apraxia and a left-hemisphere lesion (whether or not a right-hand apraxia was also present). The left-sided apraxia could be produced by a (1) disruption of the corpus callosum, from the loss of white matter that leads from the left hemisphere to the right, in which case only a unilateral left hand apraxia would occur; or (2) a disruption of the fibers of the white matter below the sensorimotor area on the left, which would prevent the flow of information across to the right hemisphere, or (3) disruption of the sensori-motor apparatus and cortical influences that direct the left hemisphere praxis system, which would no longer be intact to cross to the right hemisphere. In contrast, a lesion of the left internal capsule would not affect praxis on the left side, since the communication across the corpus callosum would remain intact. In addition, with lesions below the capsule, the right hand would have no praxis impairment, only kinetic motor impairment, since praxis capacities derived from the cortical repository of movement formulas that activate the sensorimotor central region and both of those regions would remain intact.

LIEPMANN ON APHASIA AND APRAXIA OF SPEECH

When Liepmann suggested that complex learned purposeful motor acts are directed in great part by the left hemisphere when describing praxis, it naturally led to questions about praxis and its relationship to aphasia. Liepmann concluded that apraxia occurred independently of aphasia. For example, 6 of the 20 apraxic patients in his stroke series did not have aphasia, and 4 of the 21 patients without apraxia had aphasia. In the individual cases in which aphasia and apraxia coexisted, comprehension problems could also not explain apraxia, since all patients were tested on gestures to imitation which bypassed language, and he reported that, in his series, most were not improved by imitation. In a letter to Henschen, quoted in Henry Head's book on aphasia, Liepmann wrote "not all motor aphasics suffer from apraxia, that is to say, apraxia of the extremities. Apraxia of the face muscles, inability to whistle, to wrinkle the forehead, to make a grimace, etc., is frequently combined with motor aphasia. Apraxia of the hands, though common, is less often present. There are motor aphasics, especially those with so-called "pure word-dumbness," without apraxia; conversely, I have observed apraxic patients, not only without motor aphasia, but without any form of aphasia. Graver degrees of apraxia appear occasionally with sensory aphasia, probably owing to the proximity of the temporal and parietal lobes" (Head, 1926 vol I. pp. 99–100).

Although Liepmann demonstrated that praxis difficulties were independent of aphasia, he also acknowledged that the aspects of motor aphasia which resulted in difficulty producing and articulating sounds might have something in common with apraxia. As Henry Head describes, the apractic component of a speech deficit is characterized by "mutilation of letters and syllables with great slowness and difficulty of articulation that resembles at first sight a dysarthria."Liepmann describes how the movement formula, which in the setting of limb movements is usually contained in the form of a visual image, would, in the case of speech, be contained in the form of an acoustic image or sketch, which according to his model of apraxia, would be used to guide the spatiotemporal coordination of the innervatory apparatus. Lichtheim explains: "In order for the action of speech to take place properly, the acoustic sketch must influence the kinematic of the speech muscles, just as in an apraxia of the extremities, the visual sketch influences the kinematic of the extremities." (quoted in Head 1926, Vol 1, p. 100). Head also notes that Liepmann indicated that "the analogy must not be carried to extreme lengths and all aphasic manifestation cannot be classed as forms of apraxia." (Head, 1926, Vol. I, p. 100).

Speech difficulty and apraxia were similar in the sense that both were highly complex motor gestures that were performed without the use of objects (in one case, because objects are never part of the action, and in the other case, when actions are independent of objects, the apraxia is most evident. Liepmann speculated in some of his writing that the left hemisphere specialization with regard to both speech and praxis might in some way be derived from a predisposition of the left hemisphere to have a greater underlying capacity to learn and store knowledge about actions with symbolic associations independent of concrete objects.

In Liepmann's era, the fact that functional modules could be located in the brain was not so much in dispute, since his career followed Broca, Wernicke, Lichtheim and others who created models of higher-order neurological abnormalities based on the analysis of brain injuries including stroke. But his approach to determining the anatomical relationships of apraxia to the brain differed in some respects. Most notably, he systematically studied a very large group of over 80 patients, which in his day was unusual. While he studied this large series of patients, he also was highly indebted to case studies, and in particular, his first case of Mr. T. Liepmann acknowledged at the conclusion of this third paper on Mr. T. that the value of the case lay in the very thorough clinical description and pathology of it, a value "that will last beyond the current state of our understanding and could still provide new conclusions when reviewed in the light of future discoveries and questions." (Liepmann, 1905, personal translation, p. 243)

Visual Agnosia

Heinrich Lissauer (1861–1891), also a student of Carl Wernicke, provided the first comprehensive discussion of visual agnosia that distinguished between different components of the disorder and its types (1890, 1988). His distinction between apperceptive and associative agnosia is referred to today over a hundred years after his classic publication on the topic in 1890 and remains the most influential framework for discussing visual agnosia. He died at the age of 30 and published his only work on visual agnosia the year before his death.

The concept of visual agnosia and some of its characteristics had already been described and considered theoretically before Lissauer. Hermann Munk, an experimental physiologist in Berlin, had made partial ablations of the occipital cortex in dogs, and demonstrated that certain ablations would cause dogs to fail to recognize objects in a meaningful way, even when they still were able to navigate around these objects (Munk, 1878). After these ablations, the dogs would not be excited when they saw food or familiar people or their owners. The recognition of objects and people was intact if the dogs were allowed to smell or touch them; it was only the visual input modality that was affected. Munk described the deficit as related to a loss of the memories for visual images. With the loss of visual memories, the image could still be perceived, but the image did not elicit any memory of what the object stood for. Munk called the condition "mind blindness," and showed how it differed from other forms of blindness, caused by more extensive occipital lesions. Lesions that destroyed more of the primary visual cortex left the dogs unable to see anything, and they ran right into objects.

After Munk, HermannWilbrand assembled a lengthy monograph (1897) entitled "Mind Blindness" in which he collated cases from the literature and also discussed in general how the mind established relationships between visual forms and meanings. He included a case of his own, Mrs. G., as well as the famous case of Mr. X. of Charcot. At the onset of her illness, Mrs. G. could recognize objects and people immediately by touch or by sound, but had great difficulty recognizing them visually, especially when they were in complex scenes. For example, she mistook her dog for her physician and mistook her servant for a dining table. She had trouble finding things that she had just been handling and had recently put away, even when they were right in front of her. She described having been able to see them the whole time, but not being able to recognize them. She came to realize that "one sees more with the brain than with the eye . . . because I see absolutely anything quite clearly and lucidly, but I do not recognize it, and frequently, I do not know what the thing that I am seeing could be" (Solms et al, 1996, p. 95). Mrs. G. also had difficulties with topographical orientation, even in her neighborhood, though she could imagine scenes quite well. Charcot's famous case, Mr. X., was a highly educated man who had had an exceptional visual memory prior to his illness. After his injury, he could recognize objects much better than Mrs. G., but was completely unable to imagine anything visually or even dream in visual images. The inability to imagine visual images, including in dreaming, has been called the Charcot-Wilbrand syndrome. Mr. X., like Mrs. G., had problems with topographical agnosia, which had not been as clearly distinguished at that time.

Wilbrand's theoretical discussion of the concept of "mind blindness" emphasized, as had Munk's, that the lack of recognition of visual objects had something to do with the inability to activate visual memories. Thus, even if the image coming from the retina reached the brain intact, it might not activate the memory of that object. Normally, when perceiving an object, the retinal image reaching the brain should activate a visual memory of the object, which would then activate related knowledge associated with a variety of aspects of the object. Associated knowledge might include such properties as the object's smell, the written word for the object, gestures associated with activities in response to the object, emotional attitudes toward the object, etc.; which together would constitute its meaning. In addition, Wilbrand distinguished between mind blindness and a deficit in understanding spatial relationships between objects, which he notes can occur in other cases. He also described how patients with mind blindness can have a feeling of alienation from objects they see, even when they recognize what they are. For example, a cherished or frequently used object in a bedroom might seem foreign. One explanation for this could be a failure of activation of the affective associations usually linked with the object.

Lissauer's classic work was based on a case of an 80-year-old salesman, Gottlieb L., who had a profound disturbance of object recognition that was more severe than those of either Charcot or Wilbrand's cases (Lissauer, 1890/1988). As described by Lissauer, "he was quite incapable of visually recognizing the most common objects, although he could recognize everything by touch or hearing. Furthermore . . . it was clear from the way that he was able to look at and to handle objects that he was able to perceive visual stimuli . . . the patient could be made to draw simple unfamiliar objects placed in front of him, a clear indication that he was well able to perceive form" (Lissauer, 1890/1988, 160). Mr. L. had apparently developed his visual recognition problem gradually after being blown over on a fence in a storm. Lissauer's examination of Mr. L. was more systematic than that of other cases. Mr. L.'s visual acuity was mildly reduced, but not enough to account for his difficulties. He also had a right homonymous hemianopsia. He could perceive, but not name colors. His estimation of size and relationships of size—e.g., matching distances and bisecting lines—was accurate. His immediate visual memory was preserved for simple items: when he was given a line to draw of a certain length, he did well when asked to draw it immediately on another paper from memory. Longer term memory of visual experiences seemed to be no worse than his general memory. His ability to draw was more primitive than it had been, but he could draw the outline of real objects and make line drawings, even while he could not identify afterwards what they were. It was very challenging for him to draw from memory, possibly in part, Lissauer explained, because as soon as he had drawn part of the object, he could no longer recognize that part. Quoting Lissuauer, when Mr. L. drew from memory, he drew everything in

> . . . a bit by bit fashion . . . As soon as he had drawn one part of the object according to the image in his memory, this part, like all the other objects in his environment, became strange to him. He was no longer able to comprehend it, and therefore, was unable to complete his drawing of the whole object. The problem was not one of memory impairment, but of no longer being able to recognize the object or the part of the object which he had just drawn, and therefore not being able to compare it with the original template in his memory. For example, if he attempted to draw a boot, the leg and foot part were there but the heel had then to be attached. This the patient realized well enough but where did it belong? At this moment he was unable to comprehend his own drawing. It might

> just as well have been drawn by someone else. He drew the heel first here, then there, and eventually, he commented that he had no idea where it belonged (Lissauer 1890/1988, 168)

The patient could write fluently, but could not read. Form perception was intact for simple figures, but was impaired for more complex ones. If Lissauer provided the patient with simple forms with slight differences, the patient could point them out. But if the form was more complex, Mr. L. could not detect differences immediately recognizable to an average viewer. Lissauer explained the difficulty with form perception as stemming from the difficulty with recognizing the overall form semantically. Knowledge of the meaning helps a viewer more easily see differences in complex forms. Lissauer explains: "Imagine, for example, two pictures which show human shapes identical in all details; however, in one picture, the person has a happy face, and in the other, a sad face. To most people, this difference would be immediately obvious. However, to someone for whom these human shapes were no more than a combination of meaningless squiggles requiring line-by-line comparison, this difference would be difficult to discern" (Lissauer 1890/1988, 171).

Mr. L.'s greatest problem lay in the simple recognition of common objects. Mr. L.'s responses to objects presented in front of him often appeared to take the form of guesses which could be influenced by his response to another item, even when that item had no visual features in common. He identified a pen as a light, glasses as a lamp, and a piece of paper as a handkerchief. He often was curious to know if he was right. When given the opportunity to touch or hear a sound from the item, he usually could immediately recognize it, and would correct himself, saying that he had been mistaken. His own explanation for his errors was often that his "eyes had been mistaken." When asked to explain this further, he described that the object still looked familiar when he saw it initially, but he just could not remember what it was due to his weak memory. However, he did not have a weak memory when he touched the object, or heard it, only after he viewed it. His deficit was not simply a failure to find the name for the object, since he had no idea what the object was and could not provide any semantic information about it until he had identified it through other means (the difference between optic aphasia and agnosia). An excerpt from the patient's attempt to identify items illustrates how profound Mr. L.'s inability to recognize individual objects was:

> The patient is given a purse; he responds: "A lighter to light." The full purse is shaken close to his ear so that its contents rattle. "It's a purse."
>
> The patient is given a pocket watch; he responds: "A lamp"; after a bit,"a lighter". He is requested to draw the watch and draws the watch clearly. The watch is then put to his ear. He recognizes it at once: "Oh, it's a watch."
>
> (From Lissauer, 1890/1988, 175)

This patient's preserved ability to draw the outlines of items at which he was looking without the ability to recognize the items, prompted Lissauer to formulate a model for visual recognition with two stages. In the first stage, the item is identified on a perceptual level, and in the second stage, it is connected to meanings. He postulated that Mr. L. perceived the visual form sufficiently to identify the item, but that the form was cut off from the associated knowledge and memories, such that the meaning of the item could not be ascertained. Normally, a person who could draw the outline of a watch, indicating that they could see the watch to the degree that it contained this information, would automatically call up information that would tell him immediately what the object was. Mr. L. did not activate that associated knowledge.

Lissauer explained how it might not be enough when viewing a violin just to see the visual outline or form of the item, however unique that might be, unless it was connected with the knowledge associated with it. He described how, after the form has been identified visually, "the excitation" should "spread" to memory images "distributed throughout the whole of the cortex since they involve different modalities" (Lissauer 1890/1988, 186). The sound of the violin, and the tactile experiences that go along with handling it, along with the mental image of a violinist in his or her characteristic pose should all come to mind. Without these associations, the form's meaning would not be identified. Lissauer thought his patient primarily had the inability to activate these associations, and called this a type of agnosia, where recognition of the form of the objects was relatively intact, but the associations were disrupted. Neuroanatomically, associative agnosia was posited to be caused by a disconnection or failure of linkage among transcortical tracts coming from the visual cortex where the percept was perceived.

Implied in this formulation, is that a different type of agnosia would be caused by the failure of the first stage of perceiving the form of the object. Without recognition of the basic form of the object, it would be impossible to elicit the associations for further identifying the nature of the object. In this case, the patient would not be able to copy simple outlines of the object such that it would be impossible to proceed to the next stage of activating associations. Lissauer called this type of agnosia "apperceptive agnosia." He used the term *apperceptive* as opposed to *perceptive* in an effort to indicate that this perception was at the highest level of perception, in which the global form of the object is registered as a sensory impression with conscious awareness. In these cases, as for all agnosia patients, the patient had sufficient visual acuity and visual processing to register basic sensory features.

On an operational level, Lissauer discussed how the degree of a patient's apperceptive abilities might be indexed by having the patient compare two visual forms and try to find small differences between them. He also discussed how, for complex visual forms, it was likely that anyone with associative agnosia would have some impoverishment of their apperceptive abilities (as did Mr. L.), since some analysis of form on the complex level is shaped or guided by the knowledge of its associations. Lissauer was pointing out that top-down influences from our knowledge and associations help refine our perceptual experiences. Lissauer also noted that although the apperceptive agnosias and associative agnosias are relevant for understanding the nature of the processing problem, it might be rare to find "pure forms." It would be unlikely in the case of associative agnosia, because of the importance of top-down influences on higher level perceptual processing, that one would not find some simultaneous degree of degradation of the apperceptive process, as was found with Mr. L. when he tried to find small differences in sample complex visual forms.

Lisssauer described three recognition errors: First, there are errors which have a visual similarity to the object. In such cases, a patient might identify a pencil as a candle or a swan as a giraffe because they have similar shapes. Second, there are errors with no apparent relationship on an associative or visual percept level with the objects. In these cases, responses tend to be surprising and bizarre. In this category, he included Mr. L.'s tendency to think an object was the same object he had experienced recently, even when it had nothing visually or conceptually in common. He commented that this type of error is strange when the patient has just seen the first object and therefore might be expected to distinguish it easily from the next object. Third, there is a type of error where the error has a conceptual link to the actual object, even when it is not related on the visual dimension. In this case, a patient might call a watch a clock, or a paper a pencil. These were less prevalent in his patient.

Lissauer also points out that, in many cases of visual agnosia, it is not just that the patient does not recognize what is in front of him, but rather that the patient comes up with alternative ideas, in some cases even becoming reasonably convinced that he might be seeing another object. The reason why patients would start to believe they are seeing other things, rather than feeling simply that they have difficulty identifying an object, might have something to do with top-down processing. Thus Mr. L. thinks a coat brush is a live cat, and Ms. G. mistakes her dog for her physician. Lissauer suggests that there are two possible explanations for such positive errors of misrecognition. One explanation for the positive error is that the object is truly misperceived and appears by way of a distorted perceptual processing in a form that patients identify. The other is that the associations from another object within the mind are transferred to that of the object perceived. Lissauer preferred the second explanation, that internal active associations seem to be transferred to that of the percept presented (some type of top-down misattribution). Lissauer also makes the interesting suggestion that the misplacement of the associative connections might occur based on the proximity in which they were made in time. Thus, soon after the patient has seen a live grey cat, he is presented with a coat brush, and misidentifies the brush as the live grey cat. The associations of the live grey cat had been activated and were mis-attached to the new percept (producing what one might call a conceptual visual perseveration). He describes: "From this category of errors, we may draw an even more strange conclusion that, under these same pathological conditions, a tendency exists to link ideas which have come to mind at the same time by chance and apart from this have no connection with each other whatsoever."

Lissauer's treatment of agnosia differed from that of his predecessors and later investigators. In his monograph, Lissauer used the term "mind blindness" as had his predecessors who discussed this issue. The exception was Sigmund Freud, who actually coined the term agnosia for visual agnosia (1891). Wilbrand and others were aware of the idea of an associative network as the model to understand how concepts are represented in the brain. They were also aware that the connection to this associative network was disrupted in cases of visual agnosia, but the origin of this disruption was not so clear. The degradation of visual memories had previously been considered to be the cause for visual agnosia, and it seemed that this memory was something that was located in the visual cortex or near it. Based on a reading of Wilbrand, they assumed that this visual memory was not activated because associations to that image were not activated. That left it unclear whether this visual memory was in fact just something related to a visual disturbance and not a memory at all, that is, a failure to perceive a complete form of the image, an idea that Munk and Wilbrand rejected. Lissauer's formulation helped clarify that there were two stages involved in agnosia: one, in which the highest level percept or visual form is poorly perceived, and another, in which the associations connected to other knowledge about the image are disrupted. Lissauer divorced knowledge and memory of the concept from its percept. His formulation helped to direct investigators to establish more carefully how well patients with visual agnosia perceived forms (e.g., by using copying and matching tasks) rather than only recording their mistakes in identifying objects.

Lissauer's work distinguished between the perceptual or apperceptive stage of visual recognition, and what he conceived of as the subsequent "associative stage" in which recognition of the meaning and nature of the visual object is appreciated. Lissauer's model and approach was fundamentally influenced by Wernicke's information-processing scheme. The careful attention to detail recorded in his observations were like those recorded by Wernicke in his publications on aphasia. This type of model tried to identify functional stages or processing units that might be to a greater or lesser extent localized neuroanatomically. In the case of visual agnosia, Lissauer, like Wernicke postulated that the disruption in local areas of the cortex was more likely to disrupt a single modality of processing, such as vision. The connections to the meanings and concepts would be distributed in the brain. Apperceptive agnosia would be based more on circumscribed lesions of the occipital cortices and nearby regions, whereas associative agnosia would be based on disruption of transcortical pathways that connected that percept to associations that were simultaneously represented in various perceptual modalities.

The Information Processing Model and the Connectionistic Framework of Wernicke and his Followers versus Alternative Models and Perspectives

THE INFORMATION PROCESSING MODEL AND CONNECTIONISTIC FRAMEWORK

As is apparent from this chapter, one of the dominant frameworks for understanding relationships of the brain to cognitive function in the late 1800s and early 1900s is the "connectionistic" perspective of brain organization, a conception of cognitive architecture that developed primarily out of the Wernicke school. In this framework, the brain was understood to have specialized anatomical centers that supported specialized functions that would be connected to each other to allow information flow between them. Pathological behavior could be predicted from an understanding of how information flow had been disrupted between the centers or how the centers themselves had been destroyed. Particular theories put forward within this information processing framework are well depicted by diagrams that highlight the critical anatomical centers and their directional connections of information flow (e.g., as seen for example in both Lichtheim and Liepmann's work and figures).

Some have suggested that the information-flow modeling and connectionist approach that derives from Wernicke's school represents the birth of cognitive neuroscience. Hypotheses could be tested by predicting behaviors that would be generated by disruption in the centers and their various connections. The relation of behavioral deficits to brain anatomy could be inferred. Such models also provided a useful heuristic for understanding the essential components of complex processes, one that separated out the key components for further hypothesis testing.

ALTERNATIVE PERSPECTIVES OF BRAIN ORGANIZATION FROM THE GOLDEN ERA OF BEHAVIORAL NEUROLOGY

Despite the strength of the contributions of the connectionistic approach from this era, certain aspects of mental function, including certain aspects of language and aphasia, were not well explained with this approach. For example, it was difficult to explain why aphasics might predictably utter a sentence in one context, but not in another, such as only when motivated by emotion, or when singing. It was also not clear how connectionistic models could explain positive symptomatology exhibited by aphasics, such as an increased tendency to utter expletives. The British neurologist, John Hughlings Jackson, a contemporary of Broca and Wernicke, offered different perspectives on brain organization. He emphasized hierarchical structures in the brain and dynamic interactions between levels of brain function. In his framework, when damage occurred to what he called higher levels, i.e., those that were based on functions acquired later in development, disinhibition of lower levels would result. He suggested that basic lower level functions in the brain would be more resistant to damage because they were redundantly represented by overlearning than would less strongly represented higher-level functions. This would explain how global changes in function affect some systems more than others without requiring different localized lesions. Thus, normal speakers when they are tired have reduced generalized global processing efficiency that can result in paraphasic errors like those of aphasic speakers. Jackson's perspective showed an understanding of dynamic inhibitory relationships between levels of function (Jackson, 1915).

Unfortunately, although the connectionistic modelers themselves were the first to admit that their models did not account for every fascinating finding in aphasia or in other behavioral deficits (see Wernicke), attacks against the connectionist approach led to an abandonment of important insights into cognition developed in the late 1800s and early 1900s. Starting in the early 1900s, attacks on connectionist views became frequent at the intersection of psychology and neurology. One of the first challengers was Pierre Marie in 1906. While Marie did not entirely reject localization, he argued that Wernicke's aphasia was the only true aphasia, and that aphasia was based on a unitary comprehension of language module. He argued that the motor aphasia of Broca and its localization had been improperly interpreted because of *a priori* assumptions and oversimplifications. This aphasia was a motor output disruption caused by an internal capsule lesion and was independent of Broca's area. Marie's papers led to a lively debate in France about whether the localizationists and connectionists had overreached in their models of language and other functions.

The neurologists Henry Head and Kurt Goldstein, played a further influential role in discrediting the information-flow connectionistic models. Henry Head, in his 1926 book on aphasia and kindred disorders of speech, called the legacy of the "diagram makers" (a term he coined and used derogatively) to be "chaos." He went so far as to allege that the "diagram makers" would "lop and twist their cases to fit the procrustean bed of their hypothetical conceptions." (Head, 1926, vol. 1, p. 63). Although Head contributed important insights in many areas of neurology, his particular dedication to recording phenomenology in detail (he famously cut his own nerve to record the subjective experience of aspect of pain and the time course of their resolution) may have led him to reject the connectionistic models.. Head's dedication to the details of the phenomenology may have made it more difficult for him to appreciate how larger distinctions, which might not account for every detail, could be explanatory. Head extolled the virtues of John Hughlings Jackson for providing alternative theories. Head's own theories of aphasia did not offer much greater elucidation of the topic, and many of his aphasia subtypes could be mapped fairly readily onto the aphasia subtypes of the classical connectionist era. Evidence of the general influence of Head, is apparent in the comments of Shepherd Ivory Franz, a prominent American experimental psychologist, who criticized the work of connectionists like Liepmann and Joseph Jules Déjerine as being "crowded with the mental-cerebral assumptions which have been disputed by Head, and which are not supported by careful analysis of the material" (Franz 1916, pp. 167).

Kurt Goldstein, who had been a student of Wernicke and had originally, published contributions based on localizationist and connectionist modeling principles (1908), turned against those principles in his later years after working with Gestalt psychologists and emigrating to the United States. Goldstein's major treatise, entitled "The Organism," tried to explain how the organism responds to disruption in any part of the system as a whole. While Goldstein wrote on aphasia, and deemphasized the topographical approach to identification of aphasic syndromes, he was clearly steeped in this tradition and his explanations of aphasic syndromes, located in the technical aspects of his books, still relied heavily on principles derived from the classic models (see Geschwind on *The Paradoxical Stance of Kurt Goldstein*). The strong and prominent opinions of such influential figures as Head and Goldstein led to a loss of interest in the carefully developed models of functional anatomy from the late 1800s and early 1900s.

Schools of thought in the early part of the century which promoted a more holistic view of mind were very influential in the early 20th century and also worked to reduce enthusiasm for the connectionistic models. Such schools included Gestalt psychology, Freudian psychology, behaviorism, and an experimental psychology which was coming to anti- localizationists conclusions. Gestalt psychologists, many from Germany, were interested in probing how the mind actively imposes a unified perception on external stimuli in the context of changing figure and ground relationships. They were interested more in how the mind was organized in terms of pattern recognition rules that process contiguity and context than with the identification of discrete processing stations and connections of the flow modelers. Freudian psychology developed a psychodynamic model of mind components, which relied on introspective reports of subjective experience and personal history that were impossible to reduce to mechanistic flow models. Behaviorism, which arose partly from the rejection of reliance on subjective reports, regarded the brain as a black box, and restricted itself to the measuring of inputs and outputs to understand behavior. Eschewing any discussion of internal components of mind and brain, behaviorism was remote from the concerns of connectionists. Finally, Karl Lashley, who became head of the American Psychological Association, was representative of a group of experimental psychologists who had difficulty demonstrating that specific brain lesions produced critical effects on brain functions such as memory (based on lesioning animals). He revived a view that harked back to that of the anti-localizationist stance of brain equipotentiality promoted by Flourens in his debates with Gall one hundred years earlier (e.g., *Brain Mechanisms and Intelligence*, 1929). Lashley, who concentrated on the complexity of brain organization, argued that the brain has hierarchical internal programs, a position different from that of behaviorists, but was still unconvinced that specific brain centers were dedicated to specific higher level complex functions.

NORMAN GESCHWIND AND THE REVIVAL OF INTEREST IN CLASSICAL MODELS

Norman Geschwind described how in the 1950s he proudly regarded himself a member of the "philosophically sophisticated Jackson-Head-Goldstein school of neurology," and how, like others raised in the British and American traditions in the mid-20th century, he considered the work of Wernicke and the information processing modelers to be essentially misguided, unscientific, irrelevant, and supplanted by more important theories. But Geschwind was prompted to revisit the older literature at the encouragement of a European-trained neurologist Fred Quadfasel, and discovered that neurologists at the turn of the century had been detailed in their analyses and insightful in their conclusions. They had generated models that continued to be relevant, if not more so than the ones with which he had been trained. Geschwind described how, due to his former training, he had expected the older work not to be helpful, but instead discovered the "broadside accusations of carelessness, of inadequate examination, of unconcern with psychology all unfounded" (Geschwind, 1964/1997, 54). Geschwind subsequently became a champion of these former models, bringing them to prominence again, in particular with his discussion of the work of Lichtheim, Wernicke, and Liepmann in his magnum opus "Disconnection Syndromes in Animals and Man" (Geschwind, 1965). Geschwind's later career continued to be influenced by the connectionistic approach. After him, these models once again became a starting point for modeling the cognitive architecture of the brain.

Summary

This chapter has reviewed some of the most influential models of language, apraxia, and agnosia from the beginning and the height of the classical period in behavioral neurology, a time when there was great amount of energy focused on attempting to understand the underlying functional and anatomical organization of higher mental functions in the brain. Although the contributions of Wernicke, Lichtheim, Liepmann, and Lissauer have been highlighted here, there were also many other contributors in the late 1800s and early 1900s who were involved in elucidating the modular architecture of the mind and brain (e.g., to name a few: Déjerine, Boenhoffer, Bastian, Charcot, Henschen). This prolific and rich period of behavioral neurology, sometimes referred to as the Golden

Era, left a legacy of fascinating and insightful perspectives on higher-level brain organization.

On reviewing the work from this era, one is impressed with the neuroanatomical knowledge and insight that formed the basis for hypothesizing the location of specialized centers. The neurologists typically not only utilized careful observations of behavior, but also considered cytoarchitectonic and embryological factors when they posited the neuroanoatomical location of functions, while also considering broader organisational principles of neuroanatomic function related to basic motor and sensory processes.

The connectionistic approach taken by the Wernicke school and his followers, has a surprising affinity to current approaches to modeling in cognitive neuroscience, despite hailing from over 100 years ago. While there is strong interest today in distributed networks that support functions today, there is also recognition that there is modularity on a variety of levels, with specialized anatomical centers specialized to support more specific functions.

Although there are flaws of methods based on clinical-pathological correlation, work derived from the study of neurological patients with lesions is a critical approach that helps define the limits of structural mental anatomy. Lesion-based studies, because they are not generated by experimental manipulation devised by the investigator, can challenge major psychological theories in their broader limits. Convergent evidence from a variety of methods gives us the greatest confidence in our hypotheses. The conclusions and controversies of the classical period of connectionist modeling have persisted over time and continue to frame the approach to the neural bases of cognitive systems in the modern era.

References

Bichat, F. X. (1978). Physiological researches on life and earth (F. Gold, Trans.). In D. N. Robinson (Ed.), Significant contributors to the history of psychology (pp. i–334). Ser. E. Physiological psychology: Vol 2, X. Bichat. J.G. Spurzheim., P Fluorens. Washington, DC: University Publications of America. (Original work published 1805).

Bouillaud, J. B. (1847–1848). Recherches cliniques propre à démontrer que la sens du langage articulé et le principe coordinateur de movements de la parole resident dans le lobules antérieuer du cerveau. Bulletin de l'Académie Royale de Médicine, XIII, 699–710, 778–816.

Breasted, J. H. (1930). The Edwin Smith Surgical Papyrus. Chicago: University of Chicago Press.

Broca, P. (1861). Remarques sur le siège de la faculté du langage articulé, suivie d'une observation d'aphémie (perte de la parole). Bulletins de la Société Anatomique, 6, 330–357.

Broca P. (1994). Notes on the faculty of articulated language, followed by an observation of aphemia. (incl. pp 330–336 and 342–346 of original). In P. Eling (ed.), Reader in the history of aphasia. Amsterdam/ Philadelphia: John Benjamins Publishing Company. pp. 41–55. (Original work published 1861).

Broca P. (1977). Remarks on the Seat of the Faculty of Articulate Speech, Followed by the Report of a Case of Aphemia (Loss of Speech). (incl. pp. 332–33 and 343–357 of original). Translated by C. Wasterlain and D. A. Rottenberg. In D.A. Rottenberg and F.H. Hockberg (eds.), Neurological classics in modern translation, New York: Macmillan Press. pp. 136–149. (Original work published 1861).

Broca, P. (1865). Sur le siège de la faculté du langage articulé. *Bulletins de la Société d'Anthropologie,* 6, 377–93. (laterality)

Dax, M. (1836). Lésion de la moitié gauche de l'encéphale coincident avec l'oubli des signes de la pensée (Lu a Montpellier en 1836). Gazette Hebdomadaire de Médecine et Chirurgie 11 (Sér. 2), 1865. In English Translation in The roots of psychology, ed. S. Diamond. New York: Basic Books, 1974, 29–40.

Eling, P. (Ed.). (1994). Reader in the History of Aphasia: From Gall to Geschwind. John Benjamins Publishing Company. Amsterdam.

Ellis, A.W. (1984). Bramwell's (1897) case of word meaning deafness. Cognitive Neuropsychology, 1, 245–258.

Feinberg, T. E., Rothi, L. J. G., & Heilman, K. M. (1986). "Inner Speech" in conduction aphasia. Archives of Neurology, 43(6), 591–593.

Flourens, P. P. M. (1824). Recherches experimentales sur les propriétiés et les fonctions due systéme nerveux, dans les animaux vertebres. Paris: Crevot.

Franz, S. I. (1916). The function of the cerebrum. Psychological Bulletin, 13(4), 149–173.

Gall, F. J., & Spurzheim, J. C. (1810–1819). *Anatomie et physiologie du systême nerveux en général et du cerveau en particulier.* Paris: F. Schoell.

Gall, F. J., & Spurzheim, J. C. (1835). On the functions of the brain and of each of its parts: With observations on the possibility of determining the instincts, propensities, and talents, or the moral and intellectual dispositions of men and animals, by the configuration of the brain and head (W. Lewis, Jr., trans.). Boston: Marsh, Capen, and Lyon. (Original work, Sur le Fonctions du Cerveau, published 1822–1825).

Geschwind, N. (1965). Disconnexion syndromes in animals and man. *Brain,* 88: 237–294 and 585–644.

Hagner, M. (1997). *Der Wandel von Seelenorgan zum Gehirn.* Berlin: Berlin Verlag.

Harrington, A. *Medicine, Mind, and the Double Brain.* Princeton, NJ: Princeton University Press, 1987.

Head, H. (1926). *Aphasia and kindred disorders of speech.* 2 Vols. Cambridge, UK: Cambridge University Press.

Heilman, K. M., Tucker, D. M., & Valenstein, E. (1976). A case of mixed transcortical aphasia with intact naming. *Brain,* 99, 415–525.

Heilman, K. M., Gonzalez-Rothi, L. J., McFarling, D., & Rottmann, A. Transcortical Sensory Aphasia with Relatively Spared Spontaneous Speech and Naming. *Archives of Neurology* 38: 236–239, 1981.

Jackson H. (1915). On Aphasia and kindred affections of speech, together with a complete bibliography of his publications on speech and a reprint of some of the more important papers. *Brain,* xxxviii, 1–190.

Katz, R.B., Goodglass, H. (1990). Deep dysphasia: Analysis of a rare form of repetition disorder. *Brain and Language,* 39(1), 153–185.

Kussmaul, A. (1877). *Die Störungen der Sprache.* Leipsig: Vogel.

Lichtheim, L. (1885). On Aphasia. *Brain.* 7, 433–484.

Liepmann, H. (1905). Der weitere Krankheitsverlauf bei dem einseitig Apraktischen und der Gehirnbefund auf Grund von Serienschnitten. *Monatschrift für Psychiatrie und Neurologie,* 17: 289–311; 19: 217–243.

Liepmann H, & Mass O. (1907). Fall von Linksseitiger Agraphie and Apraxie bei rechtsseitiger Lähmung. *Journal für Psychologie und Neurologie. 10,* 214–227.

Liepmann, H. *Drei Aufsätze aus dem Apraxiegebiet.* Berlin: Karger, 1908.

Lissauer, H. (1890). Ein Fall von Seelenblindheit nebst einem Beitrag zur Theorie derselben. *Archiv für Psychiatrie*. 21:222–270. In Translation in Cognitive Neuropsychology, Vol 5 (2), 1988, 157–192. (M. Jackson, transl). A case of visual agnosia with a contribution to theory.

Marie, P. (1906). The third left frontal convolution plays no special role in the function of language. *Semaine Médicale, 26*, 241–247.

Munk, H. (1878). Über der Funktionen der Grosshirnrinde: Gesammelte Mittheilungen s den Jahren 1877–90. Berlin: Hirschwald.

Trousseau, A. (1864). De l'aphasie, maladie décrite récemment sous le nom impropre d'aphémie. Gazette Hôpitaux Civils Militaires, 37, 13–14, 25–26, 37–39, 49–50.

Wernicke C. Einige neuere Arbeiten über Aphasie, Fortrshcritte der Medizin 3 (1985); 824–830; 4(1886) 371, 463–469. Reprinted in "C. Wernicke Gesammelte Aufsätze und kritische Referate zur Pathologie des Nervensystem." Berlin: Fisher, (1893). Excerpts translated in Eling P. Reader in the History of Aphasia. pp. 90–98. Eling, P (Ed.) Reader in the History of Aphasia: From Gall to Geschwind. Amsterdam: John Benjamins Publishing Company.

Wigan, A. L. (1844). *A New View of Insanity. The Duality of the Mind*. London: Longman, Brown, Green, and Longmans.

CHAPTER 3

Deconstructing Human Memory: Insights from Amnesia

Mieke Verfaellie and Margaret M. Keane

The Amnesic Syndrome

The central feature of amnesia is an impairment in new learning (anterograde amnesia) that is evident regardless of the nature of the information (i.e., verbal or visuospatial) or modality of study presentation (i.e., auditory or visual); it is typically accompanied by difficulty in the ability to retrieve memories acquired prior to the onset of illness (retrograde amnesia), but the severity of this impairment is more variable. Amnesia occurs in the context of otherwise relatively preserved intellectual functioning and cognitive abilities. Most strikingly, amnesic patients have intact immediate or short-term memory, as evidenced by the ability to follow an ongoing conversation, or to immediately repeat back a sequence of words or numbers. Following any interference or delay, however, memory for the information is lost.

Amnesia can arise from a number of different etiologies, including anoxia, herpes simplex encephalitis (HSE), stroke, Wernicke-Korsakoff syndrome (WKS), and rupture and repair of an anterior communicating artery (ACoA) aneurysm (O'Connor & Verfaellie, 2002). The amnesia is a direct consequence of damage to structures in the medial temporal lobes including the hippocampus and surrounding entorhinal, perirhinal and parahippocampal cortices (e.g., anoxia, HSE), midline diencephalon (e.g., thalamic stroke, WKS), basal forebrain (e.g., ACoA aneurysm) or the fiber tracts that connect these regions, such as the fornix. Despite the etiological heterogeneity of the syndrome, the core characteristics of amnesia are relatively consistent. Efforts to delineate qualitative differences as a function of etiology have focused on both the contribution of lesion site (e.g., diencephalon vs. medial temporal lobe (MTL) Parkin, 1993); and lesion extent (e.g., hippocampus proper vs. hippocampus and surrounding cortices; Aggleton & Brown, 1999), but such distinctions remain the focus of debate. More clearly established is the impact of disruption of frontally mediated executive functions, which is often superimposed on the core amnesia in patients with diencephalic and basal forebrain lesions. In such cases, the anterograde amnesia may be exacerbated by additional impairments in planning and organizing incoming information, as well as in the initiation and evaluation of memory search and effortful retrieval (Moscovitch & Winocur, 2002). In clinical practice, these additional impairments, when severe, can cloud the distinction between selective amnesia and more pervasive cognitive impairment.

Despite the wide-ranging nature of the long-term memory impairment in patients with amnesia, it is striking that the impairment is not uniform across all forms of long-term memory. The distinction between preserved and impaired aspects of memory has guided much cognitive neuropsychological research and has contributed greatly to our understanding of the cognitive and neural architecture of various components of memory. However, the interest in dissociations in patients' performance led to a strong focus on isolating distinct forms of memory. This effort may have overshadowed the fact that many tasks draw on multiple memory processes, not all of which are equally affected in amnesia. More broadly, distinct forms of memory may commonly interact in the service of task performance. We review below some of the salient experimental findings that have led to these insights.

Amnesia: Experimental Studies

IMPLICIT VERSUS EXPLICIT MEMORY

Patients with amnesia show severe impairments in their ability to intentionally retrieve recently acquired information, whether in recall or recognition tasks. This explicit memory impairment stands in striking contrast to their intact performance in a number of other memory tasks in which learning is expressed implicitly, through performance rather than recollection. Over the last two decades, an extensive body of research in amnesia has focused on one particular example of implicit memory, namely repetition priming (for reviews, see Moscovitch, Vriezen, & Gottstein, 1993; Verfaellie & Keane, 2001). Repetition priming is typically assessed in tasks in which subjects identify briefly presented words, complete word stems or fragments with the first word that comes to mind, freely generate words in response to cues, or make decisions about characteristics of presented words or pictures. Priming manifests as improved performance (i.e., detection, generation, or faster decision) for those stimuli to which an individual was previously exposed relative to comparable, not previously exposed, stimuli. Dissociations in amnesia between intact performance on implicit memory tasks and impaired performance on explicit memory tasks have laid the ground work for the view that memory is a not a unitary function, but rather, that there are distinct forms of memory that may have functionally and neurally different bases.

Most tasks involve a range of processes from stimulus identification to responding, and accordingly, facilitation as a result of prior experience can occur at several processing stages, including perceptual, phonological/lexical, semantic, and response stages. One particularly influential distinction has been that between perceptual and conceptual priming (Roediger & McDermott, 1993): perceptual priming is sensitive to the reinstatement of physical features of previously presented stimuli at test, whereas conceptual priming is sensitive to the reinstatement of semantic features. The preservation of both of these forms of priming in amnesia establishes that these effects are independent of MTL structures. Behavioral evidence from patients with lesions outside of the MTL implicates posterior visual areas in visuoperceptual priming effects (Gabrieli, Fleischman, Keane, Reminger, & Morrell, 1995; Keane, Gabrieli, Mapstone, Johnson, & Corkin, 1995; Kroll et al., 2003) and higher-order multimodal association areas in conceptually based priming effects (Fleischman & Gabrieli, 1998; Keane, Gabrieli, Fennema, Growdon, & Corkin, 1991). Subsequent imaging research has confirmed and refined these neuroanatomical distinctions, pointing to posterior neocortical regions that represent the perceptual form and structure of items as the neural basis of perceptual priming, and areas in inferior temporal and frontal regions that underlie the conceptual features of items as the neural basis of conceptual priming (for review, see Schacter, Wigg, & Stevens, 2007). Further, these imaging studies have generally shown reductions in cortical activity associated with priming; such activity reductions reflect the increased efficiency of processing of primed stimuli, possibly due to increased "tuning" of neocortical representations (Wiggs & Martin, 1998).

At a cognitive level, increased processing efficiency has been conceptualized as enhanced fluency or ease of processing of stimuli that were previously encountered (Jacoby, 1983). Manipulations of processing fluency influence judgments about a variety of non-memorial attributes, such as duration, perceptual clarity, and liking, but they also can impact memorial judgments. Indeed, one influential view of recognition memory suggests that recognition judgments can be based on one of two processes: recollection (i.e., retrieval of contextual detail) or familiarity (i.e., an undifferentiated sense of oldness) (Mandler, 1980). Judgments of familiarity are thought to be based on fluency of processing (Jacoby & Dallas, 1981): since prior experience enhances processing fluency, such fluency can be used as a heuristic to make decisions about prior occurrence. Consistent with this notion, a large number of cognitive studies have documented that fluency can be used as a basis for familiarity-based recognition (for review, see Yonelinas, 2002). Importantly, several patient studies similarly have shown that amnesic patients (Verfaellie & Cermak, 1999) and patients with Alzheimer's disease (Wolk et al., 2005) can use fluency as a cue for recognition. Nonetheless, the link between fluency and familiarity has remained a matter of intense debate in the neuropsychological literature, as findings of chance recognition (i.e., familiarity) in the face of intact priming (i.e., fluency) have been taken as powerful evidence for the notion that implicit and explicit memory tasks do not share underlying processes or memorial signals (Hamann & Squire, 1997; Levy, Stark, & Squire, 2004).

In our own work, we have taken a different approach to attempt to reconcile these seemingly contradictory findings. In line with the cognitive literature, we assume that fluency signals support both implicit memory and familiarity-based explicit memory, but we argue that whereas priming is a direct (unmediated) consequence of fluent processing, familiarity-based recognition requires an additional step whereby fluency is attributed to a memorial source. The need for an additional attributional process (and the potential reluctance of amnesic patients to use that process) may provide an explanation for the apparent paradox that despite the fact that priming is largely intact in amnesia, the fluency that supports implicit memory does not support more fully familiarity-based recognition in these same patients.

In several studies, we have demonstrated that amnesics' use of a fluency-heuristic in recognition can be experimentally enhanced. In one study (Verfaellie, Giovanello, & Keane, 2001), we encouraged fluency attributions through task instructions that provided participants information about the alleged proportion of old items on a recognition test (30 percent vs. 70 percent). The actual proportion of old items on the test was constant across conditions, but we hypothesized that providing participants instructions that a majority of items were old would lead them to relax their response criterion and rely to a greater extent on processing fluency. Consistent with this hypothesis, amnesic patients had higher recognition accuracy in the 70 percent than in the 30 percent condition. In another study (Keane, Orlando, & Verfaellie, 2006), we manipulated the salience of fluency cues by drawing targets and distractors from the same pool of letters (yielding high perceptual overlap between targets and distractors) or different pools of letters (yielding low perceptual overlap between targets and distractors). Amnesic patients had higher accuracy in the low- compared to the high-overlap condition, presumably because of the increased salience of the fluency "contrast" between targets and distractors in the low-overlap condition. These findings suggest that the increased salience of fluency cues promotes the use of a fluency heuristic that is ordinarily not fully engaged in amnesia. Findings such as these highlight the importance of understanding factors that influence the use of a fluency heuristic in amnesia, as a means of gaining a fuller understanding of the relationship between priming and recognition memory (see also Voss & Paller, 2009; Willems, Salmon, & Van der Linden, 2008).

So far we have focused on priming and fluency effects for single items; another area of interest concerns amnesics' performance on tasks that assess priming of associations newly established at study. The interest in new-associative priming in amnesia stems from its relevance to theories that postulate that the hippocampus is critical for computing arbitrary links between unrelated stimuli, and to theories that characterize the core deficit in amnesia as one of binding arbitrary pieces of information (Ryan, Althoff, Whitlow, & Cohen, 2000). Here, we focus specifically on implicit memory for novel perceptual associations, because at present, most research has focused on the establishment of novel associations in the context of visual perceptual tasks. Even within this restricted domain of study, different outcomes have been obtained. On the one hand, several studies have assessed priming for the association between two words by comparing performance when a target stimulus at test is presented with the same context word as at study rather than with a different (albeit also studied) context word. Using both perceptual identification and lexical decision tasks, associative priming has been found to be intact in amnesia (Gabrieli, Keane, Zarella, & Poldrack, 1997; Goshen-Gottstein, Moscovitch, & Melo, 2000; but see Yang et al., 2003). On the other hand, several studies have examined the formation of associations between visual contextual information and target items in the context of a visual search task. Whereas normal individuals show facilitation in visual search for a target embedded in repeated arrays, amnesic patients (Chun & Phelps, 1999), and specifically those with extensive MTL lesions (Manns & Squire, 2001), have not shown such contextual facilitation. In a somewhat different paradigm examining preferential looking, normal participants show enhanced eye movements to regions of a previously viewed scene that have been altered, but again, amnesic patients have failed to show this pattern (Ryan et al., 2000). Importantly, the priming effects in these tasks, reflecting the establishment of relationships between different elements of complex visual displays, occur in control subjects even in the absence of explicit memory for repeated contexts or changes in scenes, and thus appear to reflect an unaware memory mechanism (but see, Smith, Hopkins, & Squire, 2006).

How can we understand the presence of intact new associative priming for perceptual associations between two words, but impaired new associative priming for more complex visuospatial contexts? One possibility relates to the nature of the binding operations that are required in these respective tasks. Mayes and colleagues (Mayes, Montaldi, & Migo, 2007) make a useful distinction between within-domain associations (formed between the same or very similar kinds of items) and cross-domain associations (formed between items from distinct modalities or linking information spatially), and suggest that whereas the former may be mediated by activation in closely adjacent neocortical regions, the latter may be mediated by activation in distant neocortical regions that requires integration through the MTL. Although this formulation was proposed to account for findings in explicit memory, it may also provide an explanatory framework for the divergent findings concerning implicit associative memory: associations between two words may be established directly within visual word processing areas, through co-activation of the representation of individual word forms. In contrast, associations between objects and a spatial context or scene may require MTL mediation. Supporting this notion, neuroimaging studies of implicit memory point to the importance of MTL cortical regions (Goh et al., 2004; Preston & Gabrieli, 2008) and hippocampus proper (Goh et al., 2004) in the establishment of spatial and contextual representations that integrate multiple elements.

An additional consideration relates to the fact that neocortically- and hippocampally-mediated associations are qualitatively different (Eichenbaum & Cohen, 2001): whereas neocortical binding leads to the establishment of unitized representations that are inflexible and can only be accessed as a whole, hippocampal binding allows for the establishment of relational representations that can be accessed flexibly through their separate parts. Consistent with the notion that amnesic patients can only form inflexible unitized representations, studies examining implicit memory for words pairs, in which the study and/or test stimuli were presented sequentially rather than simultaneously, have yielded impaired associative priming in patients with amnesia (Carlesimo, Perri, Costa, Serra, & Caltagirone, 2005; Paller & Mayes, 1994).

SEMANTIC VERSUS EPISODIC MEMORY

The cardinal impairment in amnesia is an inability to form and retrieve memories of personally experienced events (i.e., episodic memory). Seen in contrast to patients' generally preserved intelligence and good fund of general knowledge, this led to early conceptualizations of amnesia as a selective impairment in episodic memory, with sparing of semantic memory (Cermak, 1984; Wood, Ebert, & Kinsbourne, 1982). Further research, however, has made clear that such a view is inaccurate: whereas premorbid semantic memory is largely intact in amnesia, new semantic learning is substantially impaired. Here we briefly describe findings both in the retrograde and anterograde domain, with the aim of demonstrating that, although functionally and neurally separable, episodic memory and semantic memory do not operate in isolation.

Within the domain of remote semantic memory, with the exception of information acquired within the years immediately preceding the onset of amnesia, MTL patients show sparing of general semantic and factual knowledge (Manns, Hopkins, & Squire, 2003; Verfaellie, Reiss, & Roth, 1995). This sparing stands in stark contrast to their impairment in retrieving detailed, episodic memories, an impairment that is temporally extensive and, in cases of severe amnesia, can cover the entire lifespan (Moscovitch, Nadel, Winocur, Gilboa, & Rosenbaum, 2006; Rosenbaum et al., 2008; Steinvorth, Levine, & Corkin, 2005) although this has not always been observed (Bayley, Gold, Hopkins, & Squire, 2005; Kirwan, Bayley, Galvan, & Squire, 2008). The differential impairment in amnesia in remote episodic compared to semantic memory reinforces the distinction between these two forms of memory. Further, it suggests that the permanent storage and retrieval of detailed episodic information is mediated by MTL structures, whereas the storage and retrieval of semantic memories, once consolidated, occurs neocortically, without MTL mediation.

Whether the acquisition of new semantic memories can occur independent of the MTL structures that mediate episodic learning is more controversial. The impairment of new semantic learning in amnesia is now firmly established, and it is clear that the severity of the semantic learning impairment is linked to the extent of MTL pathology (Verfaellie, 2000). However, it is equally clear that some new semantic information can be acquired even in patients with dense episodic impairment (Kitchener, Hodges, & McCarthy, 1998; Vargha-Khadem et al., 1997). These findings can be reconciled if it is assumed that the acquisition of semantic memory can occur independent of episodic memory/MTL structures, but that nonetheless, semantic learning is typically enhanced by MTL mediation. Newly acquired information is always embedded in an episodic context, and as such, episodic learning helps support semantic acquisition. Only with time and/or repeated presentation will the gist information become dissociated from its spatiotemporal context, reflecting a process of gradual neocortical transfer with the establishment and consolidation of context-free semantic representations. In patients with extensive MTL lesions, however, gradual neocortical learning may occur of necessity in isolation. Thus, whereas the acquisition of semantic and episodic memory may be tightly coupled in normal cognition, in patients with MTL lesions, this coupling is disrupted, exposing the operation of neocortical learning by itself.

The contribution of episodic memory, however, is not limited to new semantic learning. Recent evidence suggests that even in tasks measuring retrieval of long-established semantic information, episodic memory may play a role. Ryan and colleagues (Ryan, Cox, Hayes, & Nadel, 2008) observed hippocampal activation during a prototypical semantic memory task—retrieval of category exemplars. This finding suggests that the hippocampus is involved in the retrieval of semantic information, but leaves unanswered whether it is needed to do so, and if so, what role it plays. To address these questions, we (Greenberg, Keane, & Verfaellie, 2009) asked patients with MTL lesions to generate category exemplars for three types of categories that tended to elicit different retrieval strategies in control participants: categories that elicited autobiographical spatial retrieval strategies, categories that elicited autobiographical but nonspatial strategies, and categories that elicited neither autobiographical nor spatial strategies. Patients with MTL lesions were more impaired for the former two types than for the latter, and once phonemic fluency was taken into account, the impairment was selective to categories that elicited autobiographical strategies. These findings suggest that the hippocampus may contribute to semantic retrieval through the retrieval of autobiographical detail; hippocampal damage prevents this contribution of autobiographical memory to semantic retrieval in amnesia. In a similar vein, it has been shown that having a personal autobiographical experience associated with famous names (as evidenced by judgments of recollective experience) facilitates fame judgments, but amnesic patients with MTL lesions fail to show this facilitation (Westmacott, Black, Freedman, & Moscovitch, 2004). The inverse also holds: in patients with semantic dementia, relatively unimpaired autobiographical memory can help preserve or re-establish degenerating semantic knowledge (Snowden, Griffiths, & Neary, 1994; Westmacott et al., 2004). Such findings reinforce the notion that episodic memory and semantic memory do not operate in isolation.

While so far we have considered the contribution of episodic memory to semantic learning and retrieval, there is also evidence for the contribution of semantic memory to episodic learning. The "levels of processing" framework established many years ago that new information is remembered better when it is processed semantically, presumably because semantic encoding allows new information to be linked with prior knowledge (Craik & Lockhart, 1972). In keeping with this framework, patients with semantic dementia and aphasic patients with semantic impairments perform poorly on verbal learning tasks (Graham, Simons, Pratt, Patterson, & Hodges, 2000; Ween, Verfaellie, & Alexander, 1996). However, the contribution of semantic memory extends beyond the simple analysis of incoming formation. Evidence in normal individuals suggests that information is remembered better when it can be anchored to pre-existing schematic knowledge (e.g., Anderson & Pichert, 1978; Brewer & Treyens, 1981). To evaluate whether schematic activation can support episodic learning in amnesic patients, we asked patients to remember prices of everyday grocery items (Kan, Alexander, & Verfaellie, 2009). In one condition, the to-be-remembered prices were consistent with prior knowledge about the items, whereas in another condition they were not. Control subjects had higher recognition memory for prices of items in the congruent than in the incongruent condition. A similar congruency benefit was seen in patients with restricted MTL lesions, who had intact semantic systems, but patients with lesions extending into the lateral temporal lobes, who had compromised semantic systems, failed to show a congruency benefit. These findings suggest that when prior knowledge structures are intact, they can support the acquisition of new information by facilitating the integration of new information into existing knowledge structures. The contribution of pre-existing semantic memory to episodic learning illustrated by these findings provides a potential explanation for the surprising clinical observation that some amnesic patients are able to acquire a considerable amount of new information relevant to long-standing personal interests.

Lessons Learned

In the '80s and '90s, cognitive neuropsychological studies of amnesia, with their focus on demonstrating dissociations between different aspects of memory, played a critical role in laying bare distinct forms of long-term memory. The emphasis on fractionation of memory was useful in that it allowed broad distinctions, such as those between implicit and explicit memory and between semantic and episodic memory, and allowed researchers to fully characterize these distinct forms of memory. More recent patient studies have led the way to a more refined understanding of the processes that are impaired and preserved in amnesia, revealing that process-impairments associated with amnesia do not necessarily respect taxonomic boundaries. Rather, these component processes contribute to putatively different forms of memory. Moreover, selective impairments in amnesia provide a window onto functional interactions between different forms of memory in normal cognition.

This gradual shift in emphasis reflects the accumulation of critical evidence. Early studies of implicit memory in patients with amnesia, under conditions where explicit contamination was carefully avoided, were essential to elucidating the nature of the processes that underlie priming in different tasks. Similarly, systematic study of amnesics' performance on recall and recognition tasks was necessary to recognize the existence of distinct explicit memory processes that may be differentially affected in amnesia. The emphasis on processes underlying performance within each type of memory task was prerequisite to the examination of their potential overlap, leading to the recognition that a fluency process is not unique to implicit memory, but is also a critical building block for familiarity-based (explicit) recognition memory.

The recognition that there is not a one-to-one mapping between cognitive processes and categories of memory is similarly illustrated by more recent findings indicating that amnesia does not yield a uniform dissociation between binding processes in the service of implicit and explicit memory task performance. First, the finding that amnesic patients show intact performance on associative priming tasks that require the establishment of a novel association among similar items, but impaired performance on associative priming tasks that require the establishment of associations among heterogeneous items, suggests that—even within the domain of implicit memory—not all implicit binding processes are alike. Rather, they differ depending on the nature of the representations that are created, with within-domain associations being instantiated directly in the neocortex and cross-domain associations requiring hippocampal mediation. Second, the finding that hippocampal damage interferes not only with the formation of episodic memories, which inherently places high demands on associative processes, but also with some forms of implicit associative memory, challenges the notion that the hippocampus plays a selective role in binding processes that support explicit or aware memory performance. Rather, it suggests that memory representations made up of disparate, non-local elements require hippocampal mediation, regardless of whether they are accessed in the context of implicit or explicit memory tasks. Taken together, these insights have shifted the focus of memory research from an emphasis on long-term memory systems that can be differentiated according to conscious awareness, to an emphasis on the nature of the representations and processes that support performance on any particular task (see e.g., Reder, Park, & Kieffaber, 2009).

A similar emphasis on the nature of memory representations enhances our understanding of the operation of and interactions among episodic and semantic memory. While episodic representations bind together the different aspects that make up an experienced event in its contextual richness, semantic representations are acontextual abstractions formed across time and repeated experience. In many tasks, however, these representations operate in concert. As discussed above, episodic contextual information may routinely support the acquisition of new semantic knowledge, making it difficult to disentangle the two forms of learning. In this respect, the study of patients with extensive MTL lesions offers a unique opportunity to elucidate neocortical semantic learning in isolation. Such learning occurs very gradually and lacks the flexibility associated with episodic memory (Bayley, Frascino, & Squire, 2005), but its boundaries are still not fully established (Stark, Stark, & Gordon, 2005).

Perhaps even more compelling are interactions between episodic memory and already well-established semantic memory, in that they suggest continued MTL-neocortical interactions once neocortical representations are fully established. Such interactions reflect the fact that retrieval from semantic memory may be enhanced through the use of autobiographical retrieval strategies—a process that is impaired in patients with amnesia. This process may be particularly beneficial when relatively preserved autobiographical memory can help buttress degraded semantic memory, as in patients with semantic dementia. A question that remains to be addressed more fully concerns the nature of the "episodic" representations that support semantic retrieval. In some cases semantic retrieval may be supported by autobiographical retrieval strategies that lead to recovery of information pertaining to a unique past event. In other cases, semantic retrieval is more likely supported by autobiographical memory for repeated events or contexts (e.g., retrieval of a variety of past tea-making experiences when asked to identify a teapot). Such summarized events, which are highly detailed and contextualized despite the fact that they are not time-specific, may fit Neisser's (1981) concept of "repisodic memory" or Conway's (2001) "general events" level of autobiographical knowledge. Interestingly, neuroimaging work suggests that such repeated events also activate the autobiographical memory network, and that such activation is modulated by the richness of retrieved memory (Addis, Moscovitch, Crawley, & McAndrews, 2004). Such memories share with unique episodic events the quality of recollective experience (Moscovitch, 2008), and it is this recollection of details that facilitates retrieval of information from the semantic knowledge base.

Finally, there is also support for the converse interaction—semantic memory affecting episodic memory—as evidenced by the fact that the integrity of semantic memory in general, and the availability of premorbid semantic information in particular, influence new episodic learning. As illustrated in the study by Kan et al. (2009), new learning can be facilitated by the existence of an established schematic structure into which new information can be incorporated. However, the impact of pre-existing knowledge need not always be beneficial. For instance, in patients who confabulate, the content of their confabulation is often based on true personal history (Schnider, 2003). In this case, established knowledge structures may interfere with the retrieval of episodic information, leading to the production of context-inappropriate information. Nonetheless, it appears likely that such interactions can be usefully exploited in the context of memory rehabilitation. Future studies are needed to delineate the boundary conditions of such effects.

In closing, key insights about the functional and neural organization of memory have emerged from the study of patients with amnesia. These studies in turn have influenced the direction of both cognitive and neuroimaging studies of memory in normal cognition. The studies reviewed herein have highlighted the fact that complex interactions among distinct forms of memory can be elucidated by careful attention to the nature of processes and representations that mediate task performance. Systematic study of patients with well-characterized lesions will remain central in further advancing this effort.

Acknowledgments

Writing of this chapter was supported by NIMH grants MH71783 and MH70830 and the Office of Research and Development, Medical Research Service, Department of Veterans Affairs.

References

Addis, D. R., Moscovitch, M., Crawley, A. P., & McAndrews, M. P. (2004). Recollective qualities modulate hippocampal activation during autobiographical memory retrieval. *Hippocampus, 14*, 752–762.

Aggleton, J. P., & Brown, M. W. (1999). Episodic memory, amnesia, and the hippocampal-anterior thalamic axis. *Behavioral and Brain Sciences, 22*, 425–489.

Anderson, M. C., & Pichert, J. W. (1978). Recall of previously unrecallable information following a shift in perspective. *Journal of Verbal Learning and Verbal Behavior, 17*, 1–12.

Bayley, P. J., Frascino, J. C., & Squire, L. R. (2005). Robust habit learning in the absence of awareness and independent of the medial temporal lobe. *Nature, 436*, 550–553.

Bayley, P. J., Gold, J. J., Hopkins, R. O., & Squire, L. R. (2005). The neuroanatomy of remote memory. *Neuron, 46*, 799–810.

Brewer, W. F., & Treyens, J. C. (1981). Role of schemata in memory for places. *Cognitive Psychology, 13,* 207–230.

Carlesimo, G. A., Perri, R., Costa, A., Serra, L., & Caltagirone, C. (2005). Priming for novel between-word associations in patients with organic amnesia. *Journal of the International Neuropsychological Society, 11,* 566–573.

Cermak, L. S. (1984). The episodic/semantic distinction in amnesia. In L. R. Squire & N. Butters (eds.), *The Neuropsychology of Memory* (pp. 55–62). New York: The Guilford Press.

Chun, M. M., & Phelps, E. A. (1999). Memory deficits for implicit contextual information in amnesic subjects with hippocampal damage. *Nature Neuroscience, 2,* 844–847.

Conway, M. A. (2001). Sensory-perceptual episodic memory and its context: autobiographical memory. *Philosophical Transactions of the Royal Society of London: B, 356,* 1375–1384.

Craik, F. I. M., & Lockhart, R. S. (1972). Levels of processing: A framework for memory research. *Journal of Verbal Learning and Verbal Behavior, 11,* 671–684.

Eichenbaum, H., & Cohen, N. J. (2001). From conditioning to conscious recollection. New York: Oxford University Press.

Fleischman, D. A., & Gabrieli, J. D. E. (1998). Repetition priming in normal aging and Alzheimer's disease: A review of findings and theories. *Psychology and Aging, 13,* 88–119.

Gabrieli, J. D. E., Fleischman, D. A., Keane, M. M., Reminger, S. L., & Morrell, F. (1995). Double dissociation between memory systems underlying explicit and implicit memory in the human brain. *Psychological Science, 6,* 76–82.

Gabrieli, J. D. E., Keane, M. M., Zarella, M., & Poldrack, R. A. (1997). Preservation of implicit memory for new associations in global amnesia. *Psychological Science, 8,* 326–329.

Goh, J. O. S., Siong, S. C., Park, D., Gutchess, A., Hebrank, A., & Chee, M. W. L. (2004). Cortical areas involved in object, background, and object-background processing revealed with functional magnetic resonance adaptation. *Journal of Neuroscience, 24,* 10,223–10,228.

Goshen-Gottstein, Y., Moscovitch, M., & Melo, B. (2000). Intact implicit memory for newly formed verbal associations in amnesic patients following single study trials. *Neuropsychology, 14,* 570–578.

Graham, K. S., Simons, J. S., Pratt, K. H., Patterson, K., & Hodges, J. R. (2000). Insights from semantic dementia on the relationship between episodic and semantic memory. *Neuropsychologia, 38,* 313–324.

Greenberg, D. L., Keane, M. M., & Verfaellie, M. (2009). Impaired category fluency in medial temporal lobe amnesia: The role of episodic memory. *Journal of Neuroscience, 29,* 10,900–10,908.

Hamann, S. B., & Squire, L. R. (1997). Intact perceptual memory in the absence of conscious memory. *Behavioral Neuroscience, 111,* 850–854.

Jacoby, L. L. (1983). Perceptual enhancement: Persistent effects of an experience. *Journal of Experimental Psychology: Learning, Memory and Cognition, 9,* 21–38.

Jacoby, L. L., & Dallas, M. (1981). On the relationship between autobiographical memory and perceptual learning. *Journal of Experimental Psychology: General, 110,* 306–340.

Kan, I. P., Alexander, M. P., & Verfaellie, M. (2009). Contribution of prior semantic knowledge to new episodic learning in amnesia. *Journal of Cognitive Neuroscience, 21,* 938–944.

Keane, M. M., Gabrieli, J. D. E., Fennema, A. C., Growdon, J. H., & Corkin, S. (1991). Evidence for a dissociation between perceptual and conceptual priming in Alzheimer's disease. *Behavioral Neuroscience, 105,* 236–242.

Keane, M. M., Gabrieli, J. D. E., Mapstone, H. C., Johnson, K. A., & Corkin, S. (1995). Double dissociation of memory capacities after bilateral occipital-lobe or medial temporal-lobe lesions. *Brain, 118,* 1129–1148.

Keane, M. M., Orlando, F., & Verfaellie, M. (2006). Increasing the salience of fluency cues reduces the recognition impairment in amnesia. *Neuropsychologia, 44,* 834–839.

Kirwan, C., Bayley, P. J., Galvan, V., & Squire, L. R. (2008). Detailed recollection of remote autobiographical memory after damage to the medial temporal lobe. *Proceedings of the National Academy of Sciences, USA, 105,* 2676–2680.

Kitchener, E. G., Hodges, J. R., & McCarthy, R. (1998). Acquisition of post-morbid vocabulary and semantic facts in the absence of episodic memory. *Brain, 121*, 1313–1327.

Kroll, N. E. A., Yonelinas, A. P., Kishiyama, M. M., Baynes, K., Knight, R. T., & Gazzaniga, M. S. (2003). The neural substrates of visual implicit memory: Do the two hemispheres play different roles? *Journal of Cognitive Neuroscience, 15*, 833–842.

Levy, B. J., Stark, C. E. L., & Squire, L. R. (2004). Intact conceptual priming in the absence of declarative memory. *Psychological Science, 15*, 680–686.

Mandler, G. (1980). Recognizing: The judgement of previous occurrence. *Psychological Review, 87*, 252–271.

Manns, J. R., Hopkins, R. O., & Squire, L. R. (2003). Semantic memory and the human hippocampus. *Neuron, 38*, 127–133.

Manns, J. R., & Squire, L. R. (2001). Perceptual learning, awareness, and the hippocampus. *Hippocampus, 11*, 776–782.

Mayes, A., Montaldi, D., & Migo, E. (2007). Associative memory and the medial temporal lobes. *Trends in Cognitive Sciences, 11*, 126–135.

Moscovitch, M. (2008). The hippocampus as a "stupid" domain-specific module: Implications for theories of recent and remote memory, and of imagination. *Canadian Journal of Experimental Psychology, 62*, 62–69.

Moscovitch, M., Nadel, L., Winocur, G., Gilboa, A., & Rosenbaum, R. S. (2006). The cognitive neuroscience of remote episodic, semantic and spatial memory. *Current Opinion in Neurobiology, 16*, 179–190.

Moscovitch, M., Vriezen, E., & Gottstein, J. (1993). Implicit tests of memory in patients with focal lesions or degenerative brain disorders. In H. Spinnler & F. Boller (eds.), *Handbook of Neuropsychology* (Vol. 8, pp. 133–173). Amsterdam: Elsevier.

Moscovitch, M., & Winocur, G. (2002). The frontal cortex and working with memory. In D. T. Stuss & R. T. Knight (eds.), *Principles of frontal lobe function* (pp. 188–209). Oxford: Oxford University Press.

Neisser, U. (1981). John Dean's memory: A case study. *Cognition, 9*, 1–22.

O'Connor, M. G., & Verfaellie, M. (2002). The amnesic syndrome: Overview and subtypes. In A. Baddeley, B. Wilson & M. Kopelman (eds.), *Handbook of Memory Disorders* (2nd ed., pp. 145–166). Chichester, UK: Wiley.

Paller, K. A., & Mayes, A. R. (1994). New-association priming of word identification in normal and amnesic subjects. *Cortex, 30*, 53–73.

Parkin, A. J. (1993). Functional significance of etiological factors in human amnesia. In L. R. Squire & D. L. Schacter (eds.), *Neuropsychology of Memory* (3rd ed., pp. 122–129). New York: Guilford Press.

Preston, A. R., & Gabrieli, J. D. E. (2008). Dissociation between explicit memory and configural memory in the human medial temporal lobe. *Cerebral Cortex, 18*, 2192–2207.

Reder, L. M., Park, H., & Kieffaber, P. D. (2009). Memory systems do not divide on consciousness: Reinterpreting memory in terms of activation and binding. *Psychological Bulletin, 135*, 23–49.

Roediger, H. L., & McDermott, K. B. (1993). Implicit memory in normal human subjects. In H. Spinnler & F. Boller (eds.), *Handbook of Neuropsychology* (Vol. 8, pp. 63–131). Amsterdam: Elsevier.

Rosenbaum, R. S., Moscovitch, M., Foster, J. K., Schnyer, D. M., Gao, F. Q., Kovacevic, N., et al. (2008). Patterns of autobiographical memory loss in medial temporal lobe amnesic patients. *Journal of Cognitive Neuroscience, 20*, 1490–1506.

Ryan, J. D., Althoff, R. R., Whitlow, S., & Cohen, N. J. (2000). Amnesia is a deficit in relational memory. *Psychological Science, 11*, 454–461.

Ryan, L. R., Cox, C., Hayes, S. M., & Nadel, L. (2008). Hippocampal activation during episodic and semantic memory retrieval: Comparing category production and category cued recall. *Neuropsychologia, 46*, 2109–2121.

Schacter, D. L., Wigg, G. S., & Stevens, W. D. (2007). Reductions in cortical activity during priming. *Current Opinion in Neurobiology, 17*, 171–176.

Schnider, A. (2003). Spontaneous confabulation and the adaptation of thought to ongoing reality. *Nature Reviews Neuroscience, 4*, 662–671.

Smith, N. C., Hopkins, R. A., & Squire, L. R. (2006). Experience-dependent eye movements, awareness, and hippocampus-dependent memory. *Journal of Neuroscience, 26*, 11, 304–11,312.

Snowden, J. S., Griffiths, H., & Neary, D. (1994). Semantic dementia: Autobiographical contribution to preservation of meaning. *Cognitive Neuropsychology, 11*, 265–288.

Stark, C., Stark, S., & Gordon, B. (2005). New semantic learning and generalization in a patient with amnesia. *Neuropsychology, 19*, 139–151.

Steinvorth, S., Levine, B., & Corkin, S. (2005). Medial temporal lobe structures are needed to re-experience remote autobiographical memories: Evidence from H.M. and W.R. *Neuropsychologia, 43*, 479–496.

Vargha-Khadem, F., Gadian, D. G., Watkins, K. E., Connelly, A., Van Paesschen, W., & Mishkin, M. (1997). Differential effects of early hippocampal pathology on episodic and semantic memory. *Science, 277*, 376–380.

Verfaellie, M. (2000). Semantic learning in amnesia. In L. S. Cermak (ed.), *Handbook of Neuropsychology* (2 ed., Vol. 2, pp. 335–354). Amsterdam: Elsevier Science.

Verfaellie, M., & Cermak, L. (1999). Perceptual fluency as a cue for recognition judgments in amnesia. *Neuropsychology, 13*, 198–205.

Verfaellie, M., Giovanello, K. S., & Keane, M. M. (2001). Recognition memory in amnesia: Effects of relaxing response criteria. *Cognitive, Affective and Behavioral Neuroscience, 1*, 3–9.

Verfaellie, M., & Keane, M. M. (2001). Scope and limits of implicit memory in amnesia. In B. De Gelder, E. De Haan & C. Heywood (eds.), *Unconscious minds* (pp. 151–162). Oxford: Oxford University Press.

Verfaellie, M., Reiss, L., & Roth, H. (1995). Knowledge of new English vocabulary in amnesia: An examination of premorbidly acquired semantic memory. *Journal of the International Neuropsychological Society, 1*, 443–453.

Voss, J. L., & Paller, K. A. (2009). An electrophysiological signature of unconscious recognition memory. *Nature Neuroscience, 12*, 349–355.

Ween, J. E., Verfaellie, M., & Alexander, M. P. (1996). Verbal memory function in mild aphasia. *Neurology, 47*, 795–801.

Westmacott, R., Black, S. E., Freedman, M., & Moscovitch, M. (2004). The contribution of autobiographical significance to semantic memory: Evidence from Alzheimer's disease, semantic dementia, and amnesia. *Neuropsychologia, 42*, 25–48.

Wiggs, C. L., & Martin, A. (1998). Properties and mechanisms of perceptual priming. *Current Opinion of Neurobiology, 8*, 227–233.

Willems, S., Salmon, E., & Van der Linden, M. (2008). Implicit/explicit memory dissociation in Alzheimer's disease: The consequence of inappropriate processing? Neuropsychology, 22, 710–717.

Wolk, D. A., Schacter, D. L., Berman, A. R., Holcomb, P. J., Daffner, K. R., & Budson, A. E. (2005). Patients with mild Alzheimer's disease attribute conceptual fluency to prior experience. *Neuropsychologia, 43*, 1662–1672.

Wood, F., Ebert, V., & Kinsbourne, M. (1982). The episodic-semantic memory distinction in memory and amnesia: Clinical and experimental observations. In L. S. Cermak (ed.), *Human memory and amnesia* (pp. 167–193). Hillsdale, NJ: Erlbaum.

Yang, J., Weng, X., Guan, L., Kuang, P., Zhang, M., Sun, W., et al. (2003). Involvement of the medial temporal lobe in priming for new associations. *Neuropsychologia, 41*, 818–829.

Yonelinas, A. P. (2002). The nature of recollection and familiarity: A review of 30 years of research. *Journal of Memory and Language, 46*, 441–517.

CHAPTER 4

Semantic Memory

Anastasia M. Raymer and Leslie J. Gonzalez Rothi

Several decades ago, Tulving (1972) coined the term "semantic memory" to refer to "memory necessary for the use of language. It is a mental thesaurus, organized knowledge a person possesses about words and other verbal symbols, their meaning and referents, about relations among them, and about rules, formulas, and algorithms for the manipulation of these symbols, concepts, and relations." (p. 386). Semantic memory is distinguished from episodic memory for our personal autobiographical life experiences, although establishing semantic memory depends upon personal experiences for learning (Garrard et al., 1997). Over time, however, it is unlikely that the episodic circumstances through which knowledge was acquired remain closely linked with the knowledge that is stored in semantic memory. Moreover, the knowledge is likely to transform over time as our personal experiences lead to modifications in semantic memory. Whereas both semantic and episodic memory are types of declarative knowledge systems (Squire, 1982), the distinction between them is supported by studies of patients with neurologic damage who are impaired in episodic memory with retained abilities in semantic memory, or are impaired in semantic memory with retained episodic memory abilities (Buccione et al., 2008; Kopelman, 2008).

Within cognitive psychology, a good deal of interest has centered on understanding the structure and functioning of semantic memory (Shelton & Caramazza, 2001). Evidence for theories of semantic memory is obtained through studies in experimental psychology of healthy individuals, developmental changes in memory, and pharmacologic influences on memory (Nyberg & Tulving, 1996). An additional fruitful line of evidence comes from examination of acquired semantic impairments in individuals with damage to the brain (Chatterjee, 2005; Fellows et al., 2005; Tulving, 1986). Semantic memory is engaged in a variety of lexical and object-processing tasks. Therefore, impairments of semantic memory are typically represented by failure in verbal and nonverbal tasks, including spoken and written picture naming, spoken and written word/picture matching, matching associated objects, answering questions about semantic attributes of objects and words, gesturing to verbal command and to viewed objects, among others (Garrard et al., 1997; Hillis et al., 1991; Raymer & Rothi, 2008). Patterns of breakdown across language and object processing tasks provide evidence concerning the structure and functions of semantic memory.

The purpose of this chapter is to review studies of individuals with brain impairments that inform models of semantic memory. We will introduce several neurologic conditions and patterns of brain damage that are commonly associated with semantic memory impairments. We will then review evidence from brain damaged patients with semantic impairments that guide the development and modification of theories of semantic memory. In the end, the story will be quite convincing that patient studies can provide an important converging line of evidence for the refinement of theories of semantic memory.

Neural Correlates of Semantic Impairment

In Hart and colleague's (2002) review of the neural substrates of semantic memory, he noted that several regions subserve semantic processing, among them left inferior prefrontal, left inferior parietal/posterior temporal, and left fusiform regions. Neurologic conditions that impact on this distributed network can lead to semantic dysfunction and inform models of semantic processing. Several acute neurologic conditions lead to the sudden onset of semantic difficulties, whereas other conditions have a more insidious onset, leading to slowly progressive development of semantic impairments.

Studies of patients with cerebrovascular accident (CVA) or stroke, that impact on either broad left hemisphere regions or circumscribed left hemisphere cortical (e.g., Brodmann's area 37) and subcortical structures (e.g., thalamus) have been examined for semantic breakdown (Raymer et al., 1997; Foundas et al., 1998; Jeffries et al., 2007). Schwartz and colleagues (2009) used voxel-based lesion mapping in individuals with chronic stroke and further supported the role of the left middle temporal (area 37) and the inferior frontal regions (area 45/46) in semantic stages of lexical processing. In a further analysis of spoken naming errors in individuals with aphasia, Schwartz et al. (2011) distinguished the roles of the left anterior temporal lobe (ATL) and the temporal-parietal junction (TPJ), two multimodal association areas, in semantic processing. Specifically, they proposed that the left ATL represents perceptual features of an object's taxonomic category, whereas the TPJ is interconnected with the associated context for an object.

Hillis and her colleagues (DeLeon et al., 2007; Hillis, 2007; Hillis et al., 2006; Newhart et al., 2007) have studied individuals with hyperacute stroke who are examined immediately upon onset of language symptoms and then reperfused as part of their clinical care. They proposed that such studies demonstrate essential cortex subserving language functions, and have provided support for the role of the left temporal, inferior parietal, and posterior frontal lobes in semantic processing. In particular, Hillis and colleagues (Hillis et al., 2006; Cloutman et al., 2009) reported that impairment in both word comprehension and word naming, a pattern suggestive of semantic impairment, was associated with damage affecting Brodmann's area 22 on the left, that is, the left superior temporal cortex. This finding has been subject to some dispute, however, because of the lack of converging evidence in chronic aphasia and in functional neuroimaging of healthy individuals (Schwartz et al., 2009).

Models of semantic processing have also been influenced by studies in patients with acute infection of the brain from herpes simplex encephalitis (HSE). The region most vulnerable in HSE tends to be the mesial temporal cortex, leading to episodic memory impairments; to the extent that the infection also impacts upon the lateral inferotemporal regions, semantic impairments may occur as well (Garrard et al., 1997). Descriptions of HSE have contributed to discussions, in particular, of semantic category impairments and the categorical structure of semantic memory.

Several degenerative conditions also tend to impact neural regions that mediate semantic processing. Alzheimer's disease (AD) is the most common form of dementia, leading to progressive deterioration in a variety of cognitive domains in association with the earliest pathologic changes in the bilateral mesial and inferior temporal cortex (Garrard, Lambon Ralph, Patterson, Pratt, & Hodges, 2005). The most frequently reported early symptoms of AD are deficits of episodic memory and language (Cummings, Benson, Hill, & Read, 1985; Huff, Becker, Belle, Nebes, Holland, & Boller, 1987). Within language, deficits have been attributed in large part to deterioration of semantic processing (Bayles & Kazniak, 1987; Chertkow & Bub, 1990; Hodges, 2000), with preserved phonologic and grammatical functions. Many semantic ("cat" for DOG) and unrelated errors ("thing" for DOG) are observed in constrained picture naming tasks for objects (nouns) and actions (verbs) (Bayles & Tomoeda, 1983; Martin & Fedio, 1983; Williamson, Adair, Raymer, & Heilman, 1998). AD patients are often impaired in a variety of word and picture comprehension tasks (Grossman, Robinson, Biassou, White-Devine, & D'Esposito, 1998; Hier, Hagenlocker & Shindler, 1985; Huff, Mack, Mahlmann, Greenberg, 1988; Martin & Fedio, 1983), and performance is particularly degraded when distracters in matching tasks are semantically related to target responses (e.g., target: dog; distracters: cat, horse) (Diesfeldt, 1989; Raymer & Berndt, 1996). Patients with Alzheimer's disease also demonstrate conceptual apraxia, that is, impaired knowledge of action/object relationships, leading to difficulty knowing what tools, objects, and actions to use in daily activities (Ochipa, Rothi, & Heilman, 1992; Schwartz et al., 2000). These findings indicate that degradation of semantic knowledge affects processing across all modalities of processing, verbal, object, and gestural. Even in patients with mild cognitive impairment, in which episodic memory impairments are the most evident area of cognitive decline, mild impairments of semantic processing may be noted (Ahmed et al., 2008), often heralding the evolution of cognitive decline toward probable Alzheimer's disease.

Additional degenerative conditions are associated with isolated language decline, sometimes termed primary progressive aphasia (PPA). Although the prototypic form of PPA is word retrieval difficulty in association with atrophy of left anterior temporal regions leading to nonfluent aphasia (Mesulam et al., 2003), other types of degenerative language decline also have been described. Semantic dementia, in particular, refers to a disorder in which patients present with impairments of language and visual processing, thereby expanding the cognitive dimensions beyond what is seen in PPA (Hodges et al., 1992; Hodges, 2000; Garrard et al., 1997). Impairments are evident in word recognition and retrieval, as well as in recognition of objects and faces. In contrast to the pattern typical of AD, episodic memory and frontal executive functions remain intact in semantic dementia.

A variety of acute and degenerative neurologic conditions that impact critical left hemisphere regions lead to semantic deficits in language, object, and action processing. Studies of patients with neurologic conditions therefore provide a rich source of evidence for understanding the structure and functioning of semantic memory.

Structure of Semantic Memory

For more than a century, researchers have investigated the brain and its role in cognitive-linguistic processing. Wernicke (1874) developed one of the first models of "centers" involved in language abilities, and Lichtheim (1885) expanded upon this model, adding centers for reading, writing, and concepts (cited in Caplan, 1987). Whereas Lichtheim proposed only a single conceptual center, Lissauer (1890/1988) implied that semantic memory may be multimodal in nature as he proposed that meaning is derived through an association process in which there is "activation of memories laid down through different sensory modalities" (Lissauer, 1890/1988, p. 182).

In modern times, models of cognitive mechanisms are considerably more explicit than the originally proposed Wernicke-Lichtheim model. For example, a version of the model of components involved in lexical-semantic processing is shown in Figure 4.1 (Hillis & Newhart, 2008; Raymer & Rothi, 2008).

Separate modality-specific input mechanisms store structural representations, that is, memories for familiar spoken and written words, and viewed objects.

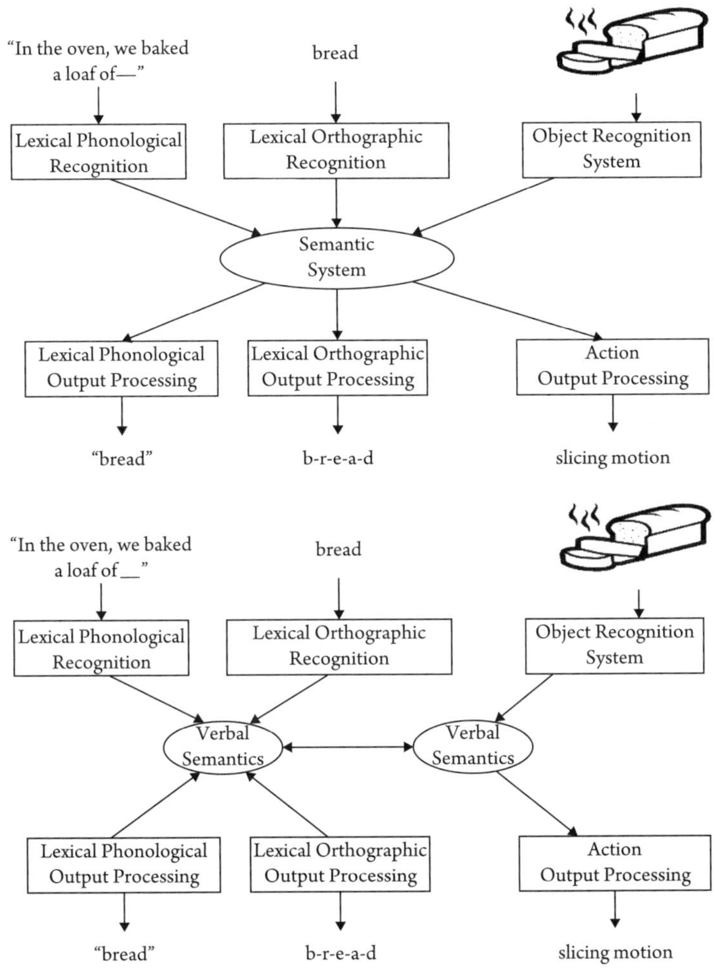

Figure 4.1 Unitary semantics model of lexical processing (upper panel); lexical processing with modality specific verbal and visual semantic subsystems (lower panel).

Activation of these modality-specific input systems allows for recognition of previously experienced items. Similarly in the output mode, components are proposed for storage and production of familiar spoken and written words and actions (gestures). These modality-specific input and output mechanisms are interconnected by way of a semantic system through which meaning is derived for words, objects, and actions. Semantic memory, in this regard, encompasses previously learned shared knowledge, including category and associated information about related objects, actions, locations, attributes, and events. Implied in these models when not explicitly stated are other sublexical assembly processes and peripheral perceptual and motor processes essential to the completion of various cognitive tasks. This discussion focuses on the central semantic system that mediates input and output mechanisms and has been the subject of considerable interest and controversy.

Unitary Semantics

As represented in Figure 4.1, an issue discussed with respect to semantic memory considers whether meaning information is stored in a single unitary semantic mechanism (upper panel) or in modality-specific semantic subsystems (lower panel). In the unitary semantics theory, a single semantic representation specifies all perceptual properties, functions, and associated knowledge relevant for the meaning of a given referent word, object, or action (Caramazza, Hillis, Rapp, & Romani, 1990; Humphreys & Riddoch, 1988; Seymour, 1973, 1979). That unitary representation is then activated to achieve meaning for spoken or written words, viewed objects and actions, and all other sensory input.

Neuropsychological evidence has been cited in support of the unitary semantics account. For example, Caramazza, Berndt, & Brownell (1982) demonstrated the relationship between failure to classify objects and impaired verbal labeling of objects in a subgroup of their patients with stroke-induced aphasia and posited a deficit to a single semantic system to represent the impairment. As further support of the unitary semantics view, Hillis, Rapp, Romani, & Caramazza (1990) described a patient with a large left hemisphere stroke who made comparable numbers of semantic errors in auditory and reading comprehension, oral and written naming, writing to dictation, and oral word reading. They argued that this quantitatively- and qualitatively-similar pattern of impairment across lexical tasks occurred because of impairment of a single semantic mechanism that was engaged across all lexical tasks.

Studies of patients with probable Alzheimer's disease (AD) also have been cited as support for a unitary semantic theory. Several studies have shown a strong association between impairments of language comprehension and limb praxis in patients with AD (Kempler, 1988; Glosser et al., 1998; Rapcsak et al., 1989). Dumont, Ska, &Joanette (2000) reported a similar pattern in that their participants with AD were impaired in both verbal and action semantic tasks to the same level of severity. They interpreted these findings as supportive of a model in which a single distributed semantic system is accessed during language and action tasks. Similarly, patients with semantic dementia who are impaired across all lexical-semantic and object-processing tasks, in the absence of episodic memory problems, provide further evidence for an impairment emanating from a unitary semantic system (Roger et al., 2004).

Consider optic aphasia. Freund (1889) reported a patient with a right homonymous hemianopsia who could not name visually presented objects, but could name them when explored through the tactile modality. Because he demonstrated recognition of objects through use of appropriate gestures, a visual agnosia was not indicated. Freund termed this disorder optic aphasia. Additional patients with optic aphasia have been described (Beauvois & Saillant, 1985; Coslett & Saffran, 1989; Hillis & Caramazza, 1995; Lhermitte & Beauvois, 1973; Riddoch & Humphreys, 1987), all with the common pattern of impaired object naming in the context of intact naming through nonvisual modalities (e.g., naming to spoken definitions), and intact recognition of objects as indicated by the ability to gesture the use of or indicate the functions of viewed objects that they are unable to name. Beauvois and Saillant (1985) argued that the prevalent unitary semantics models of lexical processing could not efficiently account for this pattern of breakdown. Therefore, modifications to the semantics model have been proposed to account for the observed dissociations noted in optic aphasia.

Privileged relationships. To account for optic aphasia, Caramazza and colleagues (1990) proposed the Organized Unitary Content Hypothesis (OUCH), later elaborated upon by Caramazza & Mahon (2006) when they noted that "certain types of input/output modalities have a privileged relationship with, or privileged access to, certain types of semantic information" (p. 14). Within this account, a semantic representation is viewed as a set of interconnected features representing the defining attributes and associated information for a given concept, whether corresponding to an object or a word. Like concepts, such as objects from the same semantic category (e.g., fruit), would have sets of shared or overlapping semantic features (outer skin, edible, sweet, juicy), that is, privileged relationships. Object-naming impairment in optic aphasia relates to a deficiency in which representations in the object recognition system fail to activate a complete semantic representation in a unitary system (Hillis & Caramazza, 1995). Some features in the object recognition system are able to access some features of the semantic representation that are relevant to the viewed object (privileged accessibility), making it is possible to retrieve the corresponding gesture or state the function of the object, yet not name the object which requires a full semantic specification.

Although privileged access and privileged relationships (Caramazza et al., 1990) provide a reasonable explanation for dissociations of performance in cases of optic aphasia, the theory may have problems accounting for other cases reported in the literature. The assumptions when applied to object processing lead one to predict that, given a semantic-level impairment, the ability to retrieve a gesture for a viewed object may be retained in spite of impaired object-naming abilities. The converse situation in which object naming exceeds gesturing abilities for the same objects would not be predicted under the privileged access account. Ochipa, Rothi, & Heilman (1989) reported a patient with precisely this pattern of performance, however, suggesting that the OUCH model is not sufficient to fully explain the pattern of impairments observed in optic aphasia and other modality-specific disorders. Other proposals have been presented to account for these varied patterns of breakdown in language, object, and gesture processing.

Modality-Specific Semantics

Beauvois (1982; Beauvois & Saillant, 1985) invoked a modality-specific semantics perspective aligned with that of Paivio (1971, 1986) to account for the visual modality-specific naming impairment observed in optic aphasia. They suggested that object naming failure in optic aphasia results from impairment in the interactions between separate visual and verbal semantic systems (Figure 4.1, lower panel). Intact processing from visual object recognition to visual semantics allows for successful completion of tasks such as gesturing to a viewed object. Intact processing from phonologic lexical stores to verbal semantics allows for successful performance on tasks such as naming to spoken definitions. That is, processing is adequate within verbal and visual modalities, but is impaired when cross-modality visual plus verbal semantic processing is necessary for successful completion of a task, such as object naming.

The situation is further complicated by the existence of modality-specific aphasias for auditory input (Denes & Semenza, 1975) and tactile input (Beauvois, Saillant, Meininger, & Lhermitte, 1978), among others. By analogy, one may propose an even more complex structure of the semantic system, with specific mechanisms for all modalities of input including tactile semantics and auditory semantics. Several researchers have invoked such an elaborate structure of the semantic system as represented in Figure 4.2a (Allport, 1985; Shallice, 1988). Hillis & Caramazza (1995) argued that the modality-specific account needed further elaboration, however, in order to adequately evaluate its viability as a hypothesis. Another compelling line of neuropsychological data, category-specific

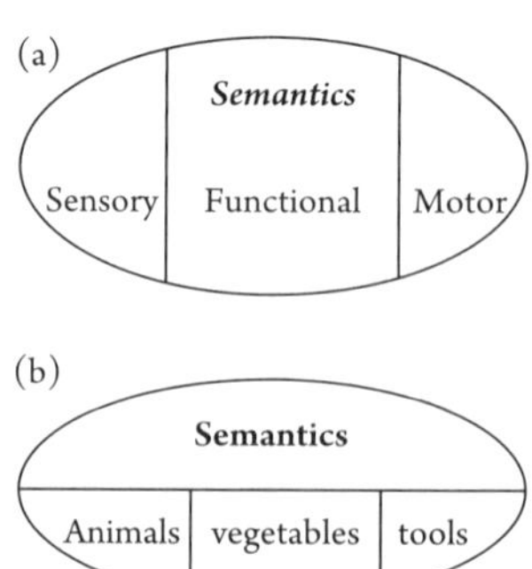

Figure 4.2 Sensory/Functional hypothesis (a) and domain specific semantic structure (b).

semantic impairments, must be considered in discussions of modality specificity in the structure of the semantic system.

Category-specific semantic impairments. Patients have been described whose spared or impaired language abilities relate to specific semantic categories, most often in the realm of living versus nonliving objects. In one of the earliest descriptions, Warrington & McCarthy (1983) described a patient with a large left hemisphere stroke who had preserved naming and comprehension abilities for living objects (foods, animals, flowers) and impaired performance for nonliving objects (tools, etc.). Warrington & Shallice (1984) then reported the opposite pattern of breakdown in four individuals with herpes simplex encephalitis (HSE), that is, greater impairment for living things than for nonliving things. Since that time, many additional studies too numerous to list have reported patients with deficits in selective semantic categories.

Capitani, Laiacona, Mahon, and Caramazza (2003) undertook a comprehensive review of the category-specific deficit literature. They identified 84 studies of patients with a variety of neurologic conditions leading to category-specific deficits or retained performance for a specific category in such categories as animals, fruits/vegetables, foods, body parts, musical instruments, and tools. A disproportionate impairment for living categories was evident in 103 patients, most commonly with a neurologic diagnosis of HSE or AD, and an inordinate impairment for nonliving categories was evident in 52 cases, most often due to stroke or AD. Further, patients have been described with even more selective impairments within the category of living things. Some patients have been described who are more impaired for living inanimate things (fruits and vegetables) than living animate things (animals) (e.g., Hart, Berndt, & Caramazza, 1985; Caramazza & Shelton, 1998) and others have displayed the converse pattern favoring animate over inanimate living categories (Farah & Wallace, 1992; Hillis & Caramazza, 1991).

Although such category dissociations may imply that the semantic system is structured according to some kinds of category relationships, researchers have attempted to propose a more principled account for these divergent category deficits. Warrington and her colleagues (Warrington & McCarthy, 1983; Warrington & Shallice, 1984; Warrington & McCarthy, 1987) explained category-specific deficits in relation to the type of semantic information that is critical for specification of that category. They proposed a distinction between functional semantic information, which is most relevant to nonliving categories like tools and transportation, versus visual sensory feature semantics which are most relevant to living categories like animals and plants. This sensory/functional hypothesis (SFH) (Figure 4.2a) is a corollary to the view proposed by Beauvois (1982) with respect to optic aphasia: modality-specific semantic systems for function information (verbal semantics) versus sensory modalities (visual semantics).

Action semantics: Warrington & McCarthy (1987) refined their proposal when they observed their patient YOT to experience more difficulty with small manipulable objects than with large objects, that is, subcategories within the broader category of nonliving objects where function information is crucial for semantic interpretation. Therefore, it was necessary to consider in addition the influence of motor information in the specification of the semantics of certain categories such as small manipulable objects, that is, a sensory/functional/motor distinction in semantic memory (Figure 4.2a)(see also Martin, Ungerleider, & Haxby, 2000, for a similar perspective). This type of motor information is a component of what Rothi, Ochipa, & Heilman (1991) called "action semantics," that is, stored knowledge about tools, including the mechanical advantage that tools provide, the objects they act upon, their functions, and associated actions (motor information). In fact, a distinction between verbal and action semantics may explain the performance of a patient described by Ochipa, Rothi, & Heilman (1989). Following a right hemisphere stroke, this left-handed patient demonstrated preserved verbal knowledge regarding tools he could not use; that is, preserved verbal semantics in the context of impaired action semantics. Ochipa, Rothi, & Heilman (1992) provided further evidence for the dissociation between verbal and action semantic knowledge in a study of patients with probable AD. A subset of AD patients who had relatively preserved verbal semantic abilities had significant impairments of tool and action knowledge as indicated by difficulty determining appropriate tools and objects to use to complete tool puzzles and matching tasks, suggesting a selective deficit of action semantics.

Domain Specific Hypothesis

One criticism of the many studies of patients with category-specific impairments is that other psycholinguistic stimulus variables were often not well controlled and may be a factor in the observed dissociations across categories. In their review of the literature on patients with category-specific semantic impairments, Capitani and colleagues (2003) found that, considering only those studies where other confounding factors were controlled, the most consistently impaired category across studies was living objects, observed for 16 cases. They also found that fractionations could be found within the category of living objects for animals (animate living objects) versus fruits/vegetables (inanimate living objects) in 12 cases. Impairments were evident for nonliving artifacts in four cases; no clear fractionations were evident within the category of artifacts. Capitani and colleagues argued that the overall patterns of category- specific deficits that emerged are contrary to predictions of the modality-specific sensory/functional hypothesis (Farah & McClelland, 1991; Warrington &

McCarthy, 1987). Importantly, there was no relationship between the category that was impaired (e.g., living things) and the type of semantic information that was impaired (e.g., visual sensory semantics), as predicted in the sensory/functional hypothesis. Most often, patients with category-specific impairments were comparably impaired for both sensory and functional semantic information. Further, the contrasting impairments observed for animals versus fruits/vegetables across at least 12 different patients is problematic for the sensory/functional hypothesis, as an impairment of visual semantics should lead to deficits for all categories that weight heavily toward visual semantic attributes for their category membership, living items, not isolated categories (e.g., animals only) within the category of living items.

Capitani et al. (2003) also noted that the observation of deficits within the category of living things is also not well explained within the OUCH privileged access perspective of unitary semantics discussed earlier. Caramazza & Shelton (1998) noted that the OUCH model does not impose constraints that explain why certain categories tend to be impaired more often, as confirmed in the systematic review (Capitani et al.). To resolve this discrepancy, Capitani and colleagues noted that the patterns of category specific semantic impairments seen in the literature are most compatible with a modification of the unitary semantics account proposed by Caramazza and colleagues (Caramazza & Shelton, 1998, 2001; Caramazza & Mahon, 2006), the domain specific hypothesis.

Caramazza & Shelton (1998; Shelton & Caramazza, 2001) proposed that, rather than certain processing or organizational principles in semantic memory, as in the sensory/functional/motor perspective, that lead to the emergence of category-specific impairments, semantic memory may indeed have subsystems for certain semantic categories (Figure 2b). Not all categories are represented. Rather, subsystems would exist only for certain categories that have advantages and adaptations for the well-being of a species, as might be claimed for categories such as plants, animals, and possibly tools. Further, these categories would be innately present. Caramazza and Shelton called this the domain specific hypothesis. They further proposed several implications of their theoretical perspective: 1) that there should be no further breakdowns within one of those domain-specific categories, say for land animals versus other types of animals; 2) the most common type of category-specific deficit should be for living things, which should be localized more proximally in the brain, and thus vulnerable to neural damage; 3) because plants and animals have an important human value as foods, it may be that other foods may be neurally-represented in close proximity to these domains, leading to possible category-specific deficits for foods in general.

In their careful review of the category-specific deficit literature, Capitani et al. (2003) found evidence in support of several of these predictions. As noted earlier, category impairments for living things occurred much more frequently than impairments for nonliving things. Further, some patients were identified who, along with impairments for living categories, demonstrated impairments for other foods as well. Capitani et al. concluded that the results of their review were most compatible with the domain specific hypothesis.

Overall Structure

The truth may lie somewhere in a blend of the strengths of the contrasting theories of semantic memory (Martin & Caramazza, 2003; Snowden, Thompson, & Neary, 2004; Tyler & Moss, 2001). Caramazza & Shelton (1998) noted that a combination of a domain-specific structure along with "domain general learning principles" (p. 20) may account for the structure of semantic memory for the full range of categories that constitute conceptual knowledge. In addition to the domain specific hypothesis, Shelton & Caramazza (2001) further proposed that other theories, such as those that discuss the relationships among features in semantic memory, also may need to be considered to encompass the representational structure within domains of semantic memory. In fact, several researchers have now recognized that that the different theoretical perspectives, unitary semantics, domain-specific semantics, modality-specific semantics, may be able to answer questions at different levels of consideration from the overall structure to the unique characteristic features of semantic representations (Martin & Caramazza, 2003; Snowden, Thompson, & Neary, 2004). Caramazza & Mahon (2006) emphasized the need to change directions in discussions of semantic memory from a focus on the overall structure of the semantic system to renewed efforts to understand the content of semantic memory. A number of recent neuropsychological studies of patients with semantic impairments have provided perspectives on the organization of semantic representations themselves.

Organization of Semantic Representations

Semantic representations are composed of networks of interconnected features corresponding to any meaningful elements that contribute to that concept (Altmann & McClung, 2008). The OUCH model reviewed earlier (Caramazza et al., 1990; Caramazza & Shelton, 1998) considered the structure of semantic representations when invoking the principles of privileged access and privileged relationships. These principles recognize that there is some texture to semantic representations, with certain features having stronger connections with other related features, leading to what has been termed a "lumpy" conceptual space. These notions have been elaborated upon in several similar theories.

Conceptual Structure Account

Tyler and colleagues (Tyler & Moss, 2001; Tyler, Moss, Durrent-Peatfield, & Levy, 2000; Tyler et al., 2003; Taylor et al., 2008) have described a connectionist account of semantic representations within a unitary semantic system (Figure 4.3). In their account, some elements of a semantic representation correspond to *perceptual* features and others are *functional* features. The relationships or interactions among these features will vary along with the fact that some of these may be *shared features* among related concepts and others are *distinctive features* that are unique to that concept. Members of a category will tend to have many shared, overlapping features among category members, along with some distinctive features. Tyler and colleagues (2000) further proposed that the category of living things tends to have more shared features that are highly interconnected; shared perceptual features tend to become connected to shared functional features. Biological motion is an important component of functional features for living things and that feature is shared across members of the category. In contrast, nonliving things tend to have distinctive functional features that are associated with distinctive perceptual features.

Under conditions of brain damage as in AD or HSE, category deficits emerge as a function of the loss of certain types of semantic features that comprise living and nonliving things and the strength of the correlations among features, with stronger relationships being maintained. Tyler et al. (2000) proposed that

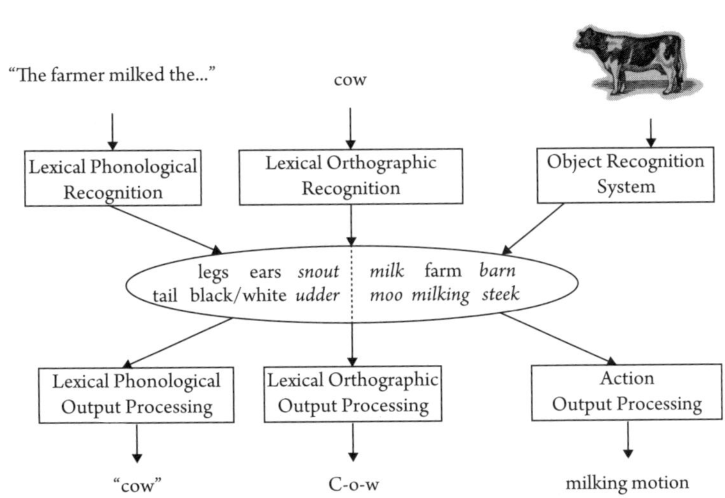

Figure 4.3 Semantic features for the Conceptual Structure Account (Tyler et al., 2008), with perceptual features (left) and functional features (right), including shared features for most animals, and distinctive features pertaining to a cow (italics).

"distinctive perceptual features for artifacts and shared perceptual features for biological kinds will be correlated with functional information and will be the most resistant to damage" (p. 204). Altmann & McClung (2008), in considering the conceptual structure account (Tyler et al., 2000), noted that living things are more susceptible to impairment than nonliving things because when the few distinctive features are lost for living things, then the remaining features tend to be shared features, which would lead to confusion across category exemplars that share those same features. If distinctive features are lost for nonliving things, they will still have many remaining distinctive features to allow for differences to exist relative to other category members and avoid confusion and errors in conditions of brain damage. Hodges (2000) noted that when patients with semantic dementia lose distinctive or "finer-grained" features due to semantic degradation, it is still possible to respond accurately in certain types of language tasks, such as making basic category judgments. Yet, these patients will be impaired in other tasks that require a full semantic specification, such as picture naming.

Some aspects of the conceptual structure account (Tyler et al., 2000) resemble the ideas proposed by Devlin, Gonnerman, Andersen, & Seidenberg (1998), including the focus on shared and distinctive features. They proposed that living things have more shared semantic features that are strongly intercorrelated than nonliving things that have more distinctive features. Their interpretation of the patterns of deficits that emerge in conditions such as AD differed from the conceptual structure account, however. They proposed that mild semantic impairments will be associated with more problems with artifacts, which rely on distinctive features that have been lost. As semantic damage becomes more severe, then sets of correlated features will tend to be lost, leading to problems with living things.

The notions of shared and distinctive perceptual and functional features allows for an account of some, though not all, categories of knowledge. Caramazza & Mahon (2006) argued that not all predictions of the conceptual structure account are supported by observations in the literature. In particular, cases have been described in which severe impairment for nonliving things has been observed in the context of spared performance for a living category, animals. This may relate in part to task demands, as how a degraded network will function will be dependent on the type of task that is attempted, whether full semantic specification is necessary, as in picture naming, or whether a basic semantic representation is sufficient, as in category judgments.

Embodied Representations

Other researchers take a decidedly different perspective on the structure of semantic representations, referred to in various places as "embodied representations" or "grounded cognition" (Barsalou, 2008; Barsalou, Breazeal, & Smith, 2007). In this view, the sensory and motor systems that are activated during learning eventually become the network that makes up the conceptual representation (Antonucci & Reilly, 2008; Martin & Chao, 2001). In fact, Wernicke's (1874) account of conceptual knowledge is consistent with such a perspective. Details of the models differ across researchers. For example, Damasio (1989; Damasio, Grabowski, Tranel, & Hichwa, 1996) does not ascribe to an actual semantic representation per se, but rather, to a semantic association *process* whereby a network of modality-specific sensory and motor representations becomes active to represent a concept by way of temporal "convergence zones" that are located in the anterior temporal lobes (Figure 4.4, upper panel).

Barsalou (2003, 2008) has written extensively on the theory of grounded cognition, noting that "cognition emerges from dependencies between all of the basic systems in the brain, including goal management, perception, action, memory, reward, affect, and learning." (Barsalau et al., 2007, p. 79) That is, Barsalou has a rich interpretation that includes some traditionally non-cognitive elements in addition to sensory and motor ones to constitute the basis of conceptual knowledge. He refers to a process of "simulation," whereby during cognitive activities, representations in the sensory, motor, and other non-cognitive systems are "re-enacted for representational use during cognitive activity" (Barsalou, 2011, p. 27). Chatterjee (2010), in contrast, advocates a weaker version of grounded cognition, recognizing that sensory and motor experiences contribute in a more "graded" manner to the development of concepts. He reviews studies in the realm of language and spatial cognition that suggest that some concepts draw upon disembodied "schemas" that develop through perceptual and motor experiences, yet lose the specificity of the original experiences, and seem to give a processing advantage during cognitive activities.

Rogers and colleagues (2004) also view abstract amodal semantic representations as developing over time through sensory/motor learning experiences. They claimed that the semantic structure that arises during learning is not feature-based and is not specialized for function or for perceptual attributes, unlike most models of semantic representations. They entertained this theory in their discussion of a connectionist model developed to account for the patterns of breakdown observed across language- and object- processing tasks (picture naming, matching, drawing) in patients with semantic dementia.

Reilly & Peele (2008) proposed a blended model of semantic representations encompassing aspects of unitary semantics along with modality-specific semantic specification (Figure 4.4, lower panel). Some aspects of the semantic representation are unitary, that is, some features of the representation are activated regardless of the modality of input and this tends to be a rather "sparse" representation of that object. Other modality-specific features can be activated as needed, based on the demands of the task at hand. That is, Reilly and Peele propose that

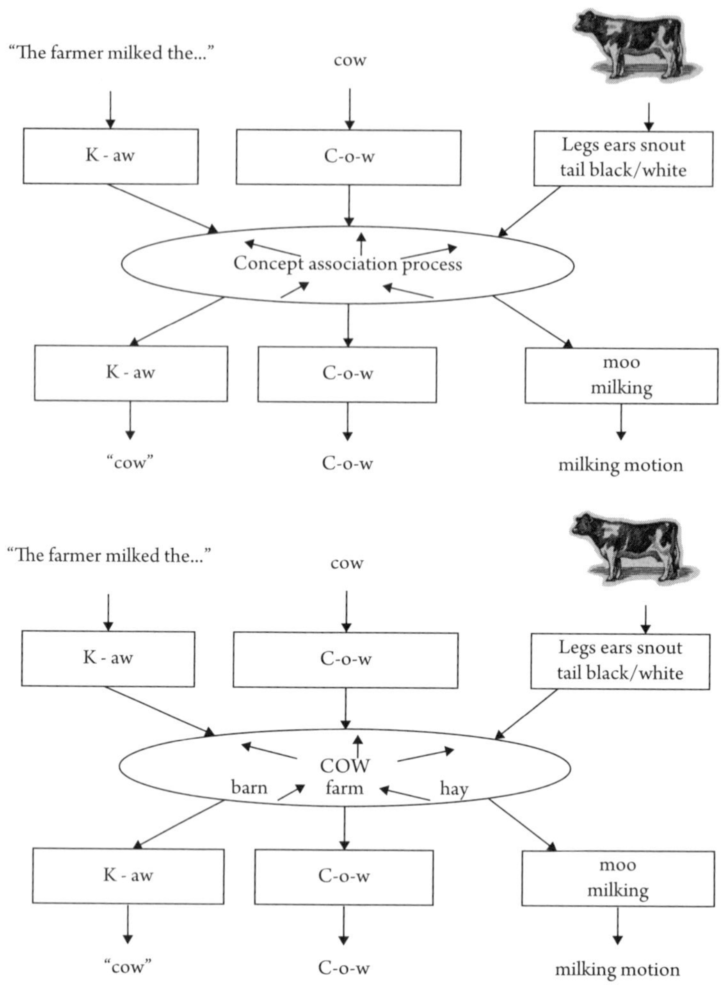

Figure 4.4 Embodied representations (upper panel) coalesced through a process that networks sensory and motor representations (e.g., Damasio et al., 1996); blended unitary semantic model (lower panel) with modality-specific semantic specifications (Reilly & Peele, 2008).

there is "dynamic interactivity in semantic memory between modality-neutral and modality-specific components" (p. 38) of semantic representations.

Summary and Conclusions

A number of neurologic conditions lead to damage affecting the left temporal region that is especially critical for the mediation of semantic memory (Hillis et al., 2006; Schwartz et al., 2009). The mesial or lateral extent of temporal damage will influence impairments evident within episodic or semantic memory. Further, within lateral temporal regions, the anterior or posterior extent of damage can impact on the patterns of impairments that emerge in semantic processing. Impairments may vary by modality of input and output, by semantic category, and by other features that are relevant in semantic processing, for example, concreteness (Reilly, Peele, & Grossman, 2007).

Many years of illustration and debate in the neuropsychological literature may be explained by the fact that semantic memory may encompass principles proposed across unitary, domain-specific, and modality-specific semantic theories (Martin & Caramazza, 2001; Shelton & Caramazza, 2001). Further, discussions that have turned toward examining the structure of semantic representations themselves (Tyler et al., 2000; Rogers et al., 2004; Barsalou, 2008) allow for an account of the richness of semantic knowledge and the dynamic interplay among features of representations as needed for daily semantic processing tasks (Reilly & Peele, 2008). Not all aspects of semantic knowledge, e.g., encyclopedic knowledge or abstract concepts, are yet encompassed in theories of semantic representations. Therefore, the enterprise of examining the performance of patients with neurologic impairments will continue in order to further our understanding of all aspects of semantic memory.

Acknowledgments

Preparation of this chapter was supported in part by NIH (NIDCD) R15 DC009690 to the first author.

References

Ahmed, S., Arnold, R., Thompson, S. A., Graham, K. S., & Hodges, J. R. (2008). Naming of objects, faces and buildings in mild cognitive impairment. *Cortex, 44,* 746–752.

Allport, D. A. (1985). Distributed memory, modular subsystems, and dysphasia. In S. Newman & R. Epstein (eds.), *Current perspectives in dysphasia* (pp. 32–60). Edinburgh: Churchill Livingstone.

Altmann, L. J. P., & McClung, J. S. (2008). Effects of semantic impairment on language use in Alzheimer's disease. *Seminars in Speech and Language, 29,* 18–31.

Antonucci, S. M., & Reilly, J. (2008). Semantic memory and language processing: A primer. *Seminars in Speech and Language, 29,* 5–17.

Barsalou, L. W. (2008). Grounded cognition. *Annual Review of Psychology, 59,* 617–645.

Barsalou, L. W. (2011). Simulation, situated conceptualization, and prediction. In M. Bar (ed.), *Prediction in the brain* (pp. 27–39). New York: Oxford University Press.

Barsalou, L. W., Breazeal, C., & Smith, L. B. (2007). *Cognitive Processes, 8,* 79–91.

Bayles, K. A., & Kazniak, A. W. (1987). *Communication and cognition in normal aging and dementia.* Boston: Little, Brown, and Company.

Bayles, K. A., & Tomoeda, C. K. (1983). Confrontation naming impairment in dementia. *Brain and Language, 19,* 98–114.

Beauvois, M.-F. (1982). Optic aphasia: A process of interaction between vision and language. Proceedings fo the Royal Society of London, Series B, 298, 35–47.

Beauvois, M. F., & Saillant, B. (1985). Optic aphasia for colours and colour agnosia: A distinction between visual and visuo-verbal impairments in the processing of colours. *Cognitive Neuropsychology, 2,* 1–48.

Beauvois, M. F., Saillant, B, Meininger, V., & Lhermitte, F. (1978). Bilateral tactile aphasia: A tacto-verbal dysfunction. *Brain, 101,* 381–401.

Buccione, I., Fadda, L., Serra, L., Caltagirone, C., & Carlesimo, G. A. (2008). Retrograde episodic and semantic memory impairment correlates with side of temporal lobe damage. *Journal of the International Neuropsychological Society, 14,* 1083–1094.

Capitani, E., Laiacona, M., Mahon, B., & Caramazza, A. (2003). What are the facts of semantic category-specific deficits? A critical review of the clinical evidence. *Cognitive Neuropsychology, 20,* 213–261.

Caplan, D. (1987). *Neurolinguistics and linguistic aphasiology*. Cambridge: Cambridge University Press.

Caramazza, A., Berndt, R. S., & Brownell, H. H. (1982). The semantic deficit hypothesis; Perceptual parsing and object classification by aphasic patients. *Brain and Language, 15,* 161–189.

Caramazza, A., Hillis, A. E., Rapp, B. C., & Romani, C. (1990). The multiple semantics hypothesis: Multiple confusions? *Cognitive Neuropsychology, 7,* 161–189.

Caramazza, A., & Mahon, B. Z. (2003). The organization of conceptual knowledge: The evidence from category-specific semantic deficits. *Trends in Cognitive Sciences, 7,* 354–361.

Caramazza, A., & Mahon, B. Z. (2006). The organization of conceptual knowledge in the brain: The future's past and some future directions. *Cognitive Neuropsychology, 23,* 13–38.

Caramazza, A., & Shelton, J. R. (1998). Domain-specific knowledge systems in the brain: The animate-inanimate distinction. *Journal of Cognitive Neuroscience, 10,* 1–34.

Chertkow, H., & Bub, D. (1990). Semantic memory loss in dementia of Alzheimer's type: What do various measures measure? *Brain, 113,* 397–417.

Chatterjee, A. (2005). A madness to the methods in cognitive neuroscience? *Journal of Cognitive Neuroscience, 17,* 847–849.

Chatterjee, A. (2010). Disembodying cognition. *Language and Cognition, 2,* 79–116.

Cloutman, L., Gottesman, R., Chaudhry, P., Davis, C., Kleinman, J. T., Pawlak, M., et al. (2009). Where (in the brain) do semantic errors comes from? *Cortex, 45,* 641–649.

Coslett, H. B., & Saffran, E. M. (1989). Preserved object recognition and reading comprehension in optic aphasia. *Brain, 112,* 1091–1110.

Cummings, J. L., Benson, D. F., Hill, M. A., & Read, S. (1985). Aphasia in dementia of the Alzheimer type. *Neurology, 35,* 394–397.

Damasio, A. R. (1989). The brain binds entities and events by multiregional activation from convergence zones. *Neural Computation, 1,* 123–132.

Damasio, H., Grabowski, T. J., Tranel, D., Hichwa, R. D., & Damasio, A. R. (1996). A neural basis for lexical retrieval. *Nature, 380,* 499–505.

DeLeon, J., Gottesman, R. F., Kleinman, J. T., Newhart, M., Davis, C., Heidler-Gary, J., Lee, A., & Hillis, A. E. (2007). Neural regions essential for distinct cognitive processes underlying picture naming. *Brain, 130,* 1408–1422.

Denes, G., & Semenza, C. (1975). Auditory modality-specific anomia: Evidence from a case study of pure word deafness. *Cortex, 11,* 401–411.

Devlin, J. T., Gonnerman, L. M., Andersen, E. S., & Seidenberg, M. S. (1998). Category-specific semantic deficits in focal and widespread brain damage: A computational account. *Journal of Cognitive Neuroscience, 10,* 77–94.

Diesfeldt, H. F. A. (1989). Semantic impairments in senile dementia of the Alzheimer type. *Aphasiology, 3,* 41–54.

Dumont, C., Ska, B., & Joanette, Y. (2000). Conceptual apraxia and semantic memory deficit in Alzheimer's disease: Two sides of the same coin? *Journal of the International Neuropsychological Society, 6,* 693–703.

Farah, M.J., McClelland, J.L. (1991) A computational model of semantic memory impairment: Modality-specificity and emergent category-specificity. Journal of Experimental Psychology: General, 120(4), 339–357.

Farah, M. J., & Wallace, M. A. (1992). Semantically-bounded anomia: Implications for the neural implementation of naming. *Neuropsychologia, 30,* 609–621.

Fellows, L. K., Heberlein, A. S., Morales, D. A., Shivde, G., Waller, S., & Wu, D. H. (2005). Method matters: An empirical study of impact in cognitive neuroscience. *Journal of Cognitive Neuroscience, 17,* 850–858.

Foundas, A. L., Daniels, S. K., & Vasterling, J. J. (1998). Anomia: Case studies in lesion localization. *Neurocase, 4,* 35–43.

Freund, C. S. (1889). Ueber optische aphasie und seelenblindheit. *Archiv fur Psychiatrie und Nervenkrankheiten, 20,* 276–297, 371–416.

Garrard, P., Perry, R., & Hodges, J. R. (1997). Disorders of semantic memory. *Journal of Neurology, Neurosurgery, and Psychiatry, 62,* 431–435.

Garrard, P., Lambon Ralph, M. A., Patterson, K., Pratt, K. H., & Hodges, J. R. (2005). Semantic feature knowledge and picture naming in dementia of Alzheimer's type: A new approach. *Brain and Language, 93,* 79–94.

Glosser, G., Wiley, M. J., & Barnoski, E. J. (1998). Gestural communication in Alzheimer's disease. *Journal of Clinical and Experimental Neuropsychology, 20,* 1–13.

Grossman, M., Robinson, K., Biassou, N., White-Devine, T., D'Esposito, M. (1998). Semantic memory in Alzheimer's disease: Representativeness, ontologic category, and material. *Neuropsychology, 12,* 34–42.

Hart, J., Moo, L. R., Segal, J. B., Adkins, E., & Kraut, M. (2002). Neural substrates of semantics. In A. E. Hillis (Ed.), *The handbook of adult language disorders* (pp. 207–227). New York: Psychology Press.

Hart, J., Berndt, R. S., & Caramazza, A. (1985). Category-specific naming deficit following cerebral infarction. *Nature, 316,* 439–440.

Hier, D. B., Hagenlocker, K., & Shindler, A. G. (1985). Language disintegration in dementia: Effects of etiology and severity. *Brain and Language, 25,* 117–133.

Hillis, A. E. (2007). Magnetic resonance perfusion imaging in the study of language. *Brain and Language, 102,* 165–175.

Hillis, A. E., & Caramazza, A. (1991). Category-specific naming and comprehension impairment: A double dissociation. *Brain, 114,* 2081–2094.

Hillis, A. E., & Caramazza, A. (1995). The compositionality of lexical semantic representations: Clues from semantic errors in object naming. *Memory, 3,* 333–358.

Hillis, A. E., & Caramazza, A. (1995). Cognitive and neural mechanisms underlying visual and semantic processing: Implications from "optic aphasia." *Journal of Cognitive Neuroscience, 7,* 457–478.

Hillis, A. E., Chaudhry, P., Davis, C., Kleinman, J., Newhart, M., & Heidler-Gary, J. (2006). Where (in the brain) do semantic errors come from? *Brain and Language, 99,* 84–85.

Hillis, A. E., & Newhart, M. (2008). Cognitive neuropsychological approaches to treatment of language disorders: Introduction. In R. Chapey (Ed.), *Language intervention strategies in aphasia and related neurogenic communication disorders* (5th ed., pp. 595–606). Baltimore: Lippincott, Williams & Wilkins.

Hillis, A. E., Rapp, B., Romani, C., & Caramazza, A. (1990). Selective impairment of semantics in lexical processing. *Cognitive Neuropsychology, 7,* 191–243.

Hodges, J. R., Patterson, K., Oxbury, S., & Funnell, E. (1992).Semantic dementia: Progressive fluent aphasia with temporal lobe atrophy. *Brain, 115,* 1783–1806.

Hodges, J. R. (2000). Memory in the dementias. In E. Tulving & F. I. M. Craik (eds.), *The Oxford handbook of memory* (pp. 441–459). New York: Oxford University Press.

Huff, F. J., Becker, J. T., Belle, S. H., Nebes, R. D., Holland, A. L., & Boller, F. (1987). Cognitive deficits and clinical diagnosis of Alzheimer's disease. *Neurology, 37,* 1119–1124.

Huff, F. J., Mack, L., Mahlmann, J., & Greenberg, S. (1988). A comparison of lexical-semantic impairments in left hemisphere stroke and Alzheimer's disease. *Brain and Language, 35,* 262–278.

Humphreys, G. W., & Riddoch, M. J. (1988). On the case for multiple semantic systems: a reply to Shallice. *Cognitive Neuropsychology, 5,* 143–150.

Humphreys, G. W., Riddoch, M. J., & Quinlan, P. T. (1988). Cascade processes in picture identification. *Cognitive Neuropsychology, 5,* 67–103.

Jeffries, E., Baker, S. S., Doran, M., & Lambon Ralph, M. A. (2007). Refractory effects in stroke aphasia: A consequence of poor semantic control. *Neuropsychologia, 45,* 1065–1079.

Kempler, D. (1988). Lexical and pantomime abilities in Alzheimer's disease. *Aphasiology, 2,* 147–159.

Kopelman, M. D. (2008). Retrograde episodic and semantic memory impairment correlates with side of temporal lobe damage. *Journal of the International Neuropsychological Society, 14,* 1081–1082.

Lhermitte, F., & Beauvois, M. F. (1973). A visual-speech disconnexion syndrome: Report of a case with optic aphasia, agnostic alexia and colour agnosia. *Brain, 97,* 695–714.

Lichtheim, L. (1885). On aphasia. *Brain, 7,* 433–484.

Lissauer, H. (1988). Ein Fall von Seelenblindheit nebst einem Beitrag zur Theorie derselben. *Cognitive Neuropsychology, 5,* 157–192, 1988. (Original work published in 1890.)

Martin, A., & Caramazza, A. (2003). Neuropsychological and neuroimaging perspectives on conceptual knowledge: An introduction. *Cognitive Neuropsychology, 20,* 195–212.

Martin, A., & Chao, L. L. (2001). Semantic memory and the brain: Structure and processes. *Current Opinions in Neurobiology, 11,* 194–201.

Martin, A., & Fedio, P. (1983). Word production and comprehension in Alzheimer's disease: The breakdown of semantic knowledge. *Brain and Language, 19,* 124–141.

Martin, A., Ungerleider, L.G., Haxby, J.V. Category specificity and the brain: The sensory/motor model of semantic represenatations of objects. In M.S. Gazzaniga (Ed.), The New Cognitive Neurosciences, MIT Press, 1999, 1023–1036.

Mesulam, M. M., Grossman, M., Hillis, A. E., Kertesz, A., & Weintraub, S. (2003). The core and halo of primary progressive aphasia and semantic dementia. *Annals of Neurology, 54* (Supplement 5), 11–14.

Newhart, M., Ken, L., Kleinman, J. T., Heidler-Gary, J., & Hillis, A. E. (2007). Neural networks essential for naming and word comprehension. *Cognitive and Behavioral Neurology, 20,* 25–30.

Nyberg, L., & Tulving, E. (1996). Classifying human long-term memory: Evidence from converging dissociations. *European Journal of Cognitive Psychology, 8,* 163–183.

Ochipa, C., Rothi, L. J. G., & Heilman, K. M. (1989). Ideational apraxia: A deficit in tool selection and use. *Annals of Neurology, 25,* 190–193.

Ochipa, C., Rothi, L. J. G., & Heilman, K. M. (1992). Conceptual apraxia in Alzheimer's disease. *Brain, 115,* 1061–1071.

Paivio, A. (1971). *Imagery and verbal processes.* New York: Holt, Rinehart, and Winston.

Paivio, A. (1986). *Mental representations: A dual coding approach.* New York: Oxford University Press.

Rapcsak, S. Z., Croswell, S. C., & Rubens, A. B. (1989). Apraxia in Alzheimer's disease. *Neurology, 39,* 664–668.

Raymer, A. M., & Berndt, R. S. (1996). Reading lexically without semantics: Evidence from patients with probable Alzheimer's disease. *Journal of the International Neuropsychological Society, 2,* 340–349.

Raymer, A. M., Foundas, A., Maher, L., Greenwald, M., Morris, M., Rothi, L. J. G., & Heilman, K. M. (1997). Cognitive neuropsychological analysis and neuroanatomic correlates in a case of acute anomia. *Brain and Language, 58,* 137–156.

Raymer, A. M., Greenwald, M. R., Richardson, L., Rothi, L. J. G., & Heilman, K. M. (1997) Optic aphasia and optic apraxia: Case analysis and theoretical implications. *Neurocase, 3,* 173–183.

Raymer, A. M., & Rothi, L. J. G. (2008). Cognitive neuropsychological approaches to assessment and treatment: Impairments of lexical comprehension and production. In R. Chapey (Ed.), *Language intervention strategies in adult aphasia* (5th ed., pp. 607–631). Baltimore: Lippincott, Williams & Wilkins.

Reilly, J., & Peele, J. E. (2008). Effects of semantic impairment on language processing in semantic dementia. *Seminars in Speech and Language, 29,* 32–43.

Reilly, J., Peele, J. E., & Grossman, M. (2007). A unitary semantics account of reverse concreteness effects in semantic dementia. *Brain and Language, 103,* 86–87.

Riddoch, M. J., & Humphreys, G. W. (1987). Visual object processing in optic aphasia: A case of semantic access agnosia. *Cognitive Neuropsychology, 4,* 131–185.

Rogers, T. T., Lambon Ralph, M. A., Garrard, P., Bozeat, S., McClelland, J. L., Hodges, J. R., & Patterson, K. (2004). Structure and deterioration of semantic memory: A neuropsychological and computational investigation. *Psychological Review, 111,* 205–235.

Rothi, L. J. G., Ochipa, C., & Heilman, K. M. (1991). A cognitive neuropsychological model of limb praxis. *Cognitive Neuropsychology, 8,* 443–458.

Schwartz, M. F., Kimberg, D. Y., Walker, G. M., Brecher, A., Faseyitan, O. K., Dell, G. S., Mirman, D., & Coslett, H. B. (2011). Neuroanatomical dissociation for taxonomic and thematic knowledge in the human brain. *Proceedings of the National Academy of Sciences, 108* (2), 8520–8524.

Schwartz, M. F., Kimberg, D. Y., Walker, G. M., Faseyitan, O., Brecher, A., Dell, G. S., & Coslett, H. B. (2009). Anterior temporal involvement in semantic word retrieval: Voxel-based lesion-symptom mapping evidence from aphasia. *Brain, 132,* 3411–3427.

Schwartz, R. L., Adair, J. C., Raymer, A. M., Williamson, D. J. G., Crosson, B., Rothi, L. J. G., Nadeau, S., & Heilman, K. M. (2000). Conceptual apraxia in probable Alzheimer's disease as demonstrated by the Florida Action Recall Test. *Journal of the International Neuropsychological Society, 6,* 265–270.

Seymour, P. H. K. (1973). A model for reading, naming, and comparison. *British Journal of Psychology, 64,* 35–49.

Seymour, P. H. K. (1979). *Human visual cognition.* New York: St. Martin's Press.

Shallice, T. (1988). Specialisation within the semantic system. *Cognitive Neuropsychology, 5,* 133–142.

Shelton, J. R., & Caramazza, A. (2001). The organization of semantic memory. In B. Rapp (ed.), *The handbook of cognitive neuropsychology* (pp. 423–443). Philadelphia, PA: Psychology Press.

Snowden, J. S., Thompson, J. C., & Neary, D. (2004). Knowledge of famous faces and names in semantic dementia. *Brain, 127,* 860–872.

Squire, L. R. (1982). The neuropsychology of human memory. *Annual Reviews of Neuroscience, 5,* 241–273.

Taylor, K. I., Salamoura, A., Randall, B., Moss, H., & Tyler, L. K. (2008). Clarifying the nature of the distinctiveness by domain interaction in conceptual structure: Comment on Cree, McNorgan, and McRae (2006). *Journal of Experimental Psychology: Learning, Memory, and Cognition, 34,* 719–725.

Tulving, E. (1972). Episodic and semantic memory. In E. Tulving & W. Donaldson, (eds.), *Organization of memory* (pp. 382–403). New York: Academic Press.

Tulving, E. (1986). What kind of a hypothesis is the distinction between episodic and semantic memory? *Journal of Experimental Psychology: Learning, Memory, and Cognition, 12,* 307–311.

Tyler, L. K., Bright, P., Dick, E., Tavares, P., Pilgrim, L., Fletcher, P., Greer, M., & Moss, H. (2003). Do semantic categories activate distinct cortical regions? Evidence for a distributed neural semantic system. *Cognitive Neuropsychology, 20,* 541–559.

Tyler, L. K., & Moss, H. E. (2001). Towards a distributed account of conceptual knowledge. *Trends in Cognitive Sciences, 5,* 244–252.

Tyler, L. K., Moss, H. E., Durrant-Peatfield, M. R., & Levy, J. P. (2000). Conceptual structure and the structure of concepts: A distributed account of category-specific deficits. *Brain and Language, 75,* 195–231.

Warrington, E. K., & McCarthy, R. (1983). Category specific access dysphasia. *Brain, 106,* 859–878.

Warrington, E. K., & McCarthy, R. (1987). Categories of knowledge: Further fractionations and an attempted integration. *Brain, 110,* 1273–1296.

Warrington, E. K., & Shallice, T. (1984). Category specific semantic impairment. *Brain, 107,* 829–854.

Williamson, D. J. G., Adair, J. C., Raymer, A. M., & Heilman, K. M. (1998). Naming impairments for objects and actions in Alzheimer's Disease. *Cortex, 34,* 601–610.

Wernicke, C. (1874). Der Aphasische Synptomenkomplex (trans.). *Boston Studies in Philosophy of Science, 4,* 34–97.

CHAPTER 5

Alexias and Agraphias

David P. Roeltgen and Elizabeth H. Lacey

Introduction

Disorders of written language (alexias and agraphias) have been studied since the 19th century. Many authors have stressed the associations between written language disorders and oral language disorders (aphasias) (Ogle, 1867) and others have stressed the dissociations between them (Nielson, 1946). Evaluation of patients with acquired disorders of written language has informed us about anatomic localization of behavior, functional systems and interactions of these systems. These evaluations have demonstrated associations of alexia and agraphia with aphasia, and with each other. They have also demonstrated that alexia and agraphia may occur independently and in isolation. Most studies focus on patients with strokes. However, studies of progressive disease, including dementia, also contribute to studies of disorders of written language.

The studies of patients with stroke have shown an evolution. From the 19th century through the mid-20th century, they focused on the clinical anatomic correlations of associations and dissociations between alexias and agraphias, and between these disorders and other cognitive functions, especially aphasia. This was probably due, at least in part, to the limits of clinical pathological correlations based on autopsy. For example, Benson and Geschwind (1969) described four alexias: hemialexia (reading of only one half of a word) from lesions of the corpus callosum; alexia without agraphia (impaired reading with the characteristics of this disorder not further defined) from lesions in the distribution of the posterior cerebral artery; alexia with agraphia (impaired reading and writing with the characteristics of these disorders not further defined) from lesions in the parietal lobe; and aphasic alexia (impaired writing dominated by spelling errors) from multiple anatomic sites associated with the aphasias. Leischner (1969) used a similar method to classify the agraphias. He delineated agraphias due to language disturbances, mostly from lesions in the temporal lobe; primary agraphias due to constructional disturbances from lesions of the parietal lobe; and apraxic agraphia often from lesions of the parietal lobe.

In contrast to the use of autopsy, clinical-anatomic analysis in the later decades of the 20th century and the first decade of the 21st century have been dominated by imaging studies. The larger numbers of analyses helped investigators make more detailed analyses of the clinical anatomic relationships. With this increased ability to do anatomic analyses, the need to utilize more detailed cognitive analyses became apparent, and studies reflected the greater insight into previously and newly described cognitive phenomena. These classifications included some disorders that are essentially unchanged in their clinical description, including pure alexia and apraxic agraphia. In contrast, others, especially those associated with aphasia, have undergone much change since the mid-20th century as analyses of aphasia, alexia, and agraphia were increasingly motivated by linguistic concepts such as phonology (organization of sounds), syntax (rules covering construction of sentences), and semantics (meaning). Simultaneously, with this evolution of cognitive analyses, the availability of structural imaging, first computed tomography (CT), then magnetic resonance imaging (MRI), allowed not only analysis of larger numbers of clinical anatomic correlations, but also analysis of these correlations in the acute and chronic phases of stroke. These changes in method have allowed significantly increased sophistication in the studies of alexia and agraphia. For example, later in this chapter, the relationships between written language behavior in acute compared to chronic lesions will be addressed in a study of agraphia.

An additional important construct is that written language is a relatively recent addition to human cognitive abilities. While oral language probably dates from 100,000 to 35,000 B.C.E. (Yule, 1996), written language probably dates from only a few thousand years B.C.E. Oral language appears to have been a biological adaptation associated with the ascent of *Homo sapiens*. Written language, however, appears to have been a societal adaptation associated with expansion and socialization within *Homo sapiens*. Therefore, although it can be argued that oral language is, at least in part, produced by brain structures that are biologically adapted specifically for that ability, it is much more likely that written language is produced by brain structures biologically adapted to other abilities. We might therefore expect a significant overlap of written-language brain-behavior relationships with non-language brain-behavior relationships.

Alexia

Alexia is traditionally divided into peripheral and linguistic alexias. Peripheral alexias are due to a disruption of systems not specific to the language network, such as vision or attention. Linguistic alexias are due to disruptions in the language network and, in that way, tend to reflect some of the constructs associated with language, including lexicality (the concept of whether a series of letters is, or is not, a word), orthography (standardized spelling), phonology, and semantics. Two of the four alexias described by Benson and Geschwind (1969) are considered peripheral alexias (hemialexia and alexia without agraphia). Pure alexia, or alexia without agraphia, may be the most well-known alexia because the behavior associated with it is so striking: patients are able to write a word, but are unable to read what they have written (Behrmann et al., 1998). Other patients are also unable to name letters and some show a mild naming impairment (Binder & Mohr, 1992; Behrmann et al., 1998). Pure alexia was attributed to a lesion in the distribution of the left posterior cerebral artery that caused right homonymous hemianopia. Dejerine described this disorder, and Geschwind applied a disconnection model in explaining the clinical-pathological associations. This model postulated that, because posterior strokes usually involve intrahemispheric connections, the visual information in the intact right hemisphere could not access the intact left hemisphere language systems. Some recent studies have argued that pure alexia results from a specific lesion location rather than a disconnection (Beversdorf, 1997). Trying to characterize the lesion that reliably causes certain aspects of the syndrome known as pure alexia has implications for which structures are involved in normal reading. If damage to intrahemispheric connections is necessary for pure alexia to result, the implication is that the right hemisphere can process the orthographic stimuli, but the damage to its connection to the left hemisphere prevents the information from reaching the language centers. If such damage is not necessary, the implication is that pure alexia results from damage to left occipital and temporal areas necessary for decoding of visually presented orthographic stimuli.

Cohen and colleagues attempted to delineate the pathophysiology of pure alexia by using an overlap technique to establish a critical lesion for causing pure alexia (2003). They suggested that the fusiform gyrus in the posterior left temporal lobe was the critical region that, when lesioned, produced pure alexia. Because of this and the region's tendency to show preferential activity for word stimuli in fMRI studies, the term Visual Word Form Area (VWFA) was coined to describe this region (Shallice and Warrington, 1980; Cohen et al., 2003). However, there is much debate about the level of specificity of this area. Some have argued that it is misleading to use the term VWFA, considering that the area is also active for other types of stimuli, and because there is evidence that damage to this area has not been shown to be specific to reading (Price & Devlin, 2003). The debate as to the specificity of this region continues (Tsapkini & Rapp, 2010; Starrfelt et al., 2010).

Studies of patients with pure alexia provide important insights about reading and its relationship to the brain. Some patients with pure alexia cannot read letters or words (Lott & Friedman, 1994; Binder & Mohr, 1992). Some can read letters, but not words and are unable to piece the word together one letter at a time. Some can read letters but not words and use a letter-by-letter strategy piecing the word together one letter at a time. Other patients with a less severe form of pure alexia can read words, but show a marked effect of length. They make errors on longer words and read longer words more slowly. Additionally, there are hemianopic patients who read words accurately, but slowly compared to normal controls. These findings suggest that these patients represent a continuum of cognitive dysfunction. There also appears to be a continuum related to the size of the lesion (larger lesions causing greater disability), but also a continuum of location, from primarily inferior and medial occipital to inferior temporal. Lesions that are primarily occipital appear to be associated with slowed reading and hemianopia (Pflugshauptet al., 2009)] and lesions that are primarily inferior temporal, with or without occipital involvement, appear to be associated with greater impairment of reading letters and words (Binder & Mohr, 1992).

The continuum of deficits in this disorder generates questions about how written language is organized in the brain. Although the most severe patients are unable to name single letters, they can be trained to do so using a tactile-kinesthetic strategy (Lott & Friedman, 1994), suggesting that an abstract representation of the letter is intact even though the decoding of the visual stimulus has been disrupted. This is consistent with studies showing that representations of orthography become increasingly abstract as the ventral processing stream moves from the occipital to temporal cortex (Vinckier, 2007).

Hemialexia, the other peripheral alexia, is a rare disorder. Typically, these are patients who have difficulty reading words in the left visual field. These patients invariably have lesions of the posterior corpus callosum, including the splenium, and perhaps the posterior aspect of the body (Sieroff and Lavidor, 2007). This relationship is best interpreted using a model similar to that used for pure alexia. Visual input to the right hemisphere has impaired access to the left fusiform gyrus.

The central or linguistic alexias (phonological, deep, and surface alexia) usually arise from lesions in or adjacent to the perisylvian area. Such lesions also typically cause aphasia, agraphia, or both. Benson and Geschwind (1969) referred to these as alexia with agraphia if patients did not have aphasia, and aphasic alexia if they did. However, Marshal and Newcombe (1966) took an alternative approach to the analysis of reading. Instead of focusing on the relationships between reading and other cognitive abilities, especially writing, they described a linguistic analysis of alexia. Their study and subsequent studies have delineated a category of what may be termed linguistic alexias. These studies support the contention that there are two routes or systems for reading, a phonological route and a lexical route. The former relies on the relationship connecting the written word to a series of sounds. Patients with an impairment of this route show an inability to read pseudowords (e.g., *nud*), but are able to read real words, including words with irregular orthographic-phonological relationships (irregular words, e.g., *yacht*). This performance demonstrates an inability to use the visual system to access word sounds. (accessing phonology from orthography). This disability is termed phonological agraphia. Patients with phonological alexia may also demonstrate reading deficits for words with low semantic value, such as function words (e.g., *it, the*) and abstract words (e.g., *truth, faith*), but good performance on reading concrete words (e.g., *dog, pencil*). This pattern is interpreted as an over-reliance on semantic systems (Friedman, 2002). A controversy similar to that involving pure alexia and the word form area is present in the literature that attempts to explain phonological alexia, Some authors have argued that patients with phonological alexia have a generalized impairment of phonological processing. The studies that support this position indicate that these patients have impaired ability on non-reading phonological tasks in addition to having impaired ability on reading of pseudowords (Coltheart, 1996). In contrast, there is one report of a patient with impaired pseudoword reading who does not have other phonological deficits (Derouesné & Beauvois, 1985). Therefore, it would appear that the transformation of novel written words into the appropriate sound sequences requires a phonological reading system that is closely tied to a more generalized phonological ability. A possible subgroup of patients with phonological alexia make semantic errors on reading real, concrete words (e.g., reading *pencil* as *scissors*) in addition to being unable to read pseudowords. They are described as having deep alexia (Coltheart et al., 1980). Whether this is a separate disorder, or similar to the continuum of severity described with pure alexia, a more severe form of phonological alexia is another area of debate.

In contrast to the group of patients who cannot read psuedowords is a group of patients who have difficulty reading orthographically irregular words (e.g., *yacht*). Additionally, they may make regularization errors, such as reading *island* as *izland*. These patients may also make lexicalization errors such as reporting that a pseudoword (e.g., *sope*) is the real word *soap*. Patients with these error patterns are described as having surface alexia. The cognitive mechanism that produces this disorder is an over-reliance on the phonological system due to the impairment of the ability to utilize links between complex or irregular orthographic sequences and their phonological relationships. We may describe this as disruption of an orthographic system. Much of the recent work on surface alexia focuses on patients with semantic dementia because of the relatively consistent pathology in the temporal lobe and the high frequency of surface alexia in this population (Woolams et al., 2007). Surface alexia can be observed after stroke, but is more common after hemorrhage or head injury (Coslett, 2003).

Lesions causing phonologic alexia are usually in the distribution of the left middle cerebral artery (MCA), often involving the superior temporal lobe, angular gyrus. and supramarginal gyrus (Coslett, 2003). It has been suggested that deep alexia is simply a more severe version of phonological alexia on a continuum of phonological reading deficits (Friedman, 1996). These patients generally have larger left perisylvian lesions (Coslett, 2003). In English reading patients with alexia, the dual route model is widely accepted. (See studies by McClelland and others for an alternative approach, arguing for a single route model.) Support for this model is also present in studies done on patients who read Japanese. The Japanese language contains both syllabograms (kana) and logograms (kanji). There are reports of patients who are severely impaired when reading words, including concrete words, in the kana script, in which symbols represent sounds, as in English. However, their reading of kanji, in which symbols directly represent concepts, is relatively preserved. The opposite may also occur. These data offer further support for a lexical and non-lexical route in reading. (Coltheart et al., 1980).

The dual route model has been quite influential in generating hypotheses about how humans accomplish the task of reading, and it would not have been possible without careful study of patients with lesions to purported anatomical areas corresponding to cognitive modules in reading. In an era of highly sophisticated imaging techniques, certain questions can still only be answered by studying stroke patients. For example, Hillis et al (2001; 2005; 2007) studied patients at the superacute stage (within 24 hours of stroke) to determine deficits to the major components of reading (orthographic input lexicon, lexical semantics, phonological output lexicon). By conducting behavioral testing and imaging the areas to which blood flow had been restored, these authors were able to determine definitive links between recovery of specific aspects of reading and reperfusion of specific brain areas. Pseudoword reading (and spelling) appears to rely on a network of areas that include Brodmann's areas 37 and 40 (supermarginal gyrus and posterior-inferior temporal/fusiform gyrus). This method gives us precise information without the confound of reorganization that is inherent in studies of chronic (and even acute) stroke patients. Also, unlike functional neuroimaging of control subjects, it gives us information about the areas *necessary* to reading as opposed to the areas *involved* in reading.

Agraphia

Similar to alexia, there are two general categories of agraphia. Agraphia is traditionally divided into linguistic and motor agraphias (Ogle, 1867). Linguistic agraphias are those that have language dysfunction as their basis. The patients with aphasic agraphia described by Leischner (1969) are roughly equivalent to the patients described as having linguistic agraphias. Similar to that described for reading, there appear to be two routes for spelling, a phonological route and a lexical route. Linguistic agraphias include phonological, lexical (or surface), and semantic agraphias in this category. (Roeltgen, and Ullrich, 2012; Roeltgen and Heilman, 1985; Roeltgen and Rapcsak, 1993; Rapcsak et al., 2009; Marien et al 2001; Henry et al., 2007). Patients with motor agraphias have impairments in output, and include primary agraphias (constructional) and apraxic agraphia. Current models also include agraphias from impairments of attention and allographic knowledge in this category.

Phonological agraphia is similar to phonological alexia and was first described by Shallice (1981). He described an agraphia characterized by relatively preserved ability to spell real words, including words that are orthographically irregular (i.e., *yacht*) but with an inability to spell pronounceable pseudowords (i.e., *nud*). Patients with this disorder usually make phonologically incorrect errors that may have a degree of visual similarity to the correct response. Shallice concluded that this patient had an impairment of phonological processing, necessary for translating sounds into letters.

In contrast to the patient described by Shallice (1981) was a patient with lexical agraphia described by Beauvois and Derouesné (1981). Their patient was able to spell pronounceable pseudowords, but had difficulty spelling orthographically irregular words compared to regular words (i.e., *thing*). Their patient also made frequent regularization errors when spelling irregular words (*yacht*->YAT). Impairment of this type is consistent with disruption of an orthographic (letter group) or lexical (whole word) route, with relative preservation of a phonological route. Although Beauvois and Derouesne(1981) were the first to describe lexical agraphia, Roeltgen and Heilman (1984) were the first to attempt to delineate the anatomy underlying it. They proposed that the junction of the posterior angular gyrus and the parietal-occipital lobule was an important anatomic substrate for this disorder. Subsequent studies have demonstrated that cortical or subcortical lesions involving multiple non-perisylvian sites are typically associated with lexical agraphia (Wolz & Roeltgen, 1989: Alexander et al., 1990; Rothi et al., 1987; Croisile et al., 1989; Rapcsak et al., 1988; Roeltgen and Rapcsak 1993, Rapcsak and Beeson, 2004). This heterogeneity is consistent with Hatfield's (1985) position that the lexical system might contain multiple cognitive components. Additionally, in a cross-sectional study, Roeltgen has found that the typical pattern of lexical agraphia appears to be more common in stroke patients who have chronic lesions than in patients who have acute lesions (Roeltgen and Ullrich, 2012). We have suggested that the ability to utilize the phonological route to spell is not necessarily an automatic process, but requires time, training (therapy), or brain reorganization to be successful in spelling real words.

Roeltgen and colleagues (Roeltgen et al., 1983; Roeltgen and Heilman, 1984) originally proposed that the supramarginal gyrus or the insula medial to it was the anatomic basis of phonological agraphia. Subsequent studies have demonstrated a degree of anatomic diversity, with lesions occurring within the entire perisylvian region resulting in phonological agraphia (Shallice, 1981; Bub and Kertesz, 1982; Nolan and Caramazza, 1982; Alexander et al., 1992; Baxter and

Warrington,1986; Bolla-Wilson et al. 1985; Rapcsak and Beeson, 2002; Henry et al, 2007; Marien et al, 2001; Rapcsak et al., 2009). Henry and colleagues (2007) have suggested that the diversity in phonological agraphia represents individual variations in cerebral architecture and functional representation (Henry et al, 2007). The association of phonological agraphia with the perisylvian area is similar to the association of phonological alexia and the perisylvian area. These findings of perisylvian involvement support the perisylvian role in phonological processing. However, studies have shown that this association does not represent a single cognitive and cerebral system that translates all symbolic visual input into sounds (phonological reading), then reverses direction to translate sounds into symbolic output (phonological writing). A few patients have been described who demonstrate dissociations between phonological alexia and agraphia (Roeltgen and Heilman, 1984 and Roeltgen,1993). Clinical and radiological presentations of phonological and lexical agraphia create a double dissociation of phonological processing and lexical (orthographic) processing, as well as a double dissociation of anatomic sites, similar to that found with alexia.

Initial reports describing phonological agraphia argued that preserved spelling utilized a lexical-semantic route (Beauvois & Derouesne, 1981; Roeltgen, Sevush, & Heilman, 1983). However, Roeltgen and colleagues (1986) described patients who were able to spell pronounceable pseudowords, and therefore had an intact phonological system, and many orthographically irregular words, and therefore had an intact lexical system, but had difficulty providing the semantically correct spelling for irregular homophones. For example, when asked to write *doe* as in "the doe ran through the forest," these patients might write "dough." Detailed patient analysis demonstrated a disruption of semantic ability or a disconnection of semantics from spelling. They termed this disorder "semantic agraphia." (Roeltgen et al., 1986). Patients with semantic agraphia lose their ability to spell and write with meaning. They may produce semantic jargon in sentence production (Rapcsak and Rubens, 1990). The pathology of the reported patients with semantic agraphia is variable, but frequently involves anatomic substrates important for accessing meaning in speech (Roeltgen and Rapcsak, 1993). Semantic agraphia is also a common finding in early Alzheimer's disease (Niels and Roeltgen, 1995a), consistent with the early semantic dysfunction in that disorder.

Models of Writing

Analysis of the three linguistic agraphias described above results in a model such as that described in Figure 1. Spontaneous writing initiates activity in the semantic region prior to utilization of the lexical, and perhaps, the phonologic systems for production of the correct word. Writing to dictation requires auditory input into either the orthographic system (writing words that one can spell, but does not

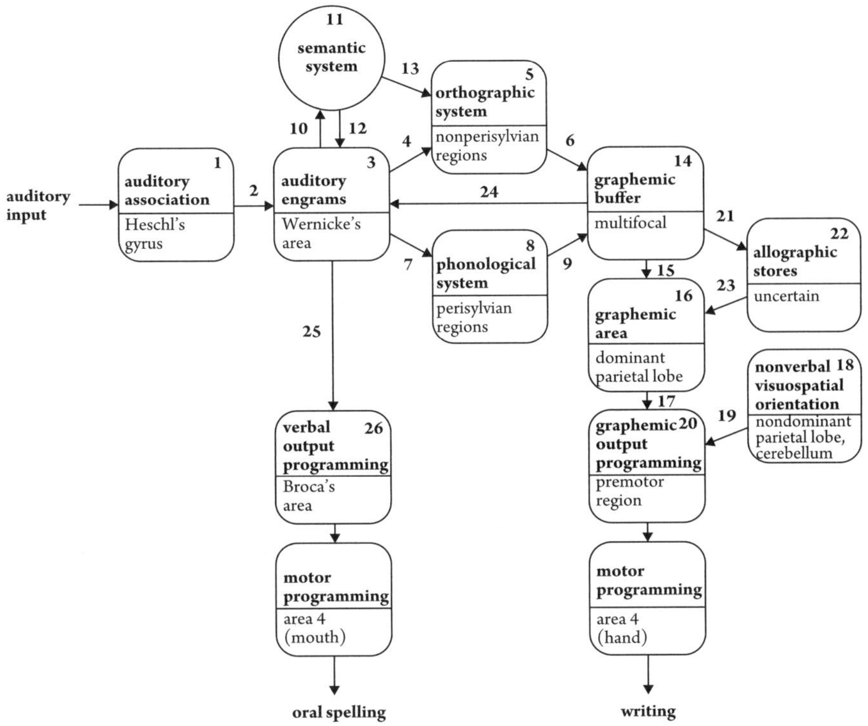

Figure 5.1 A schematic diagram of the processes involved in writing and spelling.

know the meaning of), the phonologic systems (writing words that are unknown, but orthographically regular) with or without input from the semantic system, for words whose meaning is known.

In contrast to the linguistic agraphias described above are the peripheral agraphias. Impaired attention, a common cause of peripheral agraphia, is associated with production of correctly formed but linguistically incorrect letters. Omissions, substitutions, insertions, and transpositions in pseudowords and real words in oral and written spelling are the prominent error types. Impairment occurs in spontaneous writing, writing to dictation, written naming, and delayed copying. Errors are not affected by linguistic factors (i.e., word class, regularity, and imageability). Errors are more common at the beginning and ends of and in longer words (Cantagallo and Bonazzi, 1996). If there is a lateralized impairment of attention, there may be a reflection of that lateralization, leading to a preponderance of errors on the side of the word that is contralateral to the lesion. Studies of patients with these error types have led to the conclusion that there is a graphemic buffer or working memory storage system. It has been proposed that this temporary store of information contains the abstract letter concept in preparation for processing by the output systems for oral or written spelling. Lesions associated with graphemic buffer disturbances have included the left frontal parietal region (Hillis and Caramazza, 1989; Lesser, 1990), the left parietal region (Miceli et al., 1985; Cubelli, 1991; Posteraro et al., 1988; Annoni et al., 1998), and the right frontal parietal and basal ganglia region (Hillis and Caramazza, 1989). We (unpublished observation) and M. Laine (personal communication) have each observed patients with apparent agraphia due to impairment of the graphemic buffer; these patients had relatively discrete lesions of the left posterior dorsal lateral frontal lobe. Cubelli (1991) described an instance of the disorder from a subcortical left frontal lesion. Of note, these lesions lie in regions not associated with the linguistic written language disorders.

Rothi and Heilman (1981) described a patient who had difficulty producing the correct strokes when writing and had trouble recognizing the correct strokes in letters when reading. However, this patient was able to spell aloud without difficulty, and writing improved with copying. They suggested that this represented dysfunction of a "graphemic area," a system important for assembling the proper strokes in written letter output, and utilized visuokinesthetic motor engrams. The pattern of errors is similar to the sequencing and position errors made by patients with apraxia. The disorder that these patients have is termed apraxic agraphia, and these patients may or may not have limb apraxia (Heilman et al., 1973, 1974; Valenstein and Heilman, 1979;Roeltgen and Heilman 1983; Margolin and Binder,1984;Baxter and Warrington, 1986; Carey and Heilman, 1988; Hodges, 1991; Otsuki et al., 1999; Del GrossoDestreri et al., 2000). Therefore, the graphemic area appears to be anatomically and conceptually distinct from, but closely related to, the structures important for limb praxis. Clinical-radiological correlations support the conclusion that the dominant parietal lobe is important for this function. Within the parietal lobe, lesions specific to the postcentral gyrus, the intraparietal sulcus, and the anterior intraparietal sulcus may be associated with clinically distinct types of apraxic agraphia (Sakurai et al., 2007). However, at least one patient with this disorder has had a frontal lesion (Hodges, 1991).

Other disturbances of stroke production in writing have been described. Such patients show reiteration of strokes and inability to write on a straight horizontal line, and insertion of blank spaces between graphemes. They may also write on only one side of the paper (when associated with the neglect syndrome). Patients with such findings have been described as having constructional agraphia, visuospatial agraphia or afferent "dysgraphia" (Ellis et al.,1987). This syndrome is usually due to nondominant parietal or frontal lobe lesions (Ardila & Rosselli, 1993). Ellis and colleagues (1987) emphasized the term *afferent* and suggested that it occurred due to failure to utilize visual and kinesthetic feedback. Silveri and colleagues (1997) provided support for this latter hypothesis in a patient with spatial agraphia from a cerebellar lesion. Their patient performed much better with his eyes open than with his eyes closed.

Evaluations of writing errors in normal subjects (slips of the pen) (Ellis, 1979) and patients with brain lesions may show errors of case (upper versus lower) or style (print [manuscript] versus script [cursive](Black et al., 1987; Debastiani and Barry, 1989; Kartounis, 1992; Trojano and Chichio, 1994; Del GrossoDestini et al., 2000; Menichelli et al., 2008). These errors include difficulty producing a specific case or style or substitution of one particular case or style for another. Analyses of these patients are consistent with a degree of functional and anatomic separation between letters in different formats. The abitity to direct the handwriting system to produce the specific letter form has been termed the allographic store. Insufficient subjects with this impairment have been described to allow for conclusions regarding possible anatomic localization.

Hemiagraphia is an inability to write with nondominant hand. It has, in conjunction with associated impairments, helped the understanding of laterality and interhemispheric connectivity by the corpus callosum. In the agraphias previously described, the dominant and nondominant hands are equally affected, except when one hand is paretic. Liepman and Maas (1907) and others (Geschwind and Kaplan, 1962; Bogen, 1969; Levy, et al.. 1971; Rubens et al.. 1977; Sugishita et al.. 1980; Yamadori et al., 1980; Gersh and Damasio, 1981; Watson and Heilman, 1983: Tanaka et al., 1990) have described patients who can write with their dominant hand, but are unable to with their nondominant hand. The production with the nondominant hand is usually unintelligible, but improves with copying. Some patients can type with their affected limb (Watson and Heilman, 1983) and others cannot (Geschwind and Kaplan, 1962). Watson and Heilman (1983) suggested that the difference was sparing of the genu of the corpus callosum, allowing for transmission of verbal-motor engrams to the nondominant hemisphere. Patients with hemiagraphia usually also have unilateral apraxia of the dominant hand (Watson and Heilman, 1983). However, this also is not always true (Gersh and Damasio, 1981). Additionally, the patient of Gersh and Damasio (1981) had a lesion of the posterior corpus callosum and produced aphasic-type errors. Watson and Heilman (1983) concluded that language information (correct spellings) was transferred in the posterior (splenium) of the corpus callosum and praxis in the central (body). Analysis of patients with hemiagraphia, similar to the analysis of patients with hemialexia, therefore illustrates many of the clinical dissociations that can occur in written language and gives insight into the functional localization of the corpus callosum.

Conclusions

Analyses of patients with alexia and agraphia have yielded considerable insight into brain function. Important in this regard is the need to consider that written language is a late development in human evolution. The relationships between phonological alexia and agraphia and brain localization of function are consistent with a fundamental construct regarding the linguistic processing within the left hemisphere. Structures within the perisylvian region appear to be capable of or perhaps necessary for (as suggested by the results of Hillis and colleagues) performing sound-to-letter conversion and letter-to-sound conversion. Structures distinct from those involved in phonological relationships appear important for many of the non-phonological facets of written language. These relationships are consistant with the notion that the evolution of written language abilities have depended on the presence of oral language. The apparent redundancy of brain regions associated with a specific function (multiple non-perisylvian areas associated with lexical agraphia) reflects the multiple brain systems that appear to mutually support a single behavior. Additionally, as is apparent from the issues concerning the visual word form area and the associations of agraphia with attention and praxis, the written language system has been constructed utilizing brain regions with capacities that are conducive to general relationships of cognitive systems or modules, not specific localized structures for specific written language functions.

References

Alexander, M. P., Friedman, R. B., Loverso, F., & Fischer, R. (1990). Anatomic correlates of Lexical Agraphia. *Presented at the Academy of Aphasia, Baltimore, MD.*

Alexander, M. P., Friedman, R. B., Loverso, F., & Fischer, R. S. (1992). Lesion localization of phonological agraphia. *Brain Language, 43,* 83–95.

Annoni, J. M., Lemay, M. A., de Mattos Pimenta, M. A., & Lecours, A. R. (1998). The contribution of attentional mechanisms to an irregularity effect at the grapheme buffer level. *Brain Language, 63,* 63–78.

Ardila, A., & Rosselli, M. (1993). *Spatial Agraphia. Brain and Cognition, 22,* 137–147.

Baxter, D. M., & Warrington, E. K. (1986). Ideational agraphia: A single case study. *Journal of Neurology, Neurosurgery and Psychiatry, 49,* 369–374.

Behrmann M., Nelson J., Sekuler, E. B. (1998). Visual complexity in letter-by-letter reading: "pure" alexia is not pure. *Neuropsychologia, 36(11),* 1115–1132.

Benson, D. F., & Geschwind, N. (1969). In P. J. Vinken & G. W. Bruyn (eds.), *Handbook of Clinical Neurology* (pp. 112–140). Amsterdam: North-Holland Publishing Company.

Binder J. R., & Mohr J. P. (1992). The topography of transcallosal reading pathways: a case–control analysis. *Brain, 115,* 1807–1826.

Beversdorf, D. Q., Ratcliffe, N. R., Rhodes, C. H., & Reeves, A. G. (1997). Pure alexia: clinical-pathologic evidence for a lateralized visual language association cortex. *Clinical Neuropathology, 16*(6), 328–31.

Beauvois M. F., & Derouesné J. (1981). Lexical or orthographic agraphia. *Brain, 104 (part 1),* 21–49.

Black, S. E., Behrmann, M., Bass, K., & Hacker, P. (1987). Selective writing impairment: Beyond the allographic code. *Aphasiology, 3(3),* 265–277.

Bogen, J. E. (1969). The other side of the brain I: Dysgraphia and dyscopia following cerebral commissurotomy. *Bulletin of the Los Angeles Neurological Society, 34,* 3–105.

Bolla-Wilson, K., Speedie, J. J., & Robinson, R. G. (1985). Phonologic agraphia in a left-handed patient after a right-hemisphere lesion. *Neurology, 35*, 1778–1781.

Bub, D., & Kertesz, A. (1982). Deep agraphia. *Brain Language, 17*, 146–165.

Cantagallo & Bonazzi, (1996). Acquired dysgraphia with selective damage to the graphemic buffer: a single case report. *The Italian Journal of Neurological Sciences, 17 (3)*, 249–254.

Carey, M. A., & Heilman, K. M. (1988). Letter imagery deficits in a case of pure apraxic agraphia. *Brain Language, 34*, 147–156.

Cohen L., Martinaud O., Lemer C., Lehericy, S., Samson, Y., Obadia, M...Dehaene, S. (2003). Visual word recognition in the left and right hemispheres: anatomical and functional correlates of peripheral alexias. *Cerebral Cortex, 13*, 1313–1333.

Coltheart, M., Marshall, J. C., & Patterson, K. E. (1980). Deep Dyslexia. London: Routledge & Kegan Paul.

Coltheart, M. (1996). Phonological dyslexia: past and future issues. *Cognitive Neuropsychology, 13*, 749–762.

Coslett, H,B. (2003). Acquired Dyslexia. In Heilman, K.,Valenstein, E. (eds.), *Clinical Neuropsychology* (108–125). New York, NY: Oxford University Press.

Croisile, B., Trillet, M., Laurent, B., Latombe, D., & Schott, B. (1989). Agraphie lexicale par hematoma temporo-parietal gauche. *Revista Neurologia, 145*, 287–292.

Cubelli, R. (1991). A selective deficit for writing vowels in acquired dysgraphia. *Nature, 353*, 258–260.

Debastiani, P., & Barry, C. (1989). A cognitive analysis of an acquired dysgraphic patient with an "allographic" writing disorder. *Cognitive Neuropsychology, 6*, 41–45.

Del Grosso Destreri, N., Farina, E., Alberoni, M., Pomati, S., Nichelli, P., & Mariani, C. (2000). Selective uppercase dysgraphia with loss of visual imagery of letter forms: A window on the organization of graphomotor patterns. *Brain and Language, 71(3)*, 353–372.

Derouesné, J & Beauvois, M. F. (1985). The "phonemic state" in the non-lexical reading process: Evidence from a case of phonological alexia. In K. Patterson J. C. Marshall & M. Coltheart, (eds.). *Surface dyslexia* (pp. 399–457). Hillsdale, NJ: Erlbaum.

Ellis, A. W. (1979). Slipps of the pen. *Visible Language, 113(3)*, 265–282.

Ellis, A. W., Young, W. W., & Flude, B. M. (1987). "Afferent dysgraphia" in a patient and in normal subjects. *Cognitive Neuropsychology, 4*, 465–487.

Friedman, R. B. (1996). Recovery from deep alexia to phonological alexia: points on a continuum. *Brain and Language, 52(1)*, 114–28.

Friedman, R. B. (2002). Clinical diagnosis and treatment of reading disorders. In A. E. Hillis,(ed.), *Handbook of Adult Language Disorders* (27–47). New York, NY: Psychology Press.

Gersh, F., & Damasio, A. R. (1981). Praxis and writing of the left hand may be served by different callosal pathways. *Archives of Neurology, 38*, 634–636.

Geschwind, N., & Kaplan, E. (1962). A human cerebral disconnection syndrome. *Neurology, 12*, 675–685.

Hatfield, F. M. (1985). Visual and phonological factors in acquired dysgraphia. *Neuropsychologia, 23*, 13–29.

Heilman, K. M., Coyle, J. M., Gonyea, E. F., & Geschwind, N. (1973). Apraxia and agraphia in a left hander. *Brain, 96*, 21–28.

Heilman, K. M., Gonyea, E. F., & Geschwind, N. (1974). Apraxia and agraphia in a right hander. *Cortex, 10*, 284–288.

Henry, M. L., Beeson, P. M., Stark, A. J., & Rapcsak, S. Z. (2007). The role of left perisylvian cortical regions in spelling. *Brain and Language, 100(1)*, 44–52.

Hillis, A. E., & Caramazza, A. (1989). The graphemic buffer and attentional mechanisms. *Brain and Language, 36*, 208–235.

Hillis, A. E., Wityk, R. J., Tuffiash, E., Beauchamp, N. J., Jacobs, M. A., Barker, P. B., & Selnes, O. A. (2001). Hypoperfusion of Wernicke's area predicts severity of semantic deficit in acute stroke. *Annals of Neurology, 50*, 561–566.

Hillis, A. E., Newhart, M., Heidler, J., Barker, P., Herskovits, E., & Degaonkarb, M. (2005). The roles of the visual word form area in reading. *NeuroImage, 24,* 548–559.

Hillis, A. E. (2007). Magnetic resonance perfusion imaging in the study of language. *Brain and Language, 102,* 165–175.

Hodges, J. R. (1991). Pure apraxic agraphia with recovery after drainage of a left frontal cyst. *Cortex, 27,* 469–473.

Kartsounis, L. D. (1992). Selective lower-case letter ideational agraphia. *Cortex, 28,* 145–150.

Leischner, A. (1969). Handbook of Clinical Neurology. Vinken, P. J., & Bruyn, G. W. (eds.). Amsterdam: North-Holland Publishing Company, 112–140.

Lesser, R. (1990). Superior oral to written spelling: Evidence for separate buffers? *Cognitive Neuropsychology, 7,* 347–366.

Levy, J., Nebes, R. D., & Sperry, R. W. (1971). Expressive language in the surgically separated minor hemisphere. *Cortex, 7,* 49–58.

Liepmann, H., & Maas, O. (1907). Ein Fall von linksseitiger Agraphie und bei rechtsseitiger Lahmumg. *Journal of Psychological Neurology, 10,* 214–227.

Lott, S. N., & Friedman, R. B. (1994). Rationale and efficacy of a tactile-kinaesthetic treatment for alexia. *Aphasiology, 8(2),* 181–195.

Margolin, D. I., & Binder, L. (1984). Multiple component agraphia in a patient with atypical cerebral dominance: An error analysis. *Brain and Language, 22,* 26–40.

Marien, P., Pickuta, B. A., Engelborghsa, S., Martind, J., De Deyn, P. (2001). Phonological agraphia following a focal anterior insulo-opercular infarction. *Neuropsychologia, 39 (8),* 845–855.

Marshall, J. C., & Newcombe, F. (1966). Syntactic and semantic errors in paralexia. *Neuropsychologia, 4,* 169–176.

Menichelli, A., Rapp, B., & Semenza, C. (2008). Allographic agraphia: A case study. *Cortex, 44(70),* 861–868.

Miceli, G., Silveri, M. C., & Caramazza, A. (1985). Cognitive analysis of a case of pure dysgraphia. *Brain and Language, 25,* 187–212.

Niels, J., & Roeltgen, D. P. (1995). Spelling and attention in early Alzheimer's disease: Evidence for impairment of the graphemic buffer. *Brain and Language, 49,* 241–262.

Nielson, J. M. (1946). Agnosia, apraxia, aphasia: Their value in cerebral localization. New York: Paul B. Hoeber.

Nolan, K. A., & Caramazza, A. (1982). Modality-independent impairments in word processing in a deep dyslexic patient. *Brain and Language, 16,* 236–264.

Ogle, W. (1867). Aphasia and agraphia. In *Records of St. George's Hospital, 2,* 83–122. London: Medical Research Counsel (reproduction).

Otsuki, M., Soma, Y., Aral, T., Otsuka, A., & Tsuji, S. (1999). Pure apraxic agraphia with abnormal writing stroke sequences: Report of a Japanese patient with a left superior parietal hemorrhage. *Journal of Neurology, Neurosurgery and Psychiatry, 66,* 233–237.

Pflugshaupt T., Gutbrod K., Wurtz P., von Wartburg, R., Nyffeler, T., de Haan, B., Karnath, H., & Mueri, R. M. (2009). About the role of visual field defects in pure alexia. *Brain 2009;132,* 1907–1917.

Posteraro, L., Zinelli, P., & Mazzucci, A. (1988). Selective impairment of the graphemic buffer in acquired dysgraphia. *Brain and Language, 35,* 274–286.

Price, C. J., Devlin, J. T. (2003). The myth of the visual word form area. *Neuroimage, 19,* 473–481.

Rapcsak, S. Z., & Rubens, A. B. (1990). Disruption of semantic influence on writing following a left prefrontal lesion. *Brain and Language, 38,* 334–344.

Rapcsak, S. Z., Arthur, S. A., & Rubens, A. B. (1998). Lexical agraphia from focal lesion of the left pre-central gyrus. *Neurology, 38,* 1119–1123.

Rapcsak, S. Z., & Beeson, P. M. (2002). Neuroanatomical correlates of spelling and writing. In A. E. Hillis (ed.), *Handbook on adult language disorders: Integrating cognitive neuropsychology, neurology, and rehabilitation* (pp 71–99). New York: Psychology Press.

Rapcsak, S. Z., & Beeson, P. M. (2004). The role of left posterior inferior temporal cortex in spelling. *Neurology, 62,* 2221–2229.

Rapcsak, S. Z., Beeson, P. M., Henry, M. L., Leyden, A., Kim, E., Rising, K. et al. (2009). Phonological dyslexia and dysgraphia: Cognitive mechanisms and neural substrates. *Cortex, 45(5),* 575–591.

Roeltgen, D. P., Sevush, S., & Heilman, K. M. (1983) Phonological agraphia: Writing by the lexical-semantic route. *Neurology, 33,* 733–757.

Roeltgen, D. P., & Heilman, K. M. (1983) Apraxic agraphia in a patient with normal praxis. *Brain and Language, 18,* 35–46.

Roeltgen, D. P., &.Heilman, K. M. (1984). Lexical agraphia: further support for the two-system hypothesis of linguistic agraphia. *Brain, 107,* 811–827.

Roeltgen, D. P., & Heilman, K. M. (1985). Review of agraphia and a proposal for an anatomically-based neuropsychological model of writing. *Applied Psycholinguistics, 6,* 205–230.

Roeltgen, D. P., Rothi, L. J. G., & Heilman, K. M. (1986). Linguistic semantic agraphia. *Brain and Language, 27,* 257–280.

Roeltgen, D. P. (1993) Agraphia. In K. M. Heilman & E. Valenstein (eds.), *Clinical Neuropsychology* (3rd ed., pp. 63–90). New York: Oxford University Press.

Roeltgen, D. P., & Rapcsak, S. (1993). Acquired disorders of writing and spelling. In G. Blanken (ed.). Linguistic disorders and pathologies (pp. 262–278). Berlin: Walter de Gruyter.

Rothi, L. J. G., & Heilman, K. M. (1981). Alexia and agraphia with spared spelling and letter recognition abilities. *Brain and Language, 12,* 1–13.

Rothi, L. J. G., Roeltgen, D. P., & Kooistra, C. A. (1987). Isolated lexical agraphia in a right-handed patient with a posterior lesion of the right cerebral hemisphere. *Brain and Language, 301,* 181–190.

Rubens, A. B., Geschwind, N., Mahowald, M. W., & Mastri, A. (1977). Posttraumatic cerebral hemispheric disconnection syndrome. *Archives of Neurology, 34,* 750–755.

Sakurai, Y., Onuma, Y., Nakazawa, G., Ugawa, Y., Momose, T., Tsuji, S., & Mannen, T. (2007). Parietal dysgraphia: Characterization of abnormal writing stroke sequences, character formation and character recall. *Behavioral Neurology, 18(2),* 99–114.

Shallice, T., & Warrington, E. K. (1980). Single and multiple component central dyslexic syndromes. In M. Coltheart, K. Patterson & J. C. Marshall (eds.). Deep Dyslexia (pp. 119–145). London: Routledge and Kegan Paul.

Shallice, T. (1981). Phonological agraphia and the lexical route in writing. *Brain, 104,* 412–429.

Siéroff, E., & Lavidor, M. (2007). Examination of the split fovea theory in a case of pure left hemialexia. *Cognitive Neuropsychology, 24(3),* 243–59.

Silveri, M. C., Misciagna, S., Leggio, M. C., & Moliriari, M. (1997). Spatial Dysgraphia and cerebellar lesion: A case report. *Neurology, 48,* 1529–1532.

Starrfelt, R., Habekost T., & Gerlach, C. (2010). Visual processing in pure alexia: a case study. *Cortex, 46,* 242–255.

Sugishita, M., Toyokura, Y., Yoshioka, M., & Yamada, R. (1980). Unilateral agraphia after section of the posterior half of the truncus to the corpus callosum. *Brain and Language, 9(2),* 212–223.

Tanaka, Y., Iwasa, H., & Obayashi, T. (1990). Right hand agraphia and left hand apraxia following callosal damage in a right-hander. *Cortex, 26,* 665–671.

Trojano, L., & Chiacchio, L. (1994). Pure dysgraphia with relative sparing of lower-case writing. *Cortex, 30,* 499–501.

Tsapkini, K., Rapp, B. (2010). The orthography-specific functions of the left fusiform gyrus: evidence of modality and category specificity. *Cortex, 46,* 185–205.

Ullrich, L., & Roeltgen, D. P. (2012). Agraphia. In K. Heilman, Valenstein, E. (eds.) *Clinical Neuropsychology* (pp. 126–145). New York: Oxford University Press.

Valenstein, E., & Heilman, K. M. (1979). Apraxic agraphia with neglect-induced paragraphia. *Archives of Neurology, 67,* 44–56.

Vinckier, F., Dehaene, S., Jobert, A., Dubus, J., Sigman, M., Cohen, L. (2007). Hierarchical coding of letter strings in the ventral stream: dissecting the inner organization of the visual word-form system. *Neuron, 55*, 143–156.

Watson, R. T., & Heilman, K. M. (1983). Callosal apraxia. *Brain, 106*, 391–404.

Wolz,W., & Roeltgen, D. P. (1989). Isolated lexical agraphia due to a basal ganglia lesion. *Journal of Clinical and Experimental Neuropsychology, 11(1)*, 43.

Woollams, A. M., Lambon Ralph, M. A., Plaut, D. C., & Patterson, K. (2007). SD-squared: on the association between semantic dementia and surface dyslexia. *Psychological Review, 114(2)*, 316–39.

Yamadori, A., Osumi, Y., Ikeda, H., & Kanazawa, Y. (1980). Left unilateral agraphia and tactile anomia: Disturbances seen after occlusion of the anterior cerebral artery. *Archives of Neurology, 37*, 88–91.

Yule, G. (1996). The study of Language. Cambridge: Cambridge University Press.

CHAPTER 6

Face Recognition

Steven Z. Rapcsak

Introduction

The human brain's prodigious capacity for remembering faces is an essential biological prerequisite of normal social interaction. Although we encounter hundreds, if not thousands, of different individuals in our daily lives, a quick glance at the face is usually sufficient to determine whether we know the person or not. The remarkable speed and accuracy that characterizes normal face recognition, however, can break down in dramatic ways following brain injury, resulting in significant limitations in the area of social functioning. Early descriptions of face memory impairment in neurological patients can be traced back to the 19th century (Benton, 1990). Since that time, face recognition disorders have been the focus of intense study by behavioral neurologists and cognitive neuroscientists. In the course of these investigations, it has become apparent that face memory impairments are by no means uncommon and can be associated with a variety of neurological conditions including stroke, epilepsy/temporal lobectomy, degenerative disorders (e.g., Alzheimer's disease, frontotemporal dementia), herpes encephalitis, and head trauma. Despite variations in terms of the underlying pathology, lesion-deficit correlation studies have consistently implicated certain brain structures as being critical for the processing of face identity information. Taken together, these observations provide powerful empirical validation of the basic tenet of behavioral neurology that the location, rather than the etiology, of the brain lesion determines the nature of the cognitive deficit.

From a phenomenological perspective, face recognition impairments in neurological patients can manifest either as memory loss or memory distortion (Rapcsak, 2003). The former is reflected by a striking failure to identify *familiar* faces (and a parallel impairment in remembering new faces), whereas the latter involves false recognition or misidentification of *unfamiliar* faces. Although in some individuals both types of difficulties are observed, current evidence suggests that these two recognition disorders are potentially dissociable and may have different cognitive mechanisms and neural substrates. Historically, defective recognition of familiar faces has received much more attention from investigators than false recognition of unfamiliar faces. It is clear, however, that a comprehensive neuropsychological model of face recognition must be capable of accounting for both types of memory disorders.

In this chapter, we review what neuropsychological studies have revealed about the functional architecture and cortical localization of the neural systems involved in face recognition memory. We begin our discussion by presenting a cognitive model of face processing that provides the conceptual framework for interpreting the different types of recognition disorders encountered in neurological patients. This is followed by a detailed description of the behavioral manifestations, cognitive mechanisms, and putative neural correlates of three distinct clinical syndromes characterized by prominent face memory impairment: prosopagnosia, person recognition disorders, and false recognition/misidentification of unfamiliar faces.

Cognitive Model of Face Recognition

The information-processing diagram depicted in Figure 6.1 is a modified version of the influential model of face recognition originally proposed by Bruce & Young (1986).

Central to the revised model is the notion that face recognition performance reflects the dynamic interaction of two basic cognitive operations that involve processing faces at different levels of specificity: individuation and categorization (Fiske & Neuberg, 1990; Mason & Macrae, 2004; Quinn & Macrae, 2005). Individuation entails using facial cues to recognize familiar people at the most specific taxonomic level corresponding to unique personal identity. As shown in Figure 6.1, individuation begins with the visual analysis of the face and requires the extraction of high-quality perceptual information suitable for distinguishing the face of a particular person from all other faces represented in memory. The computational difficulty inherent in this task can be appreciated by considering the fact that faces constitute a homogeneous visual category with a high level of structural similarity among exemplars. Because all faces share the same basic parts in roughly the same general arrangement (i.e., two eyes above the nose and mouth), discriminating individual faces depends critically on the efficient processing of fine-grained configural information sensitive to subtle differences in the spatial relationship among component features (Maurer et al., 2002). According to Figure 6.1, the next step in the individuation process involves activation of "face recognition units" (FRUs) that store visual memory representations

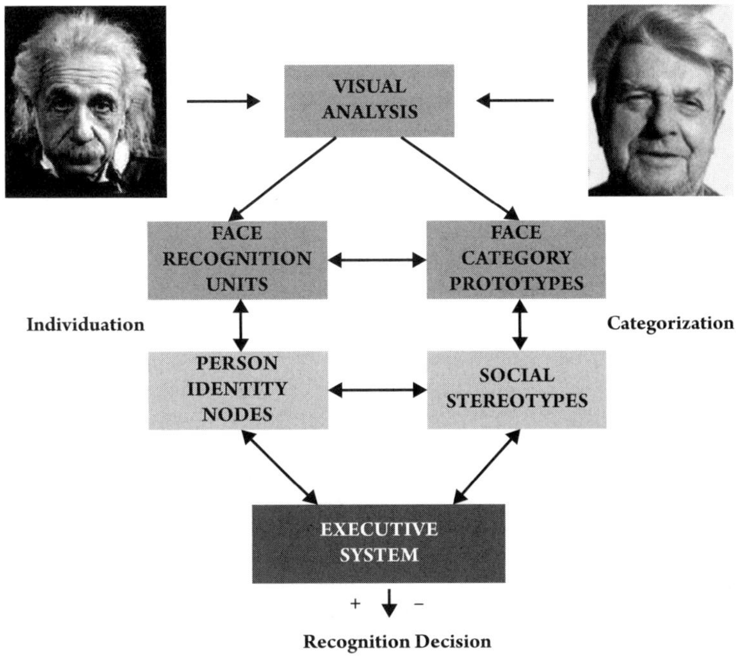

Figure 6.1 Cognitive model of face recognition memory. Recognition performance is the integrated product of individuation and categorization and involves distinct visual, (blue), semantic (yellow), and executive (magenta) operations (see color insert).

of familiar faces. The strength of FRU activation, reflecting the degree of resemblance between the current face percept and the stored memory trace, gives rise to a proportionate sense of familiarity. Under normal circumstances, the activation of FRUs is followed by the retrieval of unique identity-specific biographic information (e.g., occupation, name) from semantic memory via the activation of "person identity nodes" (PINs) that provide the appropriate context for the feeling of familiarity evoked by the face. Unlike the modality-specific visual operations involved in the processing of facial information, conceptual knowledge of familiar people is considered multimodal in nature and therefore can be accessed not only from faces but also from identity-specific cues presented through other modalities, such as hearing the voice or name of the person.

The individuation process outlined above is critical for the rapid and accurate identification of familiar people that characterizes normal face recognition performance. By relying on the encoding and retrieval of distinct and non-overlapping visual and semantic memory representations, individuation allows for maximum differentiation or "pattern separation" (McClelland et al., 1995) between memory traces and thus avoids the problem of interference that could lead to mistaking one familiar person for another. Of course, the ultimate success and efficiency of the individuation process is strongly influenced by the frequency of prior exposure to a particular person. Whereas identity-specific visual and semantic information is readily accessible in the case of highly familiar individuals, recognizing people we encounter less frequently can create difficulties as our stored knowledge of these persons is less well differentiated. Identification of individuals we are less familiar with is typically more effortful and strategic, and the process is also more error-prone due to increased susceptibility to confusions with similar representations in memory.

Although individuation provides a reliable mechanism for identifying familiar people, most persons we encounter in everyday life are in fact strangers. In these situations, the recognition system can make use of facial information to classify unfamiliar individuals into meaningful social categories (Fiske & Neuberg, 1990; Macrae & Bodenhausen, 2000; Quinn & Macrae, 2005). Categorization processes take advantage of pre-existing knowledge about salient facial characteristics shared by members of distinct social groups that are stored in memory as abstract perceptual prototypes (Figure 6.1). Face category prototypes are the result of an averaging process that extracts and preserves information about structural attributes common to many faces rather than information about the faces of specific individuals (Light et al., 1979; Cabeza et al., 1999; Valentine & Bruce, 1986; Vokey & Read, 1992). Novel faces can be assigned to one or more relevant categories based on their degree of similarity to stored prototypes. Category assignment usually reflects some combination of gender, age, and race, but it can also involve more complex social inferences based on facial attributes we associate with certain occupations (e.g., actress, politician) and personality traits (e.g., honesty, intelligence) (Klatzky et al. 1982). As shown in Figure 6.1, the activation of face category prototypes provides access to general semantic knowledge corresponding to social stereotypes that contain information about attributes ostensibly shared by members of various groups. This process has been referred to as the establishment of "visually-derived semantic codes" for the face encountered (Bruce & Young, 1986). Note that category-based recognition processes rely on visual and semantic information stored at more general or superordinate taxonomic levels of abstraction than the representations that support the recognition of individual identity. As a rule, categorization is less demanding in terms of cognitive resources and can be accomplished on the basis of more coarse-grained visual and semantic information than what is required for individuation (Gauthier et al., 1997, 2000a; Tarr & Gauthier, 2000; Tanaka, 2001; Tarr & Cheng, 2003; Cloutier et al., 2005). Although category-based recognition mechanisms have the obvious benefit of simplifying social interaction by allowing pre-existing knowledge to generalize to novel individuals, the procedure has significant intrinsic limitations due to its over-inclusiveness and lack of differentiation. Specifically, because of the emphasis on shared structure and reliance on overlapping memory representations, category-level recognition processes tend to treat all exemplars that match the generic category description as more-or-less equivalent, distinguishable only by their degree of representativeness or "typicality" with respect to the central tendency or prototype (Mervis & Rosch, 1981). Due to the strong propensity for similarity-based generalization, categorical processing cannot support the recognition of individual identity (e.g., category-level representations presumably do not discriminate between the two faces shown in Figure 6.1, treating them both as essentially interchangeable exemplars within the generic category of elderly white males). Furthermore, false recognition of novel individuals may occur when the strong feeling of familiarity evoked by "typical-looking" faces with high levels of structural similarity to stored prototypes is misattributed as evidence of specific prior exposure to the person (Rapcsak et al., 1999).

The cognitive model shown in Figure 6.1 also postulates the existence of a central executive component that interacts with and exerts strategic top-down control over the operations of the face recognition system (Rapcsak et al., 1999, 2001, 2002). Control procedures implemented by the executive system include the monitoring and verification of the information retrieved from memory in response to the face cue and the setting of appropriate response criteria for the recognition decision. Effective monitoring requires the critical evaluation of the evidence provided by activated memory traces, including the determination of whether the information available reflects the outcome of the individuation or the categorization process. Note that this type of source memory attribution cannot be made conclusively on the basis of familiarity alone, because individual and category-level face recognition processes can both give rise to feelings of familiarity. The critical difference, however, is that individuation normally results in the retrieval of additional identity-specific biographic information that provides the appropriate context for the experience of facial familiarity, whereas the general sense of familiarity associated with the categorization process is relatively undifferentiated and cannot be attributed to a specific context or source. Thus, the products of individuation versus categorization are readily distinguishable by monitoring the amount and quality of the identity-specific details retrieved. Because context recollection offers more reliable clues to personal identity than familiarity, we can improve memory accuracy by relying primarily on the output of the individuation process and using the presence or absence of detailed, identity-specific information as the appropriate criterion for recognition decisions (Rapcsak et al., 1999). It should be emphasized that extensive monitoring and memory control operations are not usually required for the recognition of highly familiar faces because for these individuals, contextual information is readily available in an automatic or bottom-up fashion. However, executive processes assume a much more critical role under conditions of uncertainty when the face cue does not directly elicit relevant identity-specific information, leaving the source of familiarity unspecified or ambiguous (i.e., when we are not sure whether a familiar-looking face is somebody we know) (Rapcsak et al., 1999).

To summarize, individuation and categorization are closely related and complementary recognition processes implemented within a single face memory system that is capable of operating at different levels of specificity. Although distinct in terms of underlying cognitive representations and computational requirements, under normal circumstances the two recognition procedures are highly interactive and may be considered to represent opposite ends of a continuum (Fiske & Neuberg, 1990). Specifically, when attending to the face of a person both processes are automatically initiated in a bottom-up fashion and both types of information are available for flexible use in recognition memory judgments. The decision to emphasize individuating versus categorical information is under strategic control and depends on the social context of the recognition task and the goals and motivations of the observer. As we have seen, familiar faces enjoy privileged status in social cognition characterized by rapid and automatic access to identity-specific biographic information via the individuation process. Although familiar faces are preferentially recognized at the most unique individual level (Tanaka, 2001) to the relative exclusion of categorical information, we can also use facial appearance to assign the famous person shown in Figure 6.1 to a number of relevant social categories. Similarly, although we may elect to rely primarily on the obligatory output of the categorization process when looking at the unfamiliar face shown in Figure 6.1 or in the course of our casual daily encounters with strangers, if sufficiently motivated, we can also decide to go beyond initial impressions and "individuate" a novel person by strategically attending to and learning about unique, identity-specific details. The dynamic flexibility of the face recognition system to shift between individuation and categorization is critical for successful functioning in everyday social settings that typically involve multiple encounters with both familiar and unfamiliar people.

Neuropsychological Disorders of Face Memory

Face memory disorders can result from damage to the visual, semantic, or executive components of the recognition system (Figure 6.1). Visual and semantic impairments are characterized by a striking failure in recognizing familiar people, combined with an equally profound inability to acquire new person-specific information. The pervasive retrograde and anterograde memory loss in these patients indicates a severe disruption of the individuation process. By contrast, executive deficits play a major role in the pathogenesis of memory distortions manifested by false recognition and misidentification of unfamiliar people. In patients with executive impairment, the breakdown of the individuation process is usually not severe and memory illusions to novel faces reflect inappropriate reliance on categorical representations in situations where the recognition task calls for identity-based processing.

PROSOPAGNOSIA

Prosopagnosia is by far the best known and most extensively studied face memory disorder in neurological patients (Damasio et al., 1982, 1990; Sergent & Signoret, 1992). The behavioral hallmark of the syndrome is the dramatic inability to recognize previously familiar faces. In severe cases, patients fail to recognize not only the faces of well-known public figures and celebrities but also the faces of close personal acquaintances and family members. Prosopagnosics do not have difficulty in distinguishing faces from other object categories, but they frequently complain that they cannot discriminate the faces of different individuals and that all faces look unfamiliar. However, prosopagnosics can recognize familiar people from their voices or names, providing evidence that semantic knowledge of these individuals is preserved. Therefore, prosopagnosia represents a modality-specific recognition disorder in which the visual appearance of the face no longer serves as a reliable clue to personal identity. It is important to emphasize that in addition to the prominent deficit in recognizing familiar faces, prosopagnosics demonstrate a severe inability to learn new faces. The combined retrograde and anterograde impairment of face identity recognition suggests damage to the visual components of the individuation process resulting in an inability to perceive and remember the unique visual attributes of different faces (Figure 6.1).

It has been proposed that prosopagnosia is not a unitary disorder and that the syndrome can be subdivided into two distinct clinical subtypes: apperceptive and associative (Damasio et al., 1990; De Renzi et al., 1991; Sergent & Signoret, 1992). In apperceptive prosopagnosia, the recognition deficit is considered to be the result of pervasive perceptual impairment caused by damage to the early visual analysis stage of face processing (Figure 6.1). Because the visual analysis stage provides perceptual input to both the individuation and the categorization process, patients with severe damage to this functional component are not only impaired in recognizing facial identity, but they also have considerable difficulty in decoding category-level facial information including gender, age, or race. By contrast, patients with associative prosopagnosia are reasonably successful in interpreting categorical information while at the same time being totally unable to recognize the individual identity of the face (Tranel et al., 1988; Sergent & Signoret, 1992). Thus, the recognition deficit in these patients cannot be attributed to low-level perceptual impairment and seems to reflect a selective disruption of face identity processing. Within the framework of our model, the retrograde and anterograde recognition memory deficit in associative prosopagnosia can be explained by postulating damage to the FRUs that store visual memory representations for the faces of familiar individuals, combined with an inability to establish new FRUs (Figure 6.1). The dissociation between severely impaired individuation and relatively preserved categorization in these patients is likely to reflect the different visual processing demands of the two recognition tasks. Specifically, the recognition of individual facial identity is perceptually more difficult because it requires the extraction and storage of fine-grained configural information sufficient to support within-category discrimination amongst structurally similar exemplars, whereas categorization can presumably be accomplished on the basis of relatively coarse-grained visual information or by attending to single diagnostic features (Gauthier et al. 1997, 2000a; Tarr & Gauthier, 2000; Tanaka, 2001; Tarr & Cheng, 2003; Mason & Macrae, 2004; Cloutier et al, 2005; Zarate et al., 2008). Consistent with this hypothesis, prosopagnosics demonstrate disproportionate impairment in processing configural facial information (Barton et al., 2002) and their approach to face recognition tasks is characterized by abnormal reliance on a slow, feature-based strategy.

Prosopagnosia is caused by damage to inferotemporal visual association areas, typically occurring in the setting of posterior cerebral artery strokes (Damasio et al., 1982, 1990; Sergent & Signoret, 1992; Bouvier & Engel, 2006). Although initial lesion-deficit correlation studies suggested that the syndrome required bilateral occipito-temporal involvement (Figure 6.2a), there are by now many cases on record where high-resolution imaging studies only revealed evidence of unilateral right-sided damage (Figures 6.2 b,c). Collectively, these observations indicate that damage to the right inferotemporal visual cortex is both necessary and sufficient to produce prominent face recognition impairment.

Neuroanatomical findings in patients with prosopagnosia are consistent with demonstrations of face-selective neural responses in inferotemporal visual cortex by single-cell recording studies in primates and by functional neuroimaging and electrophysiological studies of face processing in human subjects (for recent reviews see Tsao & Livingstone, 2008 and Duchaine & Yovel, 2008). In particular, evidence from functional imaging studies suggests that the critical neural substrate of prosopagnosia involves damage to two anatomically distinct but functionally integrated right-hemisphere extrastriate cortical regions known as the fusiform face area (FFA) and the occipital face area (OFA) (Kanwisher, McDermott, & Chun, 1997; Gauthier et al., 2000b). The FFA occupies the mid-lateral portions of the fusiform gyrus, whereas the OFA has been localized to a more posterior cortical region within the inferior occipital gyrus (Figure 6.5). These face-selective cortical areas show stronger activation when normal subjects view faces compared to other visual object categories, and the neural responses are generally more robust in the right than in the left hemisphere (for a review, see Haxby et al., 2000). It has been proposed that the processing of facial information within the extrastriate visual cortex is hierarchically organized, with the OFA primarily involved in the early perceptual analysis of facial features and the FFA more critically involved in the recognition of facial identity that requires perceptual integration of individual features into unique facial configurations (Haxby et al., 2000; Rossion et al., 2000; Liu, Harris, & Kanwisher, 2010. The central role of the FFA in the selective coding of facial identity is supported by demonstrations that the faces of different individuals elicit distinct neural response patterns

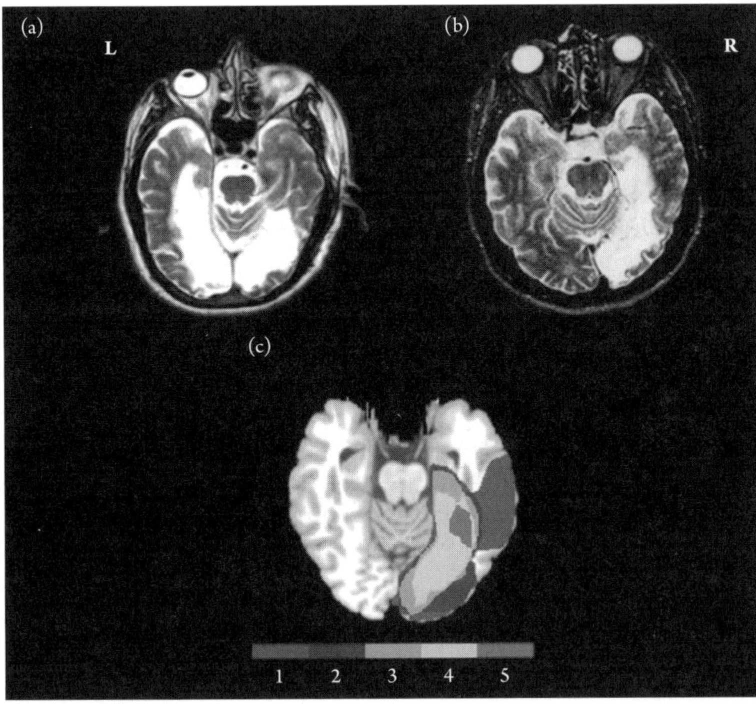

Figure 6.2 Bilateral (a) and unilateral right-sided (b) occipito-temporal lesions in patients with prosopagnosia following PCA strokes. Lesion overlap map of five patients with prosopagnosia due to unilateral right occipito-temporal damage (c). The area of maximum damage (red) includes right mid-fusiform cortex corresponding to the location of the fusiform face area (FFA) in functional neuroimaging studies (see color insert).

in this region (Gauthier et al., 2000b; Grill-Spector et al., 2004; Rothstein et al., 2005). Furthermore, FFA activation is modulated by levels of familiarity, with novel faces typically producing stronger responses than familiar faces (Rossion et al., 2001, 2003). The finding that the efficiency of neural computations within the FFA is facilitated by prior experience with a particular face is consistent with the hypothesis that this region contains visual memory representations of familiar faces. Additional support for the proposed role of the FFA in face memory storage comes from demonstrations that this region is activated not only during bottom-up perceptual processing of familiar faces, but also during mental imagery that involves top-down activation of long-term visual memory representations for the faces of familiar individuals (Ishai et al., 2002; Mechelli et al., 2004).

To summarize, converging evidence from lesion-deficit correlation studies in patients with prosopagnosia and functional imaging studies of face processing in normal subjects suggests that visual recognition of faces depends critically on a right-hemisphere network of hierarchically organized extrastriate cortical areas comprised of the OFA and the FFA. The OFA and FFA make distinct contributions to face processing and the structural and functional integrity of both cortical regions is necessary for normal performance (Rossion et al., 2003; Bouvier & Engel, 2006; Schiltz et al., 2006; Steeves et al., 2006; Sorger et al., 2007). The OFA is involved in the early visual analysis stage of face processing (Figure 6.1) and provides perceptual input to the FFA. Damage to the OFA is likely to play an important role in the pathogenesis of apperceptive prosopagnosia. By contrast, the FFA extracts and stores configural information critical for determining the individual identity of the face and this region may therefore represent the neural substrate of FRUs (Figure 6.1). Damage to the FFA results in associative prosopagnosia characterized by the loss of high-level perceptual expertise required for within-category discrimination of individual faces and the subsequent inability to activate stored biographic records about familiar people from facial cues. In patients with associative prosopagnosia, category-level recognition processes mediated by facial prototypes can be relatively preserved (Figure 6.1).

PERSON RECOGNITION DISORDERS

Memory loss for familiar faces is also a prominent finding in patients with person recognition disorders (for a review, see Gainotti, 2007). However, unlike prosopagnosics, patients with person recognition disorders demonstrate profound difficulty in identifying familiar individuals, not only from their faces, but also from voice or name cues, or when presented with verbal descriptions/biographic vignettes. The multimodal nature of the deficit suggests that the underlying mechanism of the recognition impairment involves the loss of identity-specific semantic knowledge about familiar persons. The failure to recognize familiar people is accompanied by an inability to acquire new person-specific semantic information (i.e., defective cross-modal integration of face, name, and biographic information about novel individuals) (Tsukiura et al., 2002; Moran et al., 2005). Within the framework of our model, person recognition disorders reflect disruption of the semantic components of the individuation process caused by damage to PINs (Figure 6.1).

The type of errors produced by patients with person recognition disorders on retrograde face memory tasks reflects the severity of the underlying semantic deficit. In mild cases, patients recognize that the face is familiar, but they cannot recall the person's name and can provide relatively few identity-specific biographic details (e.g., "one of the Beatles, I think he may have died"). With greater degree of impairment, one familiar person may be confused with another based on shared semantic attributes, resulting in the production of semantic errors (e.g., misidentifying John Lennon as Mick Jagger). In more severe cases, individuating semantic information can no longer be retrieved and only general or superordinate category knowledge remains (e.g., "rock musician"). Note, however, that such generic responses may reflect reliance on visually-derived semantic codes rather than indicate residual person-specific knowledge (e.g., the attractive face of a young actress could potentially be assigned to the correct occupational category without the person being recognized). Consistent with this hypothesis, category-based processing sometimes leads to incorrect semantic classification of famous persons (e.g., one of our patients identified the photograph of the African American actor Denzel Washington as a "famous athlete," reflecting the influence of face category prototypes and social stereotypes). Finally, in patients with profound semantic deficits, "don't know" recognition responses predominate, although a vague sense of familiarity with the face occasionally remains. Taken together, behavioral observations in patients with person recognition disorders provide evidence of levels of specificity effects in semantic memory (cf. Rogers & McClelland, 2004) and indicate that identity-specific knowledge of individuals is more vulnerable to neurological damage than categorical information. In particular, increasing amounts of semantic impairment seem to be accompanied by a specific-to-general deterioration of familiar person knowledge. Fine-grained information about the distinctive semantic properties of unique individuals is lost before coarse-grained similarity information about shared attributes of category members. With the erosion of individuating semantic information, recognition responses become susceptible to the influence of general or category-level knowledge about people corresponding to social stereotypes.

Person recognition disorders are associated with neurological conditions that produce damage to the anterior temporal lobes, including Alzheimer's disease (for a review, see Werheid & Clare, 2007), semantic dementia (Evans et al., 1995; Gentileschi et al., 2001; Gainotti et al., 2003; Snowden et al., 2004; Thompson et al., 2004; Josephs et al., 2008; Joubert et al., 2006), herpes encephalitis (Hanley et al., 1989; Eslinger et al., 1996), and temporal lobe epilepsy/lobectomy (Ellis et al., 1989; Seidenberg et al., 2002; Viskontas et al., 2002; Glosser et al., 2003; Moran et al., 2005). The responsible lesions typically involve anterior temporal cortex (ATC) (temporal pole, anterior fusiform, inferior/middle temporal gyri) and medial temporal lobe (MTL) structures (hippocampus, perirhinal, entorhinal, parahippocampal cortex) in various combinations (Figure 6.3). These neuroanatomical observations suggest that both ATC and MTL are necessary for the encoding and retrieval of multimodal semantic information about unique individuals.

Establishing semantic memory representations for people requires cross-modal integration of different types of person-specific information (e.g., face, voice, name) processed in distinct modality-specific cortical regions. ATC/MTL are ideally suited to accomplish this type of integration as these brain regions receive convergent sensory input from all modality-specific cortical processing areas. It is currently a matter of debate whether cross-modal semantic integration in ATC is accomplished by re-coding convergent modality-specific sensory

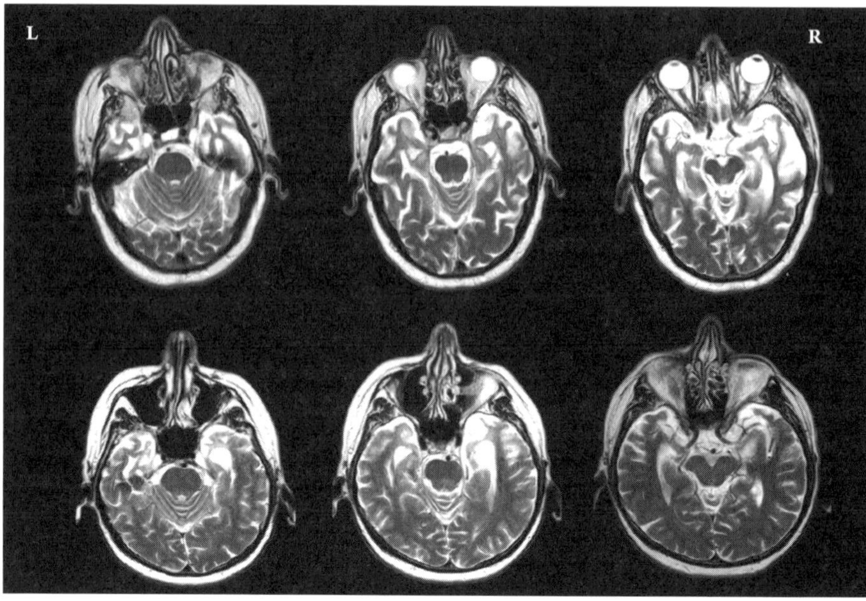

Figure 6.3 Bilateral atrophy involving anterior temporal cortex (ATC) and medial temporal lobe (MTL) structures in patients with person recognition disorders.

input into abstract amodal representations, or whether this regions acts as a relay station containing "pointers" for re-activating the entire distributed network of modality-specific cortical areas that collectively constitute our conceptual knowledge of familiar people from information presented through any sensory input channel (Damasio, 1989; Damasio et al., 2004; Barsalou et al., 2003; Rogers et al., 2004; Snowden et al., 2004; Gainotti, 2007). It is also presently unclear whether MTL memory systems have a time-limited role in the encoding and maintenance of multimodal semantic information about familiar people, or whether these structures play a life-long role in the retrieval of detailed person-specific semantic knowledge (Moscovitch et al., 2006; Squire & Bayley, 2007). Regarding the hemispheric lateralization of identity-specific semantic information, person recognition disorders can be associated with left or right anterior temporal lobe lesions, although the deficit seems both more common and more pronounced in patients with right-hemisphere pathology (Tranel et al., 1997; Damasio et al., 2004; Gainotti, 2007). While this question is far from settled, the brunt of the neuropsychological evidence seems to favor the view that semantic knowledge of familiar people is bilaterally represented, with left and right anterior temporal lobe regions playing specialized roles in storing or processing verbal versus non-verbal person-specific information (Rapcsak, 2003; Snowden et al. 2004; Damasio et al., 2004; Gainotti, 2007). In addition, retrieving the names of familiar people may be disproportionately impaired in patients with left anterior temporal lobe damage (Damasio et al., 2004; Seidenberg et al., 2002; Glosser et al., 2003; Gainotti, 2007; Tranel, 2006).

Lesion-deficit correlations in patients with person recognition disorders are consistent with the results of functional imaging studies investigating the neural substrates of identity-specific semantic knowledge in normal individuals. In particular, these studies have provided evidence that recognition of familiar people from face, voice, or name cues is accompanied by activation of ATC/MTL in addition to activation within the appropriate modality-specific cortical areas (e.g., the right FFA for faces, right superior temporal sulcus or STS for voices, left inferior temporo-occipital cortex for written names) (Sergent et al., 1992, 1994; Gorno-Tempini & Price, 2001; Leveroni et al., 2000; Damasio et al., 2004; Bernard et al., 2004; Haist et al., 2001; Douville et al., 2005; Nakamura et al., 2001; von Kriegstein & Giraud, 2004; von Kriegstein et al., 2005; Sugiura et al., 2006). The engagement of ATC/MTL regardless of the modality of the sensory input is consistent with the proposed role of these regions in cross-modal integration and in accessing multimodal semantic knowledge of familiar people. Similarly, associative learning of novel face, name, and biographic information recruits ATC/MTL, demonstrating the critical contribution of these regions to establishing new person-specific semantic representations by binding information processed in modality-specific cortical regions into a unified memory trace (Sperling et al., 2001, 2003; Zeineh et al., 2003; Tsukiura et al., 2002, 2006). Multimodal integration of person-specific semantic information, however, may not be mediated exclusively via ATC/MTL and may also involve direct crosstalk between modality-specific cortical regions (Campanella & Belin, 2007).

FALSE RECOGNITION AND MISIDENTIFICATION OF UNFAMILIAR FACES

In contrast to the defective recognition of familiar faces that characterizes prosopagnosia and person recognition disorders, in some neurological patients, the memory impairment manifests primarily as false recognition of unfamiliar faces (Rapcsak et al., 1999, 2001, 2002). Misattributions of facial familiarity in patients with false recognition can take different clinical forms. In some cases, memory illusions are revealed by the strong tendency to produce "false alarms" to novel distractor faces in anterograde memory experiments. Other patients, however, also demonstrate false recognition in retrograde memory paradigms when they are asked to judge whether they had ever seen a particular face before. In these situations, the spurious sense of familiarity triggered by novel faces may be accompanied by the retrieval of false biographic information resulting in frank misidentifications. In severe cases, patients may mistake unfamiliar individuals for famous people or personal acquaintances in real-life settings (Rapcsak et al., 1994,1996, 1998; Ward et al., 1999; Ward & Jones, 2003).

Although impaired recognition of familiar faces and false recognition of unfamiliar faces may co-exist in some patients, the two types of memory disorders are dissociable (Rapcsak et al., 1996, 1999, 2002). In particular, whereas right temporal lobe damage plays a critical role in producing memory impairment for familiar faces in patients with prosopagnosia or person recognition disorders, the most striking cases of false facial recognition have been observed in patients with damage to right prefrontal cortex (PFC) (Rapcsak et al., 1996, 1999, 2001, 2002) (Figure 6.4).

The fact that false recognition errors are more prevalent following right PFC damage than in patients with right temporal lobe lesions suggests that memory illusions are not simply the result of face memory loss (Rapcsak et al., 1999, 2002). Instead, the available evidence indicates that false recognition in frontal patients results from abnormal reliance on category-level face memory representations that cannot support the recognition of individual identity. For instance, it has been shown that following exposure to pictures of white male faces in the study phase of an anterograde memory experiment, frontal patients were much more likely to false alarm to category-consistent distractors (i.e., other white males) than to category-inconsistent distractors that differed from target faces in terms of race or gender (i.e., non-white males or white females) (Rapcsak et al., 1999). This finding can be explained by assuming that frontal patients primarily encoded

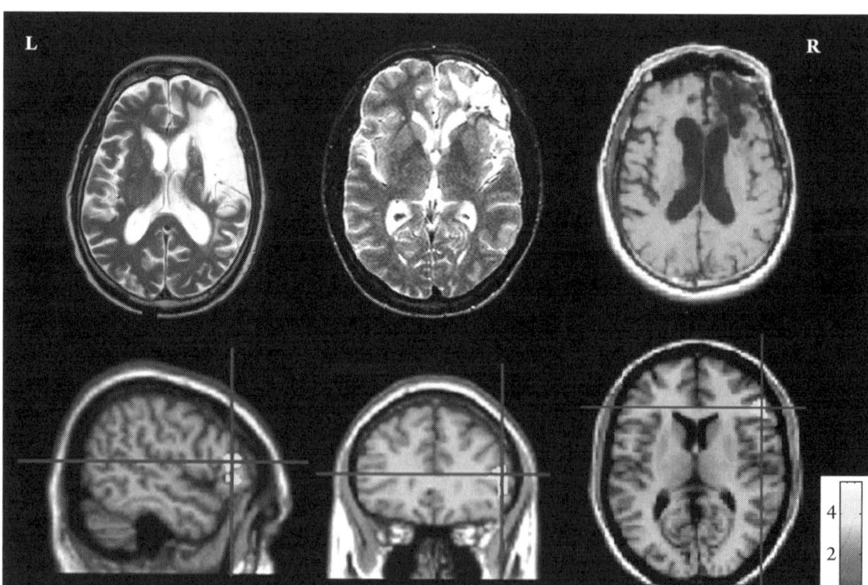

Figure 6.4 Right prefrontal cortex (PFC) lesions in patients with false facial recognition (top). Damage involves a ventrolateral frontal lobe region that shows activation during face recognition performance in normal subjects (bottom) (see color insert).

categorical information about study items and, as a result, had difficulty opposing the sense of familiarity induced by novel distractor faces that matched this general or category-level memory description of the study episode. In fact, the performance of frontal patients in this face memory experiment demonstrates all the key behavioral signatures of categorical processing: preserved between-category but poor within-category discrimination and a strong propensity for similarity-based generalization to novel items.

Category-level processing of faces may also account for false recognition errors in retrograde memory tasks (Rapcsak et al., 1999, 2001, 2002). For example, frontal patients may incorrectly claim that a novel face is familiar/famous based on strong categorical resemblance to facial prototypes that we associate with celebrity status (e.g., "actress-type"). Activation of facial prototypes automatically cues the appropriate social stereotype, leading to the establishment of visually-derived semantic codes for the novel person and setting the stage for false recognition (Figure 6.1). However, the general sense of familiarity associated with the activation of categorical memory representations can be opposed by engaging in a strategic memory search to retrieve confirmatory biographic information via the individuation process (e.g., by attempting to recollect specific movies the "actress" appeared in or by trying to remember her name). Thus, normal subjects can avoid false recognition by using the presence or absence of identity-specific contextual information as the appropriate criterion for making face memory decisions (Rapcsak et al., 1999). By contrast, frontal patients do not seem to engage in effortful and strategic context retrieval and are likely to respond on the basis of general familiarity that is the undifferentiated output of the categorization process. Due to defective monitoring, patients may fail to realize that the absence of individuating contextual information is inconsistent with a positive recognition decision and consequently mistake "looking famous" for "being famous." Consistent with the hypothesis that face memory distortions reflect the use of inappropriate decision criteria, false recognition errors in frontal patients can be dramatically reduced by asking them to call faces familiar/famous only if they can remember the profession and name of the person (Rapcsak et al., 1999). Thus, frontal patients can use the output of the individuation process to suppress false recognition once the appropriate strategy is pointed out to them.

In terms of our cognitive model (Figure 6.1), false recognition of unfamiliar faces in frontal patients can be explained by postulating damage to the executive system. In particular, the neuropsychological evidence suggests that frontal lobe structures play an important role in face recognition by implementing strategic memory retrieval, monitoring, and decision functions critical for attributing facial familiarity to a specific context or source (Rapcsak et al., 1999, 2001, 2002). Under conditions of uncertainty, when the face cue does not automatically elicit identity-specific information, effortful and strategic recollection of individuating contextual details by the frontal executive system provides the principal mechanism for suppressing false recognition by opposing the misleading influence of general or undifferentiated familiarity associated with the output of the categorization process. Consistent with the hypothesis that false recognition is based on the activation of categorical memory representations, frontal patients typically use generic descriptions to justify their claim that a novel person is familiar/famous (e.g., "saw her on TV"). However, in order to explain the more outlandish and implausible misidentifications produced by some patients, we have to assume that in severe cases dysfunctional frontal systems may exert inappropriate top-down control over the entire recognition process. In such patients, the defective frontal executive may override or ignore bottom-up information generated by temporal lobe memory systems and assign bizarre and improbable semantic contexts and identities to novel faces regardless of their physical attributes or perceived levels of familiarity, resulting in confabulatory or delusional misidentification (Rapcsak et al., 1994, 1996, 1999; Ward et al., 1999; Ward & Jones, 2003). Frontal lobe dysfunction may also lead to inappropriate questioning of the "real" identity of highly familiar persons, as occurs in the Capgras delusion (Ellis & Lewis, 2001; Devinsky, 2009). In short, false facial recognition, confabulation, and delusional misidentification may represent a clinical continuum of increasingly severe memory distortions and reality monitoring failures attributable to frontal lobe dysfunction (Rapcsak et al., 1994, 1996, 1999). Consistent with the proposed monitoring impairment, frontal patients with false recognition/misidentification exhibit anosognosia for their face memory deficit and have difficulty judging the accuracy of their recognition decisions (Rapcsak et al., 1994, 1996, 1998; Pannu et al., 2005). In terms of cognitive theory, memory distortions in patients with frontal lobe lesions underscore the fact that face recognition is not merely the automatic product of a direct match between the face cue and representations of faces stored in memory. Instead, remembering faces is more appropriately viewed as a constructive process that requires dynamic interactions between temporal lobe face memory systems and frontal executive systems involved in the strategic control of conscious recollection (Rapcsak et al., 2002).

Consistent with neuropsychological evidence of face memory impairments in patients with frontal lobe lesions, imaging studies in normal subjects have demonstrated frontal lobe activation during recognition of familiar faces (Leveroni et al., 2000), new face learning (Kelley et al., 1998; McDermott et al., 1999), and in working memory tasks that require the active maintenance and manipulation of face memory information (for reviews, see Ranganath, 2006; D'Esposito, 2007) (Figure 6.4). Collectively, the results of these studies support the view that face recognition requires functional integration between temporal lobe regions involved in face perception/memory and frontal executive systems (Figure 6.5). Furthermore, imaging evidence that levels of neural activity within temporal lobe face processing areas are modulated by top-down signals originating in PFC (Gazzaley et al., 2005; Ranganath, 2006; Johnson et al., 2007, D'Esposito, 2007) is consistent with the notion that the frontal lobes exert executive control over the operations of the face recognition system (Figures 6.1 and 6.5).

Input from PFC may serve to bias processing in temporal lobe face memory systems toward the retrieval of task-relevant information while at the same time suppressing the distracting influence of task-irrelevant or competing memory representations. For instance, when the face memory task calls for the recognition of individual identity, automatically activated categorical information is irrelevant and needs to be inhibited. In these situations, top-down signals from PFC may selectively enhance the retrieval of individuating face memory information while at the same time limiting interference by suppressing competition from categorical memory representations. According to this view, executive functions implemented by PFC improve memory accuracy by increasing the signal-to-noise ratio within the face memory system (Rapcsak et al., 2002). Determining how the various memory control operations postulated by cognitive models map onto different functional subdivisions within PFC remains an important challenge for future investigations.

Conclusions

Lesion-deficit correlation studies in neurological patients have made critical contributions to our understanding of the cognitive mechanisms and neural substrates of face recognition memory. These investigations have provided compelling evidence that face memory is not localizable to any single cortical region and is mediated instead by a predominantly right-lateralized neural network comprised of inferotemporal visual cortex (OFA/FFA), anterior and medial temporal lobe structures (ATC/MTL), and prefrontal cortex (PFC) (Figure 6.5). The various components of this distributed neural system have distinct functional roles in the recognition process, and damage to these regions results in qualitatively different types of face recognition impairments characterized by memory loss or memory distortion. Specifically, damage to the visual components of the network (OFA/FFA) gives rise to prosopagnosia, multimodal semantic impairment following damage to ATC/MTL is associated with person recognition disorders, while executive dysfunction is the primary abnormality contributing to false facial recognition in patients with PFC lesions (Rapcsak, 2003).

The neuropsychological evidence reviewed here suggests further that face recognition performance is the integrated product of two basic cognitive operations that involve processing faces at different levels of specificity: individuation and categorization. Whereas individuated memory traces emphasize unique identity-specific facial and semantic attributes that distinguish one person from another, categorical representations emphasize similarities across exemplars and thus provide information about what the person who is the current

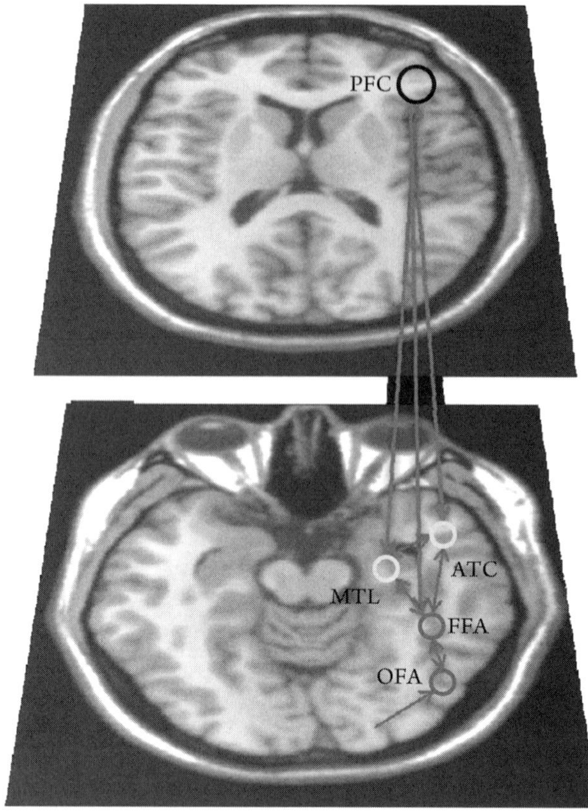

Figure 6.5 The distributed face memory network. OFA = occipital face area, FFA = fusiform face area, ATC = anterior temporal cortex, MTL = medial temporal lobe, PFC = prefrontal cortex. Circles identifying different corticalregions are color-coded with the visual, semantic, and executive components of the face recognition model depicted in Figure 6.1. Only the right-hemisphere network is shown here but it is assumed that homologous regions in the left hemisphere also contribute to face recognition.

focus of attention has in common with people we have encountered in the past. Categorization processes play a useful role in social cognition by allowing us to quickly construct a "composite identity" for a novel person based on our prior experiences with similar individuals. However, due to the strong propensity for similarity-based generalization, categorical memory representations lack specificity and cannot support the recognition of individual identity. In everyday life, individuation and categorization are used in a flexible and interactive fashion depending on the social context of the recognition task and the goals of the observer. However, individuation involves more fine-grained visual and semantic analysis than categorization. Furthermore, recollection of identity-specific information may necessitate the deployment of strategic memory retrieval, monitoring, and decision functions orchestrated by the executive system. Thus, in addition to requiring access to more detailed visual and semantic information, individuation is also more dependent on executive resources than categorization. Consistent with the notion that processing demands in recognition tasks increase with levels of specificity, functional imaging studies have documented greater activation within the face memory network during person individuation than categorization (Mason & Macrae, 2004; Turk et al., 2005). Because it is normally more difficult for the recognition system to extract identity-specific information, individuation is more vulnerable to the deleterious effects of brain damage than categorization. Applying the "levels-of-specificity" framework to the different neuropsychological syndromes discussed in this chapter, prosopagnosia and person recognition disorders can be interpreted as reflecting severe damage to the visual and semantic components of the individuation process (Figure 6.1). By contrast, in false recognition the automatic or bottom-up aspects of individuation are relatively preserved but patients show a bias toward categorical processing in situations where identity-specific information is not immediately available or is ambiguous and therefore requires the effortful and strategic expenditure of top-down executive resources. As we have seen, converging neuropsychological and imaging data indicate that individuation or identity-based recognition of faces depends critically on right-hemisphere mechanisms and requires fine-grained processing of configural information (e.g., Barton et al., 2002; Rossion et al., 2000). By contrast, it has been proposed that the left hemisphere demonstrates an intrinsic bias toward categorical or similarity-based processing of faces that involves extracting single diagnostic features useful for determining group membership (Mason & Macrae, 2004; Zarate et al., 2008). Therefore, the relative preservation of categorization in patients with right-hemisphere damage may in part reflect the preferred cognitive style of the intact left-hemisphere face recognition system in addition to any residual processing by the degraded right-hemisphere face memory network.

Finally, we wish to acknowledge that the question of whether face recognition is mediated by a dedicated or domain-specific neural system, or whether the same system is recruited in a domain-general fashion whenever non-face objects must be discriminated at the unique individual rather than at the basic category level (e.g., "my chocolate Labrador Snickers" as opposed to "dog") has been a highly contentious topic in cognitive neuropsychology. Consistent with the domain-general hypothesis, patients with prosopagnosia following damage to the OFA/FFA often have difficulty with subordinate-level identification of objects within visually homogeneous categories (e.g., cars, animals) (Damasio et al. 1982, 1990; Gauthier, Behrmann, & Tarr, 1999). Similarly, patients with damage to ATC/MTL are usually impaired not only in identifying familiar people but also in subordinate-level recognition/naming of objects, especially living things and semantically unique entities such as famous landmarks/monuments

(Ellis et al., 1989; Hanley et al., 1989; Rogers et al., 2004; Tyler et al., 2004; Moss et al., 2005; Bright et al., 2005; Damasio et al., 2004; Brambati et al., 2006; Tranel, 2006; Ahmed et al., 2008. The fact that person and object recognition deficits in patients with anterior temporal lobe lesions show similar levels of specificity effects, with better preservation of knowledge represented at the category than at the unique exemplar level, is consistent with a domain-general impairment of semantic individuation. In our experience, the tendency of frontal patients to produce false recognition errors to novel items is also not limited to faces and can be demonstrated in other anterograde visual object memory tasks that require within-category discrimination among structurally similar exemplars. Furthermore, some patients produce false recognition/misidentification errors not only to novel faces but also to unfamiliar names or voices in retrograde memory tasks involving familiarity/fame judgments (Rapcsak et al., 1994,1998; Ward et al., 1999; Ward & Jones, 2003). These observations suggest that the frontal lobe regions implicated in false facial recognition play a domain-general role in the executive control of memory. On the other hand, consistent with the domain-specific hypothesis, there are reports of prosopagnosics with recognition impairments highly specific to human faces (for a review, see Riddoch et al., 2008). Dissociations between person-specific and general object knowledge have also been documented in patients with semantic impairment following anterior temporal lobe damage (Thompson et al., 2002, 2004). Because the brain lesions that result in domain-specific versus domain-general recognition impairments are often anatomically indistinguishable, it is possible that differences in the selectivity of the deficit reflect individual variations in the cortical representation of face and object processing skills. It could also be argued that naturally occurring lesions may not be ideal for examining the question of domain-specificity, as the area of brain damage is typically large (Figures 6.2, 6.3, 6.4) and likely to involve not only regions ostensibly dedicated to face recognition but also adjacent cortical areas specialized for processing other visual object categories. Although imaging experiments in normal subjects may seem better suited for studying the fine-scale functional neuroanatomy of face and object processing, these investigations have also produced inconsistent results with evidence both for domain-specificity and for domain-generality within the face recognition network (Gauthier et al., 1997, 2000a,c; Kanwisher, 2000; Kanwisher & Yovel, 2006; Tarr & Gauthier, 2000; Tarr & Cheng, 2003; Grill-Spector et al., 2004, 2006; Haxby et al., 2001; Gorno-Tempini & Price, 2001; Grabowski et al., 2001; Haist, Lee, & Stiles, 2010). Until the resolution of this debate, it seems prudent to accept the possibility that the face recognition system we have described here may not be domain-specific and that neuropsychological observations in patients with face memory disorders may have more general implications for our understanding of the functional organization and cortical localization of the neural systems involved in recognizing objects at different levels of specificity.

Acknowledgments

This work was supported by NIH grants P30AG19610 and DC008286. The author wishes to thank Emily C. Edmonds, M.A., Maya L. Henry Ph.D., and Sarah Andersen for their help with various aspects of this project.

References

Ahmed, S., Arnold, R., Thompson S. A., Graham, K. S., Hodges, J. R. (2008). Naming of objects, faces and buildings in mild cognitive impairment. *Cortex, 46*, 746–752.

Barsalou, L. W., Simmons, W. K., Barbey, A. K., Wison, C. D. (2003). Grounding conceptual knowledge in modality-specific systems. *Trends in Cognitive Sciences, 7*, 84–91.

Barton, J. J. S., Press, D. Z., Keenan, J. P., O'Connor, M. (2002). Lesions of the fusiform area impair perception of facial configuration in prosopagnosia. *Neurology, 58*, 71–78.

Benton, A. (1990). Facial recognition 1990. *Cortex, 26*, 491–499.

Bernard, F. A., Bullmore, E. T., Graham, K. S., Thompson, S. A., Hodges, J. R., Fletcher, P. C. (2004). The hippocampal region is involved in successful recognition of both remote and recent famous faces. *NeuroImage, 22*, 1704–1714.

Bouvier, S. E., Engel, S. A. (2006). Behavioral deficits and cortical damage loci in cerebral achromatopsia. *Cerebral Cortex, 16*, 183–191.

Brambati, S. M., Myers, D., Wilson, A., Rankin, K. P., Allison, S. C., Rosen, H. J., Miller, B. L., Gorno-Tempini, M. L. (2006). The anatomy of category-specific object naming in neurodegenerative diseases. *Journal of Cognitive Neuroscience, 18*, 1644–1653.

Bright, P., Moss, H. E., Stamatakis, E. A., Tyler, L. K. (2005). The anatomy of object processing: the role of anteromedial temporal cortex. *Quarterly Journal of Experimental Psychology, 58B*, 361–377.

Bruce, V., Young, A. W. (1986). Understanding face recognition. *British Journal of Psychology, 77*, 305–327.

Cabeza, R., Bruce, V., Kato, T., Oda., M. (1999). The prototype effect in face recognition: extensions and limits. *Memory & Cognition, 27*, 139–151.

Campanella, S., Belin, P. (2007). Integrating face and voice in person perception. *Trends in Cognitive Sciences, 11*, 535–543.

Cloutier, J., Mason, M. F., Macrae, C. N. (2005). The perceptual determinants of person construal: reopening the social-cognitive toolbox. *Journal of Personality and Social Psychology, 88*, 885–894.

Damasio, A. R. (1989). Time-locked multiregional retroactivation: a systems-level proposal for the neural substrates of recall and recognition. *Cognition, 33*, 25–62.

Damasio, A. R., Damasio H., Van Hoesen, G. W. (1982). Prosopagnosia: anatomic basis and behavioral mechanisms. *Neurology, 32*, 331–341.

Damasio, A. R, Tranel, D., Damasio, H. (1990). Face agnosia and the neural substrates of memory. *Annual Review of Neuroscience, 13*, 89–109.

Damasio, H, Tranel, D., Grabowski, T., Adolphs, R., Damasio, A. (2004). Neural systems behind word and concept retrieval. *Cognition, 92*, 179–229.

D'Esposito, M. (2007). From cognitive to neural models of working memory. *Philosophical Transactions of the Royal Society B., 362*, 761–772.

De Renzi, E., Faglioni, P., Grossi, D., Nichelli, P. (1991). Apperceptive and associative forms of prosopagnosia. *Cortex, 27*, 213–221.

Devinsky, O. (2009). Delusional misidentifications and duplications. Right brain lesions, left brain delusions. *Neurology, 72*, 80–87.

Douville, K., Woodard, J. L., Seidenberg, M., Miller, S. K., Leveroni, C. L., Nielson, K. A., Franczak, M., Antuono, P., Rao, S. M. (2005). Medial temporal lobe activity for recognition of recent and remote famous names: an event related fMRI study. *Neuropsychologia*, 43, 693–703.

Duchaine, B., Yovel, G. (2008). Face recognition. In: Basbaum, A. I., Kaneko, A., Shepherd, G. M., & Westheimer, G. (eds). The senses; a comprehensive reference, vol 2, Vision II. San Diego: Academic Press. pp. 329–358.

Ellis, A. W., Young, A. W., Critchley, E. M. R. (1989). Loss of memory for people following right temporal lobe damage. *Brain*, 112, 1469–1483.

Ellis, H. D., Lewis, M. B. (2001). Capgras delusion: a window on face recognition. *Trends in Cognitive Sciences*, 5, 149–156.

Eslinger, P. J., Easton, A., Grattan, L. M., Van Hoesen, G. W. (1996). Distinctive forms of partial retrograde amnesia after asymmetric temporal lobe lesions: possible role of the occipitotemporal gyri in memory. *Cerebral Cortex*, 6, 530–539.

Evans, J. J., Heggs, A. J., Antoun, N., Hodges, J. R. (1995). Progressive prosopagnosia associated with selective right temporal lobe atrophy. A new syndrome? *Brain*, 118, 1–13.

Fiske, S. T, Neuberg, S. L. (1990). A continuum of impression formation, from category-based to individuating processes: influences of information and motivation on attention and interpretation. *Advances in Experimental Social Psychology*, 23, 1–74.

Gainotti, G. (2007). Different patterns of famous person recognition disorders in patients with right and left anterior temporal lesions: a systematic review. *Neuropsychologia*, 45, 1591–1607.

Gainotti, G., Barbier, A., Marra, C. (2003). Slowly progressive defect in recognition of familiar people in a patient with right anterior temporal atrophy. *Brain*, 126, 792–803.

Gauthier, I., Behrmann, M., Tarr, M. J. (1999). Can face recognition really be dissociated from object recognition? *Journal of Cognitive Neuroscience*, 11, 349–370.

Gauthier, I., Anderson, A. W., Tarr, M. J., Skudlarski, P., Gore, J. C. (1997). Levels of categorization in visual recognition studied with functional MRI. *Current Biology*, 7, 645–651.

Gauthier, I., Skudlarski, P., Gore, J. C., Anderson, A. W. (2000c). Expertise for cars and birds recruits brain areas involved in face recognition. *Nature Neuroscience*, 3, 191–197.

Gauthier, I., Tarr, M. J., Mylan, J., Anderson, A. W., Skudlarski, P., Gore, J. C. (2000a). Does visual subordinate-level categorization engage the functionally defined fusiform face area? *Cognitive Neuropsychology*, 17, 143–163.

Gauthier, I., Tarr, M. J., Moylan, J., Skudlarski, P., Gore, J. C., Anderson, A. W. (2000b). The fusiform "face area" is part of a network that processes faces at this individual level. *Journal of Cognitive Neuroscience*, 12, 495–504.

Gazzaley, A., Cooney, J. W., McEvoy, K., Knight, R. T., D'Esposito, M. (2005). Top-down enhancement and suppression of the magnitude and speed of neural activity. *Journal of Cognitive Neuroscience*, 17, 507–517.

Gentileschi, V., Sperber, S., Spinnler, H. (2001). Crossmodal agnosia for familiar people as a consequence of right infero-polar temporal atrophy. *Cognitive Neuropsychology*, 18:439–463.

Glosser, G., Salvucci, A. E., Chiaravalloti, N. D. (2003). Naming and recognizing famous faces in temporal lobe epilepsy. *Neurology*, 61, 81–86.

Gorno-Tempini, M. L, Price J. C. (2001). Identification of famous faces and buildings. A functional neuroimaging study of semantically unique items. *Brain* 2001, 124:2087–2097.

Grabowski, T. J., Damasio, H., Tranel, D., Boles Ponto, L. L., Hichwa, R. D., Damasio, A. R. (2001). A role for left temporal pole in the retrieval of words for unique entities. *Human Brain Mapping*, 13,199–212.

Grill-Spector, K., Knouf, N., Kanwisher, N. (2004). The fusiform face area subserves face perception, not generic within-category identification. *Nature Neuroscience*, 7, 555–562.

Grill-Spector, K., Sayres, R., Ress, D. (2006). High-resolution imaging reveal highly selective nonface clusters in the fusiform face area. *Nature Neuroscience*, 9, 1177–1185.

Haxby, J. V., Gobbini, M. I., Furey, M. L., Ishai, A., Schoute, J. L., Pietrini, P. (2001). Distributed and overlapping representations of faces and objects in ventral temporal cortex. *Science, 293,* 2425–2430.

Haxby, J. V., Hoffman, E. A., Gobbini, M. I. (2000). The distributed human neural system for face perception. *Trends in Cognitive Sciences,* 4, 223–233.

Haist, F., Gore, J. B., Mao, H. (2001). Consolidation of human memory over decades revealed by functional magnetic resonance imaging. *Nature Neuroscience,* 4, 1139–1145.

Haist, F., Lee, K., Stiles, J. (2010). Individuating faces and common objects produces equal responses in putative face processing areas in ventral occipitotemporal cortex. *Frontiers in Human Neuroscience,* 4, 181. doi:10.3389/fnhum.2010.00181.

Hanley, J. R., Young, A. W., Pearson, N. A. (1989). Defective recognition of familiar people. *Cognitive Neuropsychology,* 6, 179–210.

Ishai, A., Haxby, J. V., Ungerleider, L. G. (2002). Visual imagery of famous faces: effects of memory and attention revealed by fMRI. *NeuroImage,* 17, 1729–1741.

Johnson, M. R., Mitchell, K. J., Raye, C. L., D'Esposito, M., Johnson, M. K. (2007). A brief thought can modulate activity in extrastriate visual areas: top-down effects of refreshing just-seen stimuli. *NeuroImage,* 37, 290–299.

Josephs, K. A., Whitwell, J. L., Vemuri, P., Senjem, M. L., Boeve. B. F., Knopman, D. S., Smith, G. E., Ivnik, R. J., Petersen, R. C., Jack, C. R. (2008). The anatomic correlate of prosopagnosia in semantic dementia. *Neurology,* 71, 1628–1633.

Joubert, S., Felician, O., Barbeau, E., Ranjeva, J-P., Cristophe, M., Didic, M., Poncet, M., Ceccaldi, M. (2006). The right temporal lobe variant of frontotemporal dementia. Cognitive and neuroanatomical profile of three patients. *Journal of Neurology,* 253, 1447–1458.

Kanwisher, N. (2000). Domain specificity of face perception. *Nature Neuroscience,* 3, 759–763.

Kanwisher, N, Yovel, G. (2006). The fusiform face area: a cortical region specialized for the perception of faces. *Philosophical Transactions of the Royal Society B,* 361, 2109–2128.

Kanwisher, N., McDermott, J., Chun, M. M. (1997). The fusiform face area: a module in human extrastriate cortex specialized for face perception. *Journal of Neuroscience,* 17, 4302–4311.

Kelley, W. M., Miezin, F. M., McDermott, K. B., et al. (1998). Hemispheric specialization in human frontal cortex and medial temporal lobe for verbal and nonverbal memory encoding. *Neuron,* 20, 927–936.

Klatzky, R. L., Martin, G. L., Kane, R. A.. (1982). Semantic interpretation effects on memory for faces. *Memory & Cognition,* 10, 195–206.

Leveroni, C. L., Seidenberg, M., Mayer, A. R., Mead, L. A., Binder, J. R., Rao, S. M. (2000). Neural systems underlying the recognition of familiar and newly learned faces. *Journal of Neuroscience,* 20, 878–886.

Light, L. L., Kayra-Stuart, F., Hollander, S. (1979). Recognition memory for typical and unusual faces. *Journal of Experimental Psychology: Human Learning and Memory,* 5, 212–228.

Liu, J., Harris, A., Kanwisher, N. (2010). Perception of face parts and face configurations: an fMRI study. *Journal of Cognitive Neuroscience,* 22, 203–211.

Macrae, C. N., Bodenhausen, G. V. (2000). Social cognition: thinking categorically about others. *Annual Review of Psychology,* 5, 193–120.

Mason, M. F., Macrae, C. N. (2004). Categorizing and individuating others: the neural substrates of person perception. *Journal of Cognitive Neuroscience,* 16, 1785–1795.

Maurer, D., Le Grand, R., Mondloch, J. (2002). The many faces of configural processing. *Trends in Cognitive Sciences,* 6, 255–260.

McClelland, J. L., McNaughton, B. L., O'Reilly, R. C. (1995). Why are there complementary learning systems in the hippocampus and neocortex: insights from the successes and failures of connectionist models of learning and memory. *Psychological Review,* 102, 419–457.

McDermott, K. B., Buckner, R. L., Petersen, S. E., Kelley,W. M., Saunders, A. L. (1999). Set- and code-specific activation in the frontal cortex: an fMRI study of encoding and retrieval of faces and words. *Journal of Cognitive Neuroscience,* 11, 631–640.

Mechelli, A., Price, C. J., Friston, K. J., Ishai, A. (2004). Where bottom-up meets top-down: neural interactions during perception and imagery. *Cerebral Cortex*, 14, 1256–1265.

Mervis, C. B., Rosch, E. (1981). Categorization of natural objects. *Annual Review of Psychology*, 32, 89–115.

Moran, M., Seidenberg, M., Sabsevitz, D., Swanson, S., Hermann, B. (2005). The acquisition of face and person identity information following anterior temporal lobectomy. *Journal of the International Neuropsychological Society*, 11, 237–278.

Moscovitch, M., Nadel, L., Winocur, G., Gilboa, A., Rosenbaum. S. (2006). The cognitive neuroscience of remote episodic, semantic and spatial memory. *Current Opinion in Neurobiology*, 16, 179–190.

Moss, H. E., Rodd, J. M., Stamatakis, E. A., Bright, P., Tyler. L. K. (2005). Anteromedial temporal cortex supports fine-grained differentiation among objects. *Cerebral Cortex*, 15, 616–627.

Nakamura, K., Kawashima, R., Sugiura, M., Kato, T., et al. (2001). Neural substrates for recognition of familiar voices: a PET study. *Neuropsychologia*, 39, 1047–1054.

Pannu, J. K., Kaszniak, A. W, Rapcsak, S. Z. (2005). Metamemory for faces following frontal lobe damage. *Journal of the International Neuropsychological Society*, 11, 668–676.

Quinn, K. A., Macrae, C. N. (2005). Categorizing others: the dynamics of person construal. *Journal of Personality and Social Psychology*, 88, 467–479.

Ranganath, C. (2006). Working memory for visual objects: complementary roles of inferior temporal, medial temporal, and prefrontal cortex. *Neuroscience*, 139, 277–289.

Rapcsak, S. Z. (2003). Face memory and its disorders. *Current Neurology and Neuroscience Reports*, 3, 494–501.

Rapcsak, S. Z., Kaszniak, A. W, Reminger, S. L., Glisky, M. L., Glisky, E. L., Comer, J. F. (1998). Dissociation between verbal and autonomic measures of recognition memory following frontal lobe damage. *Neurology*, 50, 1259–1265.

Rapcsak, S. Z., Nielson, M. A., Littrell, L. D., Glisky, E. L., Kaszniak, A. W., Laguna, J. F. (2001). Face memory impairments in patients with frontal lobe damage. *Neurology*, 57, 1168–1175.

Rapcsak, S. Z, Nielsen, L., Glisky, E. L, Kaszniak, A. W. (2002). The neuropsychology of false facial recognition. In L. Squire & D. L. Schacter (eds.), *The Neuropsychology of Memory, 3rd Edition*. New York: Guilford Press, pp. 130–142.

Rapcsak, S. Z., Polster, M. R., Comer, J. F., Rubens, A. B. (1994). False recognition and misidentification of unfamiliar faces following right hemisphere damage. *Cortex*, 30, 565–583.

Rapcsak, S. Z, Polster, M. R., Glisky, M. L., Comer, J. S. (1996). False recognition of unfamiliar faces following right hemisphere damage: neuropsychological and anatomical observations. *Cortex*, 32, 593–611.

Rapcsak, S. Z., Reminger, S. L., Glisky, E. L., Kaszniak, A. W., Comer, J. F. (1999). Neuropsychological mechanisms of false facial recognition following frontal lobe damage. *Cognitive Neuropsychology* 16, 267–292.

Riddoch, J. M., Johnston, R. A., Bracewell, R. M., Boutsen, L., Humphreys, G. W. (2008). Are faces special? A case of pure prosopagnosia. *Cognitive Neuropsychology*, 25, 3–26.

Rogers, T. T., Lambon Ralph, M. A., Garrard, P., Bozeat, S., McClelland, J. L., Hodges, J. R., Patterson, K. (2004). Structure and deterioration of semantic memory: a neuropsychological and computational investigation. *Psychological Review*, 111, 205–235.

Rogers, T. T., McClelland, J. L. (2004). Semantic cognition. A parallel distributed processing approach. Cambridge, MA:MIR Press.

Rossion, B., Caldara, R., Seghier, M., Schuller, A-M., Lazeyras. F., Mayer, E. (2003). A network of occipito-temporal face-sensitive area besides the right middle fusiform gyrus is necessary for normal face processing. *Brain*, 126, 2381–2395.

Rossion, B., Dricot, L., Devolder, A., Bodart, J-M., Crommelinck, M., de Gelder, B., Zoontjes, R. (2000). Hemispheric asymmetries for whole-based and part-based face processing in the human fusiform gyrus. *Journal of Cognitive Neuroscience*, 12, 793–802.

Rossion, B, Schiltz, C., Crommerlinck, M. (2003). The functionally defined right occipital and fusiform "face areas" discriminate novel from visually familiar faces. *NeuroImage*, 19, 877–883.

Rossion, B., Schiltz, C., Robaye, L., Pirenne, D., Crommelinck, M. (2001). How does the brain discriminate familiar and unfamiliar faces? A PET study of face categorical perception. *Journal of Cognitive Neuroscience*, 13, 1019–1034.

Rothstein, P., Henson, R. N. A., Treves, A., Driver, J., Dolan, R. J. (2005). Morphing Marilyn into Maggie dissociates physical and identity face representations in the brain. *Nature Neuroscience*, 8, 107–113.

Schiltz, C., Sorger, B., Caldara, R., Ahmed, F., Mayer. E., Goebel, R., Rossion, B. (2006). Impaired face discrimination in acquired prosopagnosia is associated with abnormal response to individual faces in the right middle fusiform gyrus. *Cerebral Cortex*, 16, 574–586.

Seidenberg, M., Griffith, R., Sabsevitz, D., Moran, M., Haltiner, A., Bell, B., Swanson, S., Hammeke, T., Hermann, B. (2002). Recognition and identification of famous faces in patients with unilateral temporal lobe epilepsy. *Neuropsychologia*, 40, 446–456.

Sergent, J., MacDonald, B., Zuck, E. (1994). Structural and functional organization of knowledge about face and proper names: positron emission tomography study. In C Umlita and M Moscovitch (eds). Attention and Performance XV: Conscious and Nonconscious Information Processing. MIT Press, Cambridge MA, pp. 203–228.

Sergent, J., Ohta, S., MacDonald, B. (1992). Functional neuroanatomy of face and object processing: a positron emission tomography study. *Brain*, 115, 15–36.

Sergent, J., Signoret, J-L. (1992). Varieties of functional deficits in prosopagnosia. *Cerebral Cortex*, 2, 375–388.

Snowden, J. S., Thompson, J. C., Neary, D. (2004). Knowledge of famous faces and names in semantic dementia. *Brain*, 127, 860–872.

Sorger, B., Goesbel, R., Schiltz, C., Rossion, B. (2007). Understanding the functional neuroanatomy of acquired prosopagnosia. *NeuroImage*, 35, 836–852.

Squire, L., Bayley, P. J. (2007). The neuroscience of remote memory. *Current Opinion in Neurobiology*, 17, 185–196.

Sperling, R. A., Bates, J. F., Cocchiarella. A. J., Schacter, D. L., Rosen, B. R., Albert, M. S. (2001). Encoding novel face-name associations: a functional MRI study. *Human Brain Mapping*, 14, 129–139.

Sperling, R., Chua, E., Cocchiarella, A., Rand-Giovanetti, E., Poldrack, R., Schacter, D. L., Albert, M. (2003). Putting names to faces: successful encoding and associative memories activate the anterior hippocampal formation. *NeuroImage*, 20, 1400–1410.

Steeves, J. K. E., Culham, J. C., Duchaine, B. C., Pratesi, C. C., Valyear, K. F., Schindler, I., Humphrey, G. K., Milner, D. A., Goodale, M. A.. (2006). The fusiform face area is not sufficient for face recognition: evidence from a patient with dense prosopagnosia and no occipital face area. *Neuropsychologia*, 44, 594–604.

Sugiura, M., Sassa, Y., Watanabe, J., Akitsuki, Y., Maeda, Y., Matsue, Y., Fukuda, H., Kawashima, R. (2006). Cortical mechanisms of person representation: recognition of famous and personally familiar names. *NeuroImage*, 31, 853–860.

Tanaka, J. W. (2001). The entry point of face recognition: evidence for face expertise. *Journal of Experimental Psychology: General*, 130, 534–543.

Tarr, M. J., Cheng, Y. D. (2003). Learning to see faces and objects. *Trends in Cognitive Sciences*, 7, 23–30.

Tarr, M. J.,Gauthier, I. (2000). FFA: a flexible fusiform area for subordinate-level visual processing automatized by expertise. *Nature Neuroscience*, 3, 764–769.

Thompson, S. A., Graham, K. S., Williams, G., Patterson, K., Kapur, N., Hodges, J. R. (2004). Dissociating person-specific from general semantic knowledge: roles of the left and right temporal lobes. *Neuropsychologia*, 42, 359–370.

Thompson, S. A., Shaikan, B. J., Graham. K. S., Patterson. K., Hodges, J. R.. (2002). Is knowledge of famous people disproportionately impaired in patients with early and questionable Alzheimer's disease? *Neuropsychology*, 16, 344–358.

Tranel, D. (2006). Impaired naming of unique landmarks is associated with left temporal polar damage. *Neuropsychology*, 20, 1–10.

Tranel, D., Damasio, A. R., Damasio, H. (1988). Intact recognition of facial expression, gender, and age in patients with impaired recognition of face identity. *Neurology*, 38, 690–696.

Tranel, D., Damasio, H., Damasio, A. R. (1997). A neural basis of the retrieval of conceptual knowledge. *Neuropsychologia*, 10, 1319–1327.

Tsao, D. Y., Livingstone, M. S. (2008). Mechanisms of face perception. *Annual Review of Neuroscience*, 31, 411–437.

Tsukiura, T., Fujii, T., Fukatsu, R., et al. (2002). Neural basis of the retrieval of people's names: evidence from brain damaged patients and fMRI. *Journal of Cognitive Neuroscience*, 14, 922–937.

Tsukiura, T., Mochizuki-Kawai, H., Fujii, T. (2006). Dissociable roles of the bilateral anterior temporal lobe in face-name associations: an event-related fMRI study. *NeuroImage*, 30, 627–626.

Turk, D. J., Rosenblum, A. C., Gazzaniga, M. S., Macrae, C. N. (2005). Seeing John Malkovich: the neural substrates of person categorization. *NeuroImage*, 24, 1147–1153.

Tyler, L. K., Stamatakis, E. A., Bright, P., Acres, K., Abdallah, S., Rodd, J. M., Moss, H. E.. (2004). Processing objects at different levels of specificity. *Journal of Cognitive Neuroscience*, 16, 351–362.

Valentine, T., Bruce, V. (1986). The effects of distinctiveness in recognising and classifying faces. *Perception*, 15, 525–535.

Viskontas, I. V., McAndrews, M. P., Moscovitch, M. (2002). Memory for famous people in patients with unilateral temporal lobe epilepsy and excisions. *Neuropsychology*, 16, 472–480.

Vokey, J. R., Read, J. D. (1992). Familiarity, memorability, and the effect of typicality on the recognition of faces. *Memory & Cognition*, 20, 291–302.

von Kriegstein, K., Giraud, A-L. (2004). Distinct functional substrates along the right superior temporal sulcus for the processing of voices. *NeuroImage*, 22, 948–955.

von Kriegstein, K., Kleinschmidt, A., Sterzer, P., Giraud, A-L. (2005). Interaction of face and voice areas during speaker recognition. *Journal of Cognitive Neuroscience*, 17, 367–376.

Ward, J., Jones, L. (2003). Inappropriate association of semantics and context to novel stimuli can give rise to the false recognition of unfamiliar people. *Neuropsychologia*, 41, 538–549.

Ward, J., Parkin, A. J., Powell, G., Squires, E. J., Townshend, J., Bradley, V. (1999). False recognition of unfamiliar people: "seeing film stars everywhere." *Cognitive Neuropsychology*, 16, 293–315.

Werheid, K., Clare L. (2007). Are faces special in Alzheimer's disease? Cognitive conceptualization, neural correlates, and diagnostic relevance of impaired memory for faces and names. *Cortex*, 43, 898–906.

Zarate, M. A., Stoever, C. J., MacLin, M. K., Arms-Chavez, C. J. (2008). Neurocognitive underpinnings of face perception: further evidence of distinct person and group perception processes. *Journal of Personality and Social Psychology*, 94, 108–115.

Zeineh, M. M., Engel, S. A, Thompson, P. M., Bookheimer, S. Y. (2003). Dynamics of the hippocampus during encoding and retrieval of face-name pairs. *Science*, 299, 577–580.

CHAPTER 7

Arousal, Attention, and Perception

Mark Mennemeier

Overview

Underlying this chapter is a proposal that symptoms of several different types of clinical disorders, including the neglect syndrome (neglect), can be attributed to altered psychophysical processes regulating the perception of stimulus intensity. Overestimating the intensity of a stimulus leads to excessive behavioral responses, and underestimating its intensity to inefficient behavioral responses. This proposal was initially prompted by studies of patients with spatial neglect, but it is not limited to neglect or to stimuli with inherent spatial properties. In fact, the same alteration might account for symptoms of two different clinical disorders in the same patient, such as the failure to recognize weakness in a limb and/or symptoms of dysphagia which are both common comorbidities in neglect, and so this alteration can be thought of as a trans-disorder process. The primary responsibility for the altered psychophysical function observed in these patients is likely to be found in changes in cortical arousal following brain injury. Thus, this proposal may link two classical theories of normal perception: the Yerkes-Dodson law, relating arousal and sensory discrimination, and the psychophysical power law, concerning perception of stimulus intensity.

In the examination of neglect in this chapter, the emphasis falls on the relationship between psychophysical processes and quantitative features of performance. Examining neglect in this way adds precision to a disorder known for its heterogeneity. Additionally, whereas psychophysical concepts add a new and necessary theoretical parameter to spatial theories of neglect, altered perception of stimulus intensity appears to influence behavior independently of spatial attention, and to also manifest as symptoms of other clinical disorders.

The first section of this chapter presents a general description of neglect and observations from patient studies that warrant the integration of psychophysical concepts and neglect theory. The second section examines the relationship between sensory perception and arousal and describes a brain mechanism that integrates arousal and sensory information. The final section reviews evidence from patient studies bearing on the functional and anatomical architecture related to perception of stimulus intensity.

Section 1. Perceptual Breakdown

NEGLECT PHENOMENOLOGY

Patients suffering with neglect act as if portions of their world do not exist. They often fail to acknowledge stimuli directed to the side of their body opposite their brain lesion (i.e., contralesional inattention), although neglect for the side of the body on which the brain injury occurred (i.e., ipsilesional) has also been observed. Sensory and motor dysfunction is common in patients with neglect, but primary sensory and motor deficits do not explain inattention (Heilman, Watson, & Valenstein, 1985). Neglect for the contralesional side of the body often contrasts sharply with preserved awareness for the ipsilesional side of the body. Patients with neglect may eat from only the ipsilesional side of plates or shave or apply makeup to only the ipsilateral side of their face. They may be able to identify objects in contralesional space when their attention is drawn to them, but then fail to notice the same objects spontaneously or when competing stimuli are present. On behavioral tests, they may fail to draw contralesional parts of pictures or to detect targets located on the contralesional side of a page. They may bisect a line as if they were not aware of the contralesional half of the line. While the separation of neglected from non-neglected space is not sharp, neglect is almost always more severe contralesional to a brain injury. Neglect behavior is heterogeneous, both across patients and within patients over time, and it typically coexists with other cognitive and behavioral abnormalities. For example, the eyes and head of a patient with neglect are often turned in an ipsilesional direction; these patients are typically slow to respond to stimulation and they may appear sleepy or even fail to stay awake during a conversation or a therapy session. The neglect syndrome; therefore, likely represents a combination of behavioral deficits, any one of which alone would be insufficient to produce it.

NEGLECT ANATOMY

Neglect is more frequent, severe, and persistent when the right rather than the left cerebral hemisphere is injured (Ringman, Saver, Woolson, Clarke, & Adams, 2004) (for reviews see (Heilman et al., 1985; Vallar & Perani, 1987; Karnath, Ferber, & Himmelbach, 2001; Ogden, 1987). Neglect follows damage to a cortical system involving heteromodal association areas in the prefrontal, anterior cingulate, inferior parietal, insular and lateral temporal cortices. Neglect also ensues when the injury involves subcortical structures, including the thalamus, striatum, and mesencephalic reticular formation and white matter pathways connecting cortical structures and subcortical structures (Watson, Valenstein, & Heilman, 1981; Mesulam, 1981; Rizzolatti & Berti, 1993; Karnath, Himmelbach, & Rorden, 2002a; Watson, Heilman, Miller, & King, 1974). Lesions that affect cortical structures appear to account for the majority of cases of neglect (greater than 50 percent), whereas, lesions restricted to subcortical structures like the striatum and thalamus account for relatively fewer cases (Karnath, Himmelbach, & Rorden, 2002b). Neglect following mesencephalic lesions in humans is rarely witnessed because the patients may not survive or be testable. Close anatomical interconnections among these different cortical areas and subcortical structures reflect the multifaceted nature of neglect, which includes deficits of attention, movement (intention), representation, and arousal.

Neglect Theory: Attention

The major theories concerning neglect syndrome have attempted to explain how neglect is more common and severe after right rather than left hemisphere damage and how left-sided neglect occurs after right hemisphere damage. Several theories focus on deficits in spatial attention. Kinsbourne (Kinsbourne, 1970) postulated that each hemisphere generates a vector of spatial attention toward contralateral space; that the two hemispheres were mutually inhibitory of each other; and that the left hemisphere's attentional vector is normally stronger than that of the right. Right hemisphere damage disinhibits the left hemisphere, resulting in a strong vector of attention to the right side of space that is not mirrored when similar damage occurs to the left hemisphere. Heilman et al. (Heilman et al., 1985) proposed a right hemisphere dominance model for spatial attention, in which the right hemisphere directs attention to both contralateral and ipsilateral hemispaces (defined relative to the body midline). The left hemisphere only directs attention to contralateral hemispace. Right hemisphere injury causes inattention to left hemispace because the intact left hemisphere cannot direct attention to left hemispace. In contrast, neglect is infrequent following left hemisphere injury because the intact right hemisphere directs attention to both right and left hemispaces. Finally, Posner (Posner & Dehaene, 1994) postulated that damage to the parietal lobe caused selective disengagement from stimuli in ipsilesional space. Neglect is explained as an inability to shift attention to contralesional space.

Neglect Theory: Intention

Theories of neglect also postulate deficits of spatial movement and intention. Watson,Valenstein, and Heilman (Heilman et al., 1985; Watson, Valenstein, & Heilman, 1978) argued that neglect patients were either disinclined to initiate movements in or toward contralesional hemispace or that they were biased to act in ipsilesional hemispace. Intentional disorders include the absence of movement, hypometric movement, motor extinction, and motor impersistence. Intentional disorders are dissociable from deficits in spatial attention, and this suggests that they contribute independently to neglect (Adair, Na, Schwartz, & Heilman, 1998; Na et al., 1998; Tegner & Levander, 1991b; Bisiach, Geminiani, Berti, & Rusconi, 1990; Coslett, Bowers, Fitzpatrick, Haws, & Heilman, 1990).

Neglect Theory: Representation

Bisiach explained neglect behavior as an inability to form mental representations of contralateral space and of objects in that space (Bisiach & Luzzatti, 1978; Bisiach, 1993). Although representational accounts of neglect have been viewed as distinct from attentional and intentional theories, each account may be valid and aimed at different components or levels of analysis of neglect behavior (Chatterjee & Mennemeier, 1998).

Neglect Theory: Arousal

Watson, Valenstein, and Heilman also proposed that attentional and intentional aspects of neglect were related to deficits in arousal (Heilman & Valenstein, 1972; Watson et al., 1981; Watson et al., 1974; Heilman & VanDenable, 1980; Heilman et al., 1985). Unilateral lesions of the reticular activating system (RAS) may cause contralesional inattention either by failing to activate the ipsilesional cortex in response to sensory stimulation or by reducing sensory transmission to the cortex via decreased inhibition of the ipsilesional nucleus reticularis, or by both mechanisms. Additionally, unilateral lesions of heteromodal association areas that project to the RAS and to the reticular nucleus of the thalamus may similarly induce contralesional inattention (Heilman et al., 1985).

Arousal involves several physiological systems in both cerebral hemispheres that regulate wakefulness, alertness, and conscious perception. Waking states of consciousness depend on neural pathways that project from the ascending reticular activation system (ARAS) to the cerebral cortex and from the cerebral cortex to the thalamus and ARAS (reviewed in Section 2). These systems regulate the general tone of cortical activation (tonic arousal) and the activation of the cerebral cortex in response to a stimulation (phasic arousal). Clinically, focal brain injury can disrupt arousal in very different ways ranging from coma to hypervigilance (reviewed in (Bassetti, 2001). Lesions in the same cerebral hemisphere can also have different effects on arousal. Thalamic, subthalamic, midbrain, and upper pontine strokes, where fibers of the RAS can be affected by a single lesion, cause the most severe and persisting disturbances of wakefulness. Large cortico-subcortical strokes associated with hypersomnia[1], particularly those with vertical and horizontal displacement of the brain secondary to edema, are often accompanied by ipsilesional gaze and head deviation, contralesional inattention and sensori-motor impairment, decreased motor and speech production, and flat affect. Hypersomnia without significant edema may be more common following anterior than posterior stroke. Some evidence based on observations of stroke patients suggested that hypersomnia was more likely after left than right hemisphere lesions (Albert, Silverberg, Reches, & Berman, 1976) but a larger, controlled study did not find laterality differences related to waking and consciousness (Cucchiara et al., 2003). Additionally, lesions of the right cerebral hemisphere are often associated with decreased indicators of arousal, such as decreased heart rate and galvanic skin response; whereas, those of the left hemisphere may actually *increase* arousal possibly via disinhibition of the intact right hemisphere or of the reticular activating system (Heilman, Blonder, Bowers, & Valenstein, 2003).

Neural systems, particularly those of the right cerebral hemisphere, control intensity aspects of attention i.e., the regulation of arousal by attentional processes[2]. These networks are commonly damaged in patients with neglect. Intensity aspects of attention include alertness, both tonic alertness measured by simple reaction time and phasic alertness measured by reaction time following a warning cue, and vigilance and sustained attention in which arousal and alertness are sustained over time (for reviews see (Posner & Dehaene, 1994; Sturm & Willmes, 2001; Posner & Boies, 1971; Robertson & Garavan, 2004). A dramatic increase in simple reaction time is associated with lesions of the right hemisphere (Posner & Rafal, 1987; Ladavas, 1987) and in patients with neglect (Anderson, Mennemeier, & Chatterjee, 2000) but reaction time improves in these patients when warning cues are provided(Posner & Rafal, 1987; Tartaglione, Bino, Spadavecchia, & Favale, 1986). This suggests that tonic rather than phasic alertness may be critically altered by right hemisphere lesions.

Hypoarousal is a term used to describe arousal deficits associated with neglect (Heilman, Schwartz, & Watson RT, 1978; Watson et al., 1981). Clinically, hypoaroused patients would appear similar to those with hypersomnia, but hypoarousal in neglect has not been evaluated systematically in large series of stroke patients, so its prevalence, specificity, and even its operational definition is not well established. Arousal deficits have been measured in studies of neglect by monitoring changes in (1) galvanic skin response and heart rate (Heilman et al., 2003; Morrow, Vrtunski, Kim, & Boller, 1981), (2) pupillary response (Kim, Schwartz, & Heilman, 1999), (3) theta- and beta-wave frequency on electroencephalography (Storrie-Baker, Segalowitz, Black, McLean, & Sullivan, 1997), (4) behavioral change following manipulations of arousal (Kerkhoff, 2001; Pierce & Buxbaum, 2002), and (5) the ability to perform two tasks simultaneously (Coslett, Bowers, & Heilman, 1987). In rehabilitation settings, hypoaroused patients are very dependent on therapists for guidance, and they often fail to transfer gains made in therapy to other settings. Studies using reaction time as a measure of tonic alertness suggest that decreased alertness is associated with disability and can persist chronically, even after spatial deficits related to neglect have improved (Robertson, 2001; Samuelsson, Hjelmquist, Jenson, Ekholm, & Blomstrand, 1998; Farne et al., 2004).

COUNTERCURRENTS TO SPATIAL THEORIES OF NEGLECT

In addition to performance deficits lateralized primarily to one side of space, neglect involves deficits that cause behavioral impairment, but are not necessarily worse on one side of the body midline than on the other (i.e., nonlateralized features of neglect) (Samuelsson et al., 1998; Robertson, 2001; Husain & Rorden, 2003). Examples include increased reaction times for detecting new stimuli, poor sustained attention, impaired spatial working memory (Robertson, 2001; Husain & Rorden, 2003), and, as discussed later in this chapter, systematic bias in the estimation of the intensity of sensory stimulation. Lateralized and nonlateralized features of neglect appear to be independent of one another and to explain different aspects of neglect behavior. Whereas lateralized deficits typically refer to "where" neglect occurs in space, nonlateralized features address performance deficiencies that are often referred to as capacity limitations. One such deficiency concerns "how much" of something is neglected or, in some cases, exaggerated.

Neglect occurs for stimuli that must be recognized at a conscious level of awareness, but information processed below a level of conscious recognition can influence and even predict neglect behavior. In one study, for example, patients with neglect were asked to make same/different judgments about pairs of pictures briefly presented to the right and left visual fields. They performed above chance, but they were no better than chance at identifying the picture on the left when it differed from the one on the right (Volpe, Ledoux, & Gazzaniga, 1979). Systematic relationships between the total amount of stimulation presented to a patient and the amount neglected by the patient have been observed on bedside tests of neglect examining the number of targets presented on cancellation tests (Chatterjee, Mennemeier, & Heilman, 1992b; Chatterjee, Mennemeier, & Heilman, 1992a; Mennemeier, Rapcsak, Dillon, & Vezey, 1998); the length of words in tests of reading (Chatterjee, 1995); the length of lines in bisection tasks (Tegner & Levander, 1991a; Chatterjee, 1995; Mennemeier et al., 2005); and even the weight of objects in extinction tests (Chatterjee, Thompson, & Ricci, 1998). In fact, when neglect behavior is expressed as a power function (a log-log plot) of the total amount of stimuli presented to a patient, the power function accounts for extremely large amounts of variance in neglect performance. Power functions appear to uniquely capture the quantitative features of neglect or how much of a stimulus was neglected.

Power function relationships reveal counterintuitive findings in neglect. During cancellation tests, patients are shown a page with target items distributed across it and asked to mark out all the items that they see. In the vast majority of cases, patients with a right hemisphere lesion and neglect cancel more targets on the right side than on the left side of the page (Albert, 1973). In one study, however, a patient with a stable pattern of left neglect on cancellation tasks was instructed to cancel targets in an alternating fashion, marking out one first on the left side of the page and then one on the right side, until she had finished (Chatterjee et al., 1992b). She cancelled the same number of targets as when performing the task during the standard administration of the test, but she neglected targets in the middle of the page rather than on the left side. Her performance could not be explained by leftward inattention, representation, or movement, but it was well accounted for by a power function that related the number of targets cancelled to the total number presented (Chatterjee et al., 1992a). The power function relationship revealed a counterintuitive finding because her neglect was systematically tied to the total number of targets presented. This observation confirmed that the patient was aware, at an implicit level, of *all* the stimuli presented to her.

Power function relationships add another parameter to spatial theories of neglect which helped to resolve a paradox known as the crossover effect (Halligan & Marshall, 1988; Marshall & Halligan, 1989). Crossover describes a pattern of performance on line bisection tasks, in which long lines (e.g., greater than 10 cm) are bisected on the ipsilesional side of true center and short lines (e.g., less than 2 cm) are bisected on the contralesional side. Crossover bisections on short lines are paradoxical for theories designed to explain contralesional neglect(Bisiach, Rusconi, Peretti, & Vallar, 1994) because they look like ipsilesional neglect. Three findings from patient studies, however, helped resolve this paradox. First, it was shown that estimates of line length by patients with neglect were biased, so that the length of long lines was underestimated and that of short lines *overestimated*. Power function relationships help confirm that crossover bisections on short lines relate to perceiving more of the line than was present rather than on perceiving less of the line, as is the case for long lines (Tegner & Levander, 1991a; Mennemeier et al., 2005; Chatterjee, 1995). Second, the crossover effect was shown to be a normal phenomenon of line bisection that was only exaggerated in neglect (Mennemeier, Vezey, Lamar, & Jewell, 2002), so it is not "caused" by deficits in spatial attention, even though attentional deficits may strengthen the crossover effect. Third, crossover bisections were shown to stem from two forms of bias that are independent of each other (Mennemeier et al., 2005). The direction of crossover, which is opposite in patients with left and right hemisphere lesions and can be experimentally reversed, is due to bias in spatial orientation that anchors attention to one end of a line. This aspect of crossover conforms to spatial theories of neglect and makes the crossover effect robust in patients with neglect. Bias in length estimation, underestimation of long lines, and overestimation of short lines produce the crossover effect. A psychophysical concept known as contextual bias (described below) might explain this aspect of crossover. Contextual effects are exaggerated in patients with neglect (Marshall, Lazar, Krakauer, & Sharma, 1998), but like the crossover effect, they are not specific to neglect and occur normally (Hollingworth, 1909; Cross, 1973). Other explanations of crossover have been proposed, but they are predicated on neglect and do not explain crossover in normal subjects (for reviews (Monaghan & Shillcock, 1998; Mennemeier et al., 2005).

NEGLECT DISABILITY AND COMORBIDITY

Neglect is a leading predictor of poor outcome following stroke rehabilitation (Mohr & Barnett, 1986; Stone et al., 1991); however, neglect rarely occurs in isolation. Comorbid problems such as sensory and motor impairment, altered awareness of deficit, and dysphagia are common and contribute to morbidity. Sensory deficits after stroke include delayed perception, uncertainty of responses, changes in sensory thresholds, fatigue, altered time sense for sensory adaptation, sensory persistence, and altered nature of sensation (Hunter & Crome, 2002; Robertson & Jones, 1994)[3]. Like neglect, sensory perceptual impairment is more common after right (37 percent) than left hemisphere injury (25 percent) (Sullivan & Hedman, 2008) and on the contralesional side of the body, although ipsilesional sensory impairment occurs with surprising frequency (Carey, 1995) (Kent, 1965); it is also associated with poor functional outcome (Carey, 1995; Rand, Gottlieb, & Weiss, 2001; Yekutiel, 2000) and with other comorbidities, including poor balance, increased vulnerability to falls, regional pain syndromes, anosognosia, hand swelling, shoulder subluxation, burns, and other injuries (Sullivan & Hedman, 2008).

Disorders of awareness, such as a lack of appropriate concern about limb weakness (anosodiaphoria) or lack of awareness of weakness (anosognosia), are associated with neglect and related to complications such as falls (Vlahov, Myers, & Al-Ibrahim, 1990; Nyberg & Gustafson, 1997; Webster et al., 1995; Rapport et al., 1993). Dysphagia, a deficit of swallowing, is a major cause of morbidity, mortality, and disability (Barer, 1989) after stroke that affects between 25 percent and 50 percent of patients (Veis & Logemann, 1985; Gordon, Hewer, & Wade, 1987). It is common to see neglect and dysphagia co-occur in clinical settings; although this observation is not well documented in the literature concerning neglect and dysphagia. One study observed neglect and dysphagia in as many as 10 of 12 patients with right hemisphere injury and in 1 of 12 patients with left hemisphere injury (Andre, Beis, Morin, & Paysant, 2000).

Theories of neglect address some of these comorbidities. Sensory extinction has been explained as attentional imbalance (Kinsbourne, 1993; Heilman et al., 1985). Anosodiaphoria and anosognosia are discussed in combination with certain forms of neglect, like personal neglect, although these disorders appear to overlap rather than cause one another, and it is not clear how they relate to neglect pathophysiology (Adair, Schwartz, & Barrett, 2003). Dysphagia is rarely viewed as related to neglect, but it may be more common in neglect patients than anosognosia (Andre et al., 2000). It is proposed here that altered perception of stimulus intensity may be a deficit that contributes to neglect and to these comorbid problems. Evidence for this postulate is examined in section 3 after some background information on arousal and perception.

Section 2: Perceptual Order

A classical experiment relating arousal and sensory perception was reported by Yerkes and Dodson in 1908 (Yerkes & Dodson, 1908). When arousal was manipulated by the delivery of varying degrees of electric shock during a luminance discrimination test, mice were observed to perform the easy discrimination tasks best during high levels of arousal, and the hard discriminations best during low levels of arousal. The Yerkes-Dodson law, now extended to the effect of stress on performance in complex behavioral tests, proposes that an optimal level of arousal is required for optimal performance. Increasing or decreasing arousal from this level negatively affects performance. It stands to reason that any task requiring sensory discrimination should be sensitive to changes in arousal and that a large fluctuation in arousal, such as that occurring after brain injury, could degrade, bias, or fundamentally alter perception.

This section reviews psychophysical concepts and methods concerning perception of stimulus intensity and the neural processes that regulate arousal. This background information is a necessary primer for the patient studies presented in section 3. Additionally, the method of measuring stimulus intensity, which is also described, is consistent with a neural mechanism that promotes conscious sensory perception.

PERCEPTION OF STIMULUS INTENSITY: THE PSYCHOPHYSICAL POWER LAW

The psychophysical power law describes a quantitative relationship between physical stimulus intensity and sensory experience (Stevens & Galanter, 1957; Stevens, 1971), based on a theoretical principle known as ratio scaling[4] (i.e., equal stimulus ratios produce equal sensation ratios (Stevens, 1975b). An example of ratio scaling is that doubling the apparent brightness of a light requires an eightfold increase in energy regardless of the original brightness of the light. Ratio scaling applies to judgments of *prothetic* perceptual continua,[5] those concerning amount or intensity, as opposed to judgments of kind, quality, location, and sort, which are called *metathetic* perceptual continua (Stevens, 1975a). Judgments of area and loudness are considered to be prothetic because they fit power functions and correspond to ratio scaling, whereas estimates of spatial location and pitch are considered to be metathetic because they fit linear functions and correspond to category scaling.

The mathematical form for the psychophysical power law is power function (a log-log plot) written as follows:

$$\Psi = \kappa\Phi^{\beta},$$

where Ψ is the sensation magnitude and Φ is the stimulus magnitude. The constant κ depends on the unit of measurement. The exponent β serves as a kind of "signature" that often differs from one sensory continuum to another. When stimulus magnitude is plotted against sensation magnitude, the fitted line assumes a curvature, or growth rate, that can vary for different sensory continua (Figure 7.1 top). Log transformation of the data also allows observations from different subjects to be averaged by geometric means. An advantageous feature of the power function is the form that it assumes when the data are plotted in logarithmic scales on both axes (log-log coordinates). The fitted line is straight, its coefficient of determination (r^2) value is a measure of variability, its slope is a direct measure of the power function exponent, and its *y* intercept is equal to the power function constant (Figure 7.1 bottom). Power function parameters, the exponent, constant and r^2 values, serve as convenient summary variables for comparison across groups and within subjects.

MAGNITUDE ESTIMATION

Four methods are commonly used to assess ratio scaling (Stevens, 1975a). Magnitude estimation requires a subject to match stimulus intensity to a number scale (e.g., between 10 and 99). Magnitude estimation is examined in more detail here because it is well suited for work with stroke patients. Other methods of ratio scaling, such as cross-modal matching, ratio production, and magnitude production (Gescheider, 1997b) are not as easy to use with stroke patients; however, after adjustment for procedural differences, all methods of ratio scaling can be expected to yield similar results (Stevens, 1975a).

Magnitude estimation requires participants to rate the intensity of a range of stimuli. Five to eight intensities are typically required to assess ratio scaling (less than five intensities may encourage participants to categorize stimuli rather than engage in ratio scaling). Stimulus intensities are presented in random order, and each intensity is repeated at least two or three times. A standard stimulus, such as a midrange value, can be presented in advance to provide a perceptual anchor for subjects, but is not necessary because the data are log-transformed and all stimuli are repeated several times during the experiment (Stevens, 1975a).

Experimental factors, such as stimulus context, broadness of the range of stimuli used, and ability of subjects to categorize stimuli, can alter the size of the

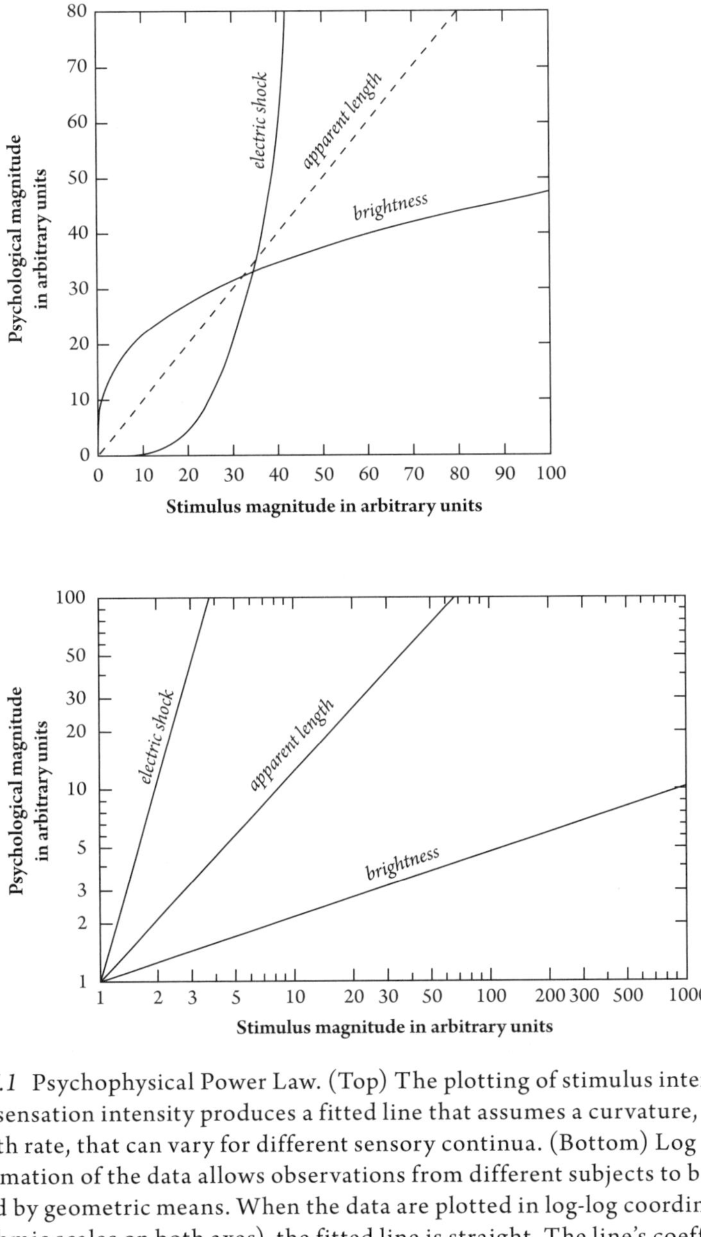

Figure 7.1 Psychophysical Power Law. (Top) The plotting of stimulus intensity against sensation intensity produces a fitted line that assumes a curvature, or growth rate, that can vary for different sensory continua. (Bottom) Log transformation of the data allows observations from different subjects to be averaged by geometric means. When the data are plotted in log-log coordinates (logarithmic scales on both axes), the fitted line is straight. The line's coefficient of determination (r^2) value is a measure of variability, its slope is a direct measure of the power function exponent, and its y intercept is equal to the power function constant (Stevens, S.S., Psychophysics; Introduction to its perceptual, neural, and social prospects, figures 5 & 6, pages 16 and 17, respectively © 1975 by John Wiley & Sons, signatory to STM).

power function exponent in normal subjects (Poulton, 1968; Algom & Marks, 1990; Cross, 1973; Hollingworth, 1909; Poulton, 1979). Contextual effects refer to an influence of the previous stimulus on perception of the current stimulus. Contextual bias[6] may restrict the range of perception and lower the power function exponent. The broadness of the range of stimulus intensities presented to a subject can dramatically alter the size of the power function exponents in normal subjects. Narrow ranges produce large exponents (steeper slopes), and broad ranges produce small exponents (flatter slopes). Categorizing stimuli with the use of only a few numbers to rate stimulus intensity also lowers the power function exponent (Gescheider, 1997a).

NEUROPSYCHOLOGY OF MAGNITUDE ESTIMATION

Brain injury, particularly in association with neglect, has a large effect on magnitude estimation and the form of power functions relative to normal subjects (Chatterjee et al., 1992a; Chatterjee, 1995; Mennemeier et al., 1998; Chatterjee et al., 1998; Mennemeier et al., 2005). Figure 7.2 illustrates the significance of a *lower power function exponent and higher constant in neglect.* Two regression lines are shown: one for normal subjects having an exponent of 1.0 and a constant of.2, and the other for neglect patients having an exponent of.76 and a constant of.38. The regression line flattens as the slope decreases. If the constant is also elevated, this means that stimuli at the high end of the magnitude scale are underestimated and that magnitude of stimuli at the low end of the scale is actually overestimated.

Magnitude estimation might be lateralized preferentially to the right hemisphere, but both hemispheres appear to calculate estimates of stimulus

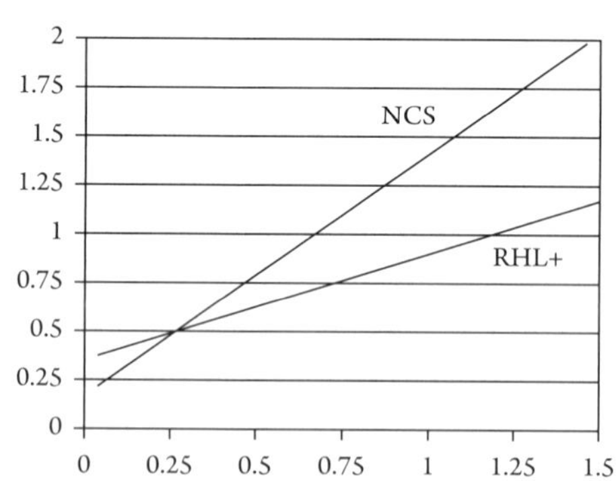

Figure 7.2 Significance of a lower power function exponent and a higher constant in neglect syndrome.The regression line for normal subjects has a power function exponent of 1.0 and a constant of .2, whereas the regression line for neglect patients has an exponent of .76 and a constant of .38. The regression line flattens as its slope decreases.

magnitude. Walsh (Walsh, 2003) proposed that human and animal studies point to a common magnitude system (for space, time, and number) localized in the inferior parietal cortex of the right hemisphere. However, Pinel et al. (Pinel, Piazza, Biham, & Dehaene, 2004) reported functional magnetic resonance imaging results from human subjects on comparative judgments of size, luminance, and number that showed overlap in cerebral activation bilaterally for each type of comparison and particularly when performance of one task interfered with that of another. Additionally, low frequency, repetitive transcranial magnetic stimulation delivered over the intraparietal sulcus of the right hemisphere, shown to be activated in the Pinel et al study, interfered with magnitude estimates of numerosity (Cappelletti, Barth, Fregni, Spelke, & Pascual-Leone, 2007). Further, patient studies indicate that magnitude estimation is disrupted by both right and left hemisphere injury (Woods et al., 2006; Taylor-Cooke et al., 2006; Mennemeier et al., 2005). Right hemisphere injury appears to have a greater effect, consistent with the notion that it is specialized for magnitude estimation, but evidence described in section 3 suggests that right and left hemisphere injury might even have opposite effects on magnitude estimation. An alternative to hemispheric specialization is that each hemisphere may have different sensitivities to factors that bias magnitude estimation, such as contextual effects that are exaggerated in neglect (Marshall et al., 1998) (less is known about the influences of range broadness and categorization in brain-injured subjects). Alternatively, arousal processes may differ between hemispheres and produce different effects on magnitude estimation.

AROUSAL SYSTEMS

Arousal systems provide a platform on which cognitive systems operate. A normal intact cerebrum is incapable of functioning in a conscious manner by itself. Bilateral damage to neurons of the midbrain reticular formation and fibers passing though it results in prolonged coma. Sustaining input from the brainstem reticular formation is required for conscious perception (Nolte, 2009).

The ARAS is a part of the brainstem reticular core that is involved in movement control, sensory transmission (including pain modulation and transmission), and autonomic regulation. Its pattern of connectivity is such that a single cell may respond to multiple sensory modalities and that functional areas within the core can exhibit considerable overlap (Nolte, 2009). Thus, the architecture of the reticular formation lends itself to changes in arousal secondary to activity in motor, sensory, and autonomic neural systems.

Arousal and the cortical desynchrony of wakefulness are mediated by several neuronal populations in the ARAS via projections to the thalamus and basal forebrain (reviewed in (Fuller, Gooley, & Saper, 2006; Garcia-Rill, 2009a). The RAS is composed of three principal cell groups: the (mainly) cholinergic pedunculopontine nucleus (PPN) and laterodorsal tegmental nucleus (LTN); the (mainly) noradrenergic locus coeruleus (LC); and the (mainly) serotonergic raphe nucleus (RN). Ascending cholinergic (PPN) and monoaminergic (LC and RN) projections from the RAS to the intralaminar thalamus activate cortex via nonspecific *thalamocortical projections*. This pathway also collaborates with those from a series of wakefulness-promoting monoaminergic cell groups constituting a massive *ventral projection system* that bypasses the thalamus and terminates diffusely throughout the cortex to modulate cortical activity. Ventral pathways include projections from the noradrenergic LC, dopaminergic neurons of the ventral periaqueductal gray matter, serotonergic dorsal and median RN, and histaminergic neurons in the tuberomammillary nucleus. Noradrenergic neurons may play a role in phasic changes related to vigilance (Robertson & Garavan, 2004; Nolte, 2009) and serotonergic neurons in tonic arousal related to pain control; however, in general, these different projection systems act in a coordinated manner to regulate arousal.

Neural fibers which either go to or come from the cerebral cortex form a structure called the internal capsule (Carpenter, 1976). One part of the internal capsule, which borders the lateral caudate nucleus, contains fibers or thalamic radiations which reciprocally connect the thalamus and the cortex. Thalamocortical fibers project from the thalamus to the cortex and corticothalamic fibers project from the cortex to the thalamus. Another part of the internal capsule contains efferent cortical fibers that arise from the cerebral cortex and converge and descend toward the brain stem (i.e., the corona radiata). These fibers connect the entire cerebral cortex with nuclei in the brain stem, including those in the reticular formation, and in the spinal cord.

Oscillatory or "rhythmic" activity is a property of thalamocortical projection systems (reviewed in (Bazhenov & Timofee, 2006) and sleep-wake rhythms are generated by mesopontine activation of thalamocortical projections (Garcia-Rill, 2009b). Normal thalamocortical rhythms include slow (.3–1 Hz frequency), delta (1–4 Hz), sleep spindle (7–14 Hz) and beta-gamma EEG oscillations (15–30 and 30–80 Hz, respectively). With regard to sleep, oscillations below 10 Hz are considered slow wave sleep[7], oscillations greater than 10 Hz are evident in waking and REM sleep[8]. ARAS inputs excite thalamocortical projections and they inhibit neurons in the reticular nucleus of the thalamus (Steriade, McCormick, & Sejnowski, 1993). Thalamocortical projections activate cortical neurons, setting up cortical processes that return descending activity to thalamocortical neurons (Pare Denis & Llinas, 1995). In the absence of ARAS inputs, the reticular nucleus of the thalamus, made up of gabaergic neurons, sets up slow oscillations in thalamocortical pathways, leading to lower frequencies and sleep (Steriade, Curro, Pare, & Oakson, 1991). Synchronous synaptic activity in cortical and thalamic neurons is largely absent during slow oscillations. Whereas peripheral sensory stimuli might reach the cerebral cortex during sleep; the timing of relay cell activity necessary for conscious perception is lost and conscious perception is impaired as a result.

The waking state is characterized by low amplitude, fast EEG oscillations in the 15–80 Hz range. Fast rhythms are synchronized between neighboring cortical sites and they are associated with normal conscious states like attentiveness, focused arousal, sensory perception, movement and prediction and with "altered" consciousness associated with some forms of anesthesia, slow wave and REM sleep (Bazhenov & Timofee, 2006).

A MECHANISM FOR CONSCIOUS PERCEPTION OF STIMULUS INTENSITY

The method of magnitude estimation requires repetitive discriminations among a range of stimulus intensities that follow one another in random succession. One neural mechanism theorized to mediate conscious sensory perception by integrating arousal and sensory information simultaneously may be particularly well suited to account for the process of magnitude estimation.

The ARAS receives input from afferent sensory systems that conduct information about the presence, absence, quality, and intensity of sensory stimulation via specific sensory thalamocortical projections. Therefore, two parallel thalamocortical projection systems arise from the ARAS: a *nonspecific system* that influences cortical neuronal responsiveness to further stimulation via projections from the intralaminar thalamus, and *specific thalamocortical projections* that convey sensory information via primary sensory relay thalamic nuclei (Figure 7.3). Both projection systems appear to fire rhythmically in relation to intrinsic oscillatory properties of thalamic cells (Llinas, Ribary, Contreras, & Pedroarena, 1998), and cells in both of these projection systems have been shown to oscillate at gamma-band frequency (between 30–50 Hz; referred to as the "40 Hz rhythm") and to be capable of recursive activation[9]. Although the mechanisms of conscious perception are uncertain, this recursive action, or resonance, could be a basis for conscious perception, such that, for a transient sensory input to be perceived or consciously appreciated, it must generate a lasting reverberation or reentrant signaling in thalamocortical systems. Thus, the ARAS modulates these oscillations both through its ascending projections to the thalamus, and through the more numerous corticothalamic projections, which outnumber the thalamocortical by a factor of 10, and may act to amplify these oscillations.

Synchronous activation of the specific and nonspecific thalamic projection systems is hypothesized to support conscious perception and to bind disparate sensory signals into one percept (Llinas, 2001). Whereas neither circuit alone may be capable of producing conscious sensory experience, concurrent summation of nonspecific and specific gamma-band activity (or resonance) may bind the context (nonspecific) and content (specific) of conscious sensory experience into one

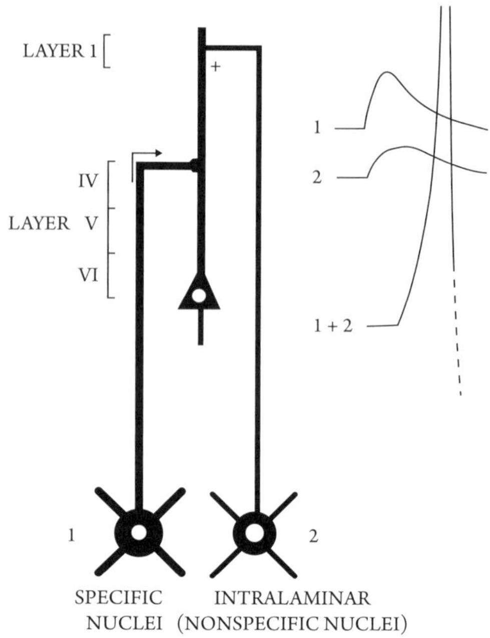

Figure 7.3 Generation of temporal binding due to coincident 40-Hz bursting activity within parallel thalamocortical projection systems arising from the RAS. A *nonspecific system* influences the responsiveness of cortical neurons to further stimulation via projections from the intralaminar thalamus to cortical layer VI, and *specific thalamocortical projections* convey sensory information via primary sensory relay thalamic nuclei to cortical layer IV. Pyramidal cells in layer V return projections to intralaminar nuclei via the reticular nucleus, forming a nonspecific thalamocortical loop, and those in layer VI return projections to sensory relay nuclei forming specific thalamocortical loops. (Llinás, Rodolfo R., *I of the Vortex: From Neurons to Self*, figure 6.2, p. 125, © 2001 Massachusetts Institute of Technology, by permission of The MIT Press.)

percept. Parallel activation of both pathways in the gamma-band range is required for optimal perception. Cortical and subcortical strokes that interfere with the coherence and resonance frequencies of specific and nonspecific processes may alter magnitude estimation. Increasing reticular input to intralaminar thalamus, either via sensory stimulation or medication, to increase arousal may help restore coherence and optimal performance(Woods et al., 2012; Meador, Ray, Day, & Loring, 2000). In fact, both sensory stimulation and arousal-enhancing medications can improve magnitude estimation and neglect.[10]

We now turn attention to studies in patients that inform understanding of the functional and anatomical architecture of magnitude estimation in neglect syndrome and other disorders.

Section 3. Contribution of Patient Studies to the Understanding of Functional and Anatomical Architecture of Magnitude Estimation and its Significance in Stroke

Investigators have known for decades that size perception is altered in patients with neglect (Gainotti & Tiacci, 1971; Milner, Harvey, Roberts, & Forster, 1993; Halligan & Marshall, 1991; Bisiach, Bulgarelli, Sterzi, & Vallar, 1983). This has been explained as a magnifying effect of focused attention on size perception and as unspecified "perceptual factors" that work to alter size estimation across a horizontal axis of space.

Magnitude estimation is at least one, if not the primary, perceptual factor accounting for altered size perception in neglect. Although, bias in magnitude estimation is exaggerated in neglect, it is not specific to patients with neglect or dependent on spatial attention. Both cerebral hemispheres calculate estimates of stimulus magnitude; however, factors such as arousal may produce different estimates of stimulus intensity that result in different behavioral abnormalities. Finally, altered perception of stimulus intensity may be a trans-disorder process that can help explain comorbidities in neglect. We now turn to the evidence for these statements in studies of stroke patients with neglect.

MAGNITUDE ESTIMATION IS ALTERED ACROSS SPATIAL AND NONSPATIAL PROTHETIC PERCEPTUAL CONTINUA FOLLOWING UNILATERAL STROKE

Prothetic refers to "how much" of something is perceived. A series of experiments in our laboratory examined how unilateral stroke alters estimates of stimulus magnitude. Results for several of these studies are summarized here for the first time. We reasoned that if magnitude estimation operates independently of spatial attention, representation, or movement, then it should be altered across prothetic perceptual continua regardless of whether they have inherent spatial qualities.

Magnitude estimates for 12 perceptual continua spanning six sensory modalities were examined in four groups of subjects (Table 7.1). Normal control subjects (NCS) included a total sample of 79 participants stratified by age (young = 19–34; middle = 35–65; and older = 65–80 years); however, stroke patients were statistically compared only with NCS between the ages of 35 and 80 (n=39). After screening stroke patients for sensory thresholds and the cognitive ability to perform magnitude estimation tests, the patient sample (n=34) included 13 participants with a unilateral right hemisphere lesion (RHL) due to stroke who *did not* have neglect (RHL^-) as defined by the Behavioral Inattention Test (Wilson, Cockburn, & Halligan, 1987), nine RHL participants

Table 7.1 **Magnitude Estimate Ranges for 12 Perceptual Continua Spanning Six Sensory Domains in Four Groups of Subjects**

Sensory Domain	*Perceptual Continua*	*Stimulus Description*	*Ranges of Stimulus Magnitudes*
Visual	Line length	Line lengths on a 94-×-555 cm sheet	10, 32, 60, 115, 170, 280, 390, 500 cm
	Area	Squares on a 240-×-240 cm sheet	100; 299; 605; 1,537; 2,894; 6,889; 12,589; 20,000 cm^2
	Numerosity	Dots on a 265-×-330 cm sheet	6, 10, 15, 22, 36, 50, 71, 90 dots
	Reflectance	Chips of light reflectance material 75 × 125 cm	84.2, 63.6, 46.8, 33, 22.19, 13.7, 7.7, 3.8% light reflectance
Tactile	Pressure (R & L)	Pressure cuff applied to forearm	20, 37, 54, 71, 88, 105, 122, 139 mmHg
	Von Frei (R & L)	Monofilaments applied to forefinger	0.6, 2, 6, 10, 26, 60, 100, 180 grams of force
	Roughness (R & L)	Textures of sand paper applied to fingertips	300; 700; 1,100; 1,280; 1,350; 1,400; 1,440; 1,476 grit
Proprio-ceptive	Finger span (R & L)	Wooden spacers between thumb and forefinger	4, 8, 14, 24, 34, 44, 54, 63 cm
Thermal	Temperature (R & L)	Heated disk (3.2 × 3.2 cm) presented to forearm	36, 38, 40, 42, 44, 46, 48, 50 ° F
Auditory	Loudness (R & L)	Tones presented to one ear- 1000Hz	35, 42, 49, 56, 63, 70, 77, 84 dB
Gustatory	Sweetness	Sugar concentrations diluted in water	0.15, 0.30, 0.60, 0.70, 0.80, 0.90, 1.05, 1.20 M
	Saltiness	Salt concentrations diluted in water	0.19, 0.25, 0.32, 0.46, 0.60, 0.74, 0.87, 1.00 M

who did have neglect (RHL$^+$), and 12 participants with a unilateral left hemisphere lesion (LHL) who did not have neglect. All stroke participants were tested at least one month after lesion onset. All four comparison groups were statistically equivalent with regard to gender, race, handedness, age, and education composition. General cognitive function was assessed with standardized tests of IQ (Axelrod, 2002), memory (Wechsler Memory Scale-Revised), language (Western Aphasia Battery), and executive functions. For each perceptual continuum, subjects rated the intensity of eight stimuli presented three times in random order, using numbers between 10 and 99 (low and high, respectively) without a modulus. Absolute and difference thresholds were tested for each continuum to ensure that subjects could both perceive and distinguish among all stimulus intensities presented and data were excluded if subjects did not meet criteria for sensory thresholds. Power function exponents, constants, and (r^2) values were derived for each subject in each continuum. Data were excluded if the r2 value was non-significant; indicating they did not fit a power function; this occurred in only a few subjects. Brain lesions were analyzed using subtraction techniques and volume analysis (Karnath, Fruhmann Berger, Kuker, & Rorden, 2004; Golay, Schnider, & Ptak, 2008) with the MRIcro and MRIcron software programs.

The following observations can be made concerning the results of the series of experiments involving normal control subjects and unilateral stroke subjects:

1. Power function parameters in normal control subjects (young, middle and older age groups) were not altered by age or gender. African American subjects had lower r^2 values (or greater variability in magnitude estimation) than non-African Americans. (Figure 7.4). Neither IQ nor education related to the size of exponents or constants. In general, lower scores on cognitive tests were associated with lower r^2 values.
2. Power function parameters were significantly different between normal control subjects and the patient groups. A significant between-group effect was found for the power function exponent ($F(3,69) = 7$, $p<.0001$). Planned contrasts showed that patients with right hemisphere lesions had lower exponents than normal control subjects and that the RHL+ group had lower exponents than RHL- group. A significant between group effect was also found for the constant ($F(3,69) = 6.4$, $p=.01$). Patients with right hemisphere lesions had significantly higher constants than did normal control subjects; however, the RHL+ group did not differ from the RHL- group. There was no difference between the LHL and NCS groups with regard to the exponent and constant. Finally, a significant between-group effect was found for the r^2 values ($F(3,69) = 22.1$, $p<.0001$). Whereas all patient data were determined to fit power functions prior to statistical analyses; all stroke patient groups had lower r^2 values than did the NCS group. Further, the RHL+ group had lower r2 values than any other group. (Figure 7.5).
3. Right hemisphere injury altered magnitude estimation across spatial and nonspatial perceptual continua (Figure 7.6). Interestingly, whereas effect sizes for visuo-spatial stimuli were small and moderate those for kinesthetic and some gustatory stimuli were very large. Large effect sizes were also observed

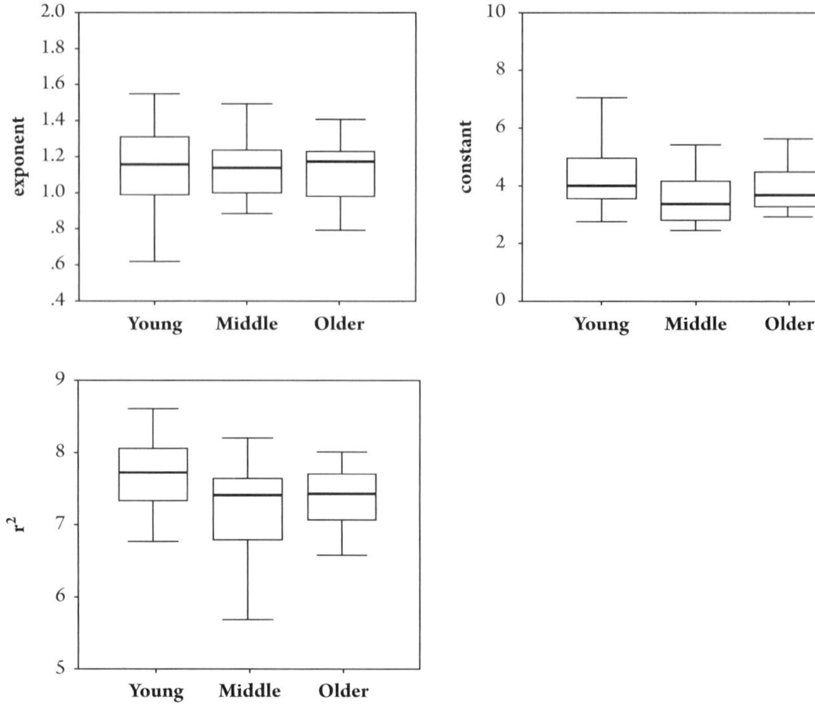

Figure 7.4 No alteration of power function parameters in normal control subjects by age. Box plots are shown for exponent, constant, and r^2 values across all 12 continua for all age groups. Error bars represent the highest and lowest values. The three horizontal lines forming the boxes represent the 25th, 50th, and 75th percentiles. Median values (dark lines) for exponent, constant, and r^2 values are similar across the age groups.

for stimuli presented to the ipsilesional as well as the contralesional side of the body.

4. Group differences in magnitude estimation were not simply due to cognitive impairment. Although LHL patients were impaired on tests of verbal IQ, executive function, memory, and language, compared to normal control subjects, they had normal power function exponents and constants. Conversely, RHL^- patients had close to normal cognitive scores, even though their power function parameters were altered relative to those of both NCS and LHL patients.
5. Lesion volume and subtraction analyses were completed using a total of 17 MRI and CT images obtained from patients with right hemisphere lesions. Lesion volume was approximately 2.5 times greater for the patients with right hemisphere lesions and neglect that for those without neglect (t=1.99, df=15, P<.06); however, no difference in lesion volume was associated with a decreased

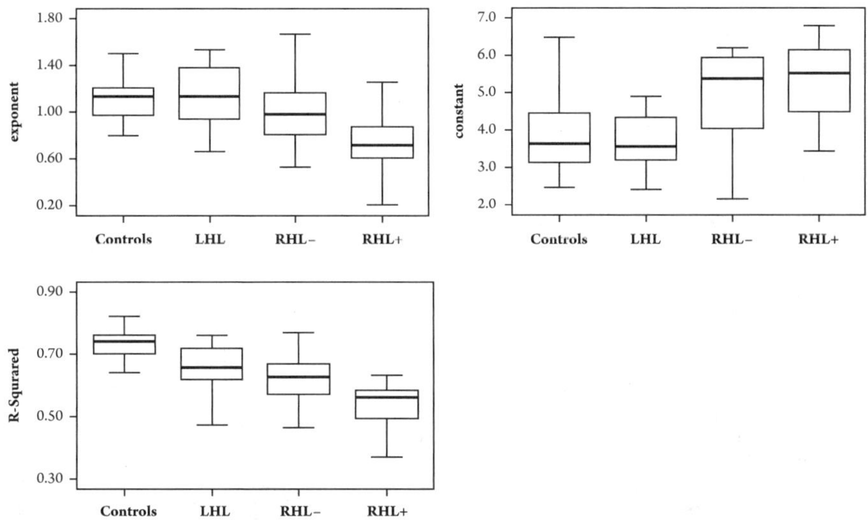

Figure 7.5 Power function parameters are significantly different between subject groups. Box plots of power function parameters are shown for each subject group. Unilateral stroke patients had lower r^2 values than controls and RHL$^+$ patients had lower r^2 values than any other group. Both RHL$^+$ and RHL$^-$ patients had lower exponent and higher constant values than normal controls and LHL patients who were not different from each other. The RHL+ group had significantly lower exponents that the RHL- group. (The details of the box plots are the same as those described in Figure 7.4.)

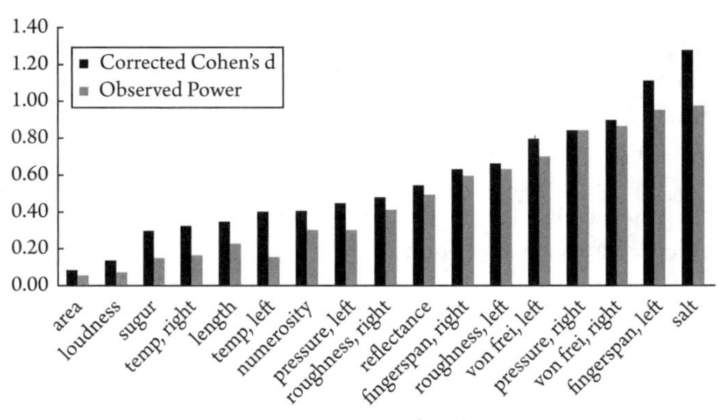

Figure 7.6 Magnitude estimation is altered across spatial and nonspatial perceptual continua following right hemisphere injury. Effect sizes (Cohen's *d corrected for sample size*) and the observed experimental power, calculated for the power function exponent, to discriminate between patients with right hemisphere lesions and normal control subjects is shown for each perceptual continuum. Moderate to large effect sizes were observed across a wide variety of kinesthetic, gustatory, somatosensory, and visual judgments.

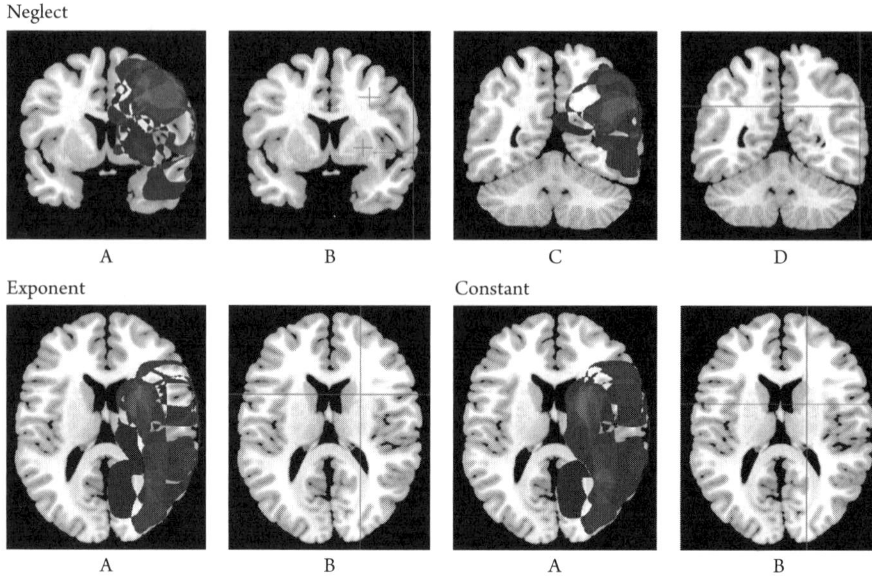

Figure 7.7 Results of a lesion subtraction analysis for 17 patients with right hemisphere lesions. The top row of pictures (Neglect) shows subtraction of RHL- from RHL+ scans. Brighter red areas indicate lesions common to RHL+ but not RHL-. Brighter blue indicates the opposite. Figure A shows brighter red areas—one involving white matter beneath BAs 6, 4 and 3 and another involving BA 38/21 in the anterior temporal lobe – and one area of brighter blue centered on the putamen. Crosshairs in figure B show the center of these areas, respectively. Figure C shows area of red overlap involving BA 39 with corresponding crosshair in Figure D. The bottom row of pictures (Exponents) show scans of RHL patients with normal or high power function exponents subtracted from those with decreased exponents and (Constants) of patients with normal or low constants subtracted from those with high constants. Figure A under exponent shows a brighter red area centered on the anterior limb of the internal capsule. [Similar involvement of the thalamic radiations was observed in higher slices (not shown).] Figure A under constant shows a brighter red area centered on the anterior limb and genu of the internal capsule (see color insert).

exponent (or an increased constant) independent of neglect status. Lesions involving Brodmann's Area (BA) 39 in the posterior parietal and BA 38/21 in the anterior temporal cortex and the white matter pathways beneath BA 6, 4, and 3 were more common among patients with neglect than patients without neglect. Lesions involving the putamen were more common among patients without neglect than those with neglect. (Figure 7.7). With regard to the power function exponent, lesions involving the anterior limb of the internal capsule and the superior thalamic radiations were more common among patients with a decreased power function exponent than those with either a normal or a high exponent. For the constant, lesions involving the anterior limb and genu of the internal capsule were more common in patients who had an increased constant but not in those patients who had either a normal or a decreased constant.

In summary, perception of stimulus intensity was altered across multiple perceptual systems and on both sides of the body. Whereas left and right hemisphere injury lead to greater variability in magnitude estimation; the power function constant was increased and the exponent decreased only in association with right hemisphere injury. Neglect was associated with a combination of deficits including an increased power function constant and an exponent that was significantly lower than in right hemisphere patients without neglect. Whereas neglect was associated with large lesions affecting cortical structures and white matter pathways, altered perception of stimulus intensity was associated with damage to fiber pathways that affect thalamocortical, corticothalamic, and corticofugal projections.

NEGLECT INVOLVES A COMBINATION OF DEFICITS IN PROTHETIC (NONSPATIAL) AND METATHETIC (e.g., SPATIAL) PERCEPTUAL CONTINUA

Robertson (Robertson, 1993) proposed that chronic unilateral neglect may require deficits in two types of attentional systems: one for spatial orientation and another for vigilance. A similar type of proposal can be made with regard to psychophysical judgment. In fact, psychophysical distinctions between judgments of "where" (metathetic) versus "how much" (prothetic) reveal conceptual problems for neuropsychological studies of neglect. Whereas most theories of neglect are designed to explain where neglect occurs in space (a metathetic continuum), most studies actually measure the amount of stimuli neglected (a prothetic continuum) as a dependent variable in experiments. This issue was addressed by Jewell (Jewell, 2003), working in our laboratory, by examining whether neglect represents a combination of deficits in estimating space and stimulus intensity. Magnitude estimates and category scales for the pitch and loudness of 1,000 Hz tones and for the area and spatial location of visual stimuli were examined in a prospective study of 32 subjects: 12 normal control subjects, 7 LHL, 6 RHL^-, and 7 RHL^+. Estimates of spatial location and pitch are considered metathetic because they fit linear functions and correspond to category scaling. In contrast, judgments of area and loudness are considered prothetic because they fit power functions and correspond to ratio scaling (Stevens & Galanter, 1957). Results of the prospective study indicated that neglect was associated with magnitude estimation deficits in both metathetic and prothetic continua (space, size, and loudness), whereas right hemisphere injury without neglect (RHL^-) was associated only with deficits in prothetic continua (loudness and size) (Figure 7.8). Effect sizes (Cohen's *d*) distinguishing normal control subjects from RHL subjects

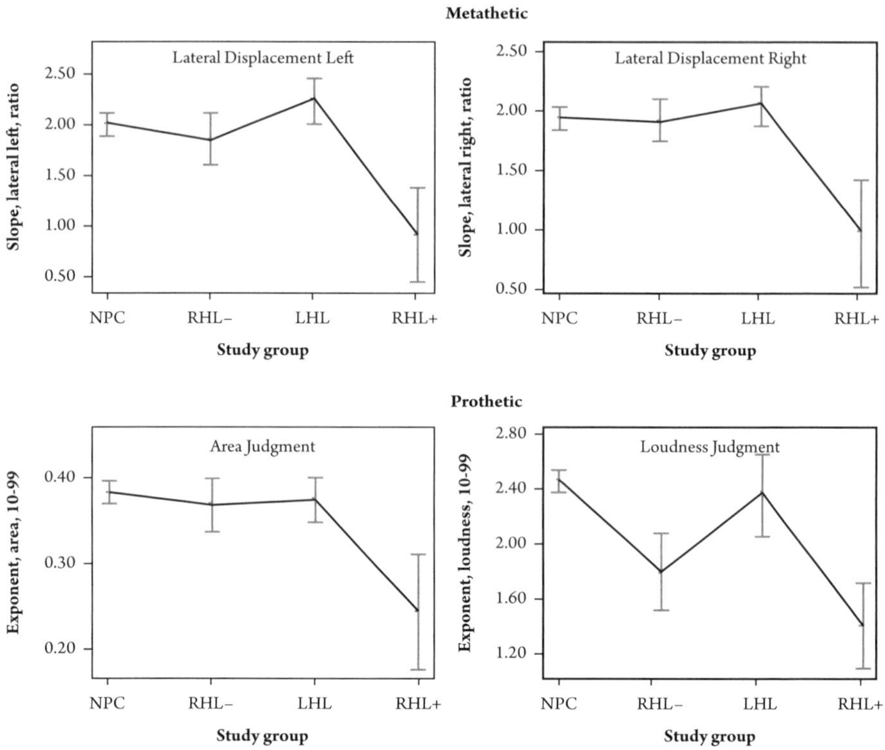

Figure 7.8 Deficits in both prothetic and metathetic perceptual continua are a distinguishing feature of neglect. Results of a prospective study involving 32 subjects (12 normal control subjects, 7 LHL, 6 RHL$^-$, and 7 RHL$^+$) indicated that neglect was associated magnitude estimation deficits in both metathetic and prothetic continua (space, size, and loudness); in contrast, RHL$^-$ was associated only with deficits in prothetic continua (loudness and size).

on the basis of loudness, area, and lateral displacement were .96, 1.25, and 1.6, respectively. All subject groups were equally adept at categorizing stimuli. Unfortunately, however, no subject group could distinguish pitch. Right hemisphere lesion volume and involvement of heteromodal association cortex were positively associated with both neglect and deficits in magnitude estimation. A combination of deficits in prothetic and metathetic perceptual continua may distinguish those with clinical signs of neglect from those without these signs.

THE LEFT CEREBRAL HEMISPHERE CONTRIBUTES TO MAGNITUDE ESTIMATION

Aphasia prevents many patients with large left hemisphere lesions from performing magnitude estimation studies. Consequently, it is not possible to create groups of RHL and LHL subjects who are equated on the basis of lesion location and volume. This issue was addressed in two case studies of magnitude estimation following left hemisphere injury (Woods et al., 2006).

Case 1. Patient B.G. was a 45-year-old, right-handed woman, a former registered nurse, who had expressive aphasia one year following a large, posterior middle cerebral artery infarction (Figure 7.9). She did not have neglect according to the Behavioral Inattention Test, but her brain lesion was typical of those associated with neglect following right hemisphere injury. She completed 7 of 12 perceptual continua tests by writing her responses. Her r^2 values fell below the 95 percent confidence limits of r^2 values obtained from normal control subjects (from the above mentioned study) in six of the seven continua that she completed. Additionally, values for her power function exponents fell below those of controls on four of the seven continua and exceeded these values on two of the seven. Sizes of the power function constants fell below those for controls on three of the seven continua and also exceeded these sizes on three of the seven.

Case 2. Patient J.W. was a 39-year-old, right-handed man with 13 years of education who had neglect acutely, without aphasia, following a following a putaminal hemorrhage of the left hemisphere. (Figure 7.10). His r^2 values were lower than those of normal control subjects in 11 of 12 perceptual continua tests. Sizes of his power function exponents fell below those of controls in 7 of 12 continua but exceeded 95 percent confidence limits on 2 of 12 continua. Power function

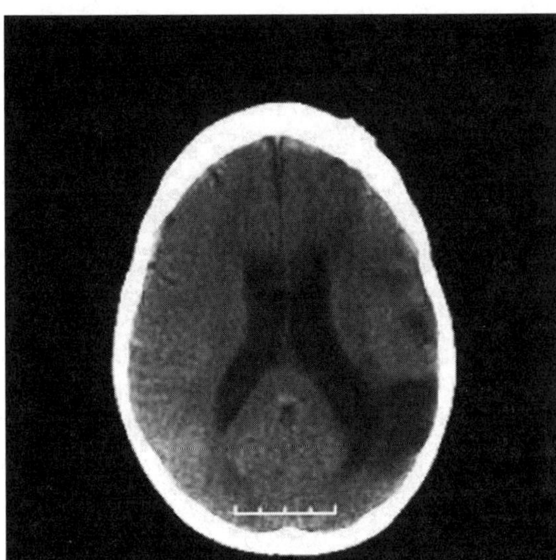

Figure 7.9 A large, posterior middle cerebral artery infarction in a 45-year-old, right-handed woman with expressive aphasia 1 year post-infarction.

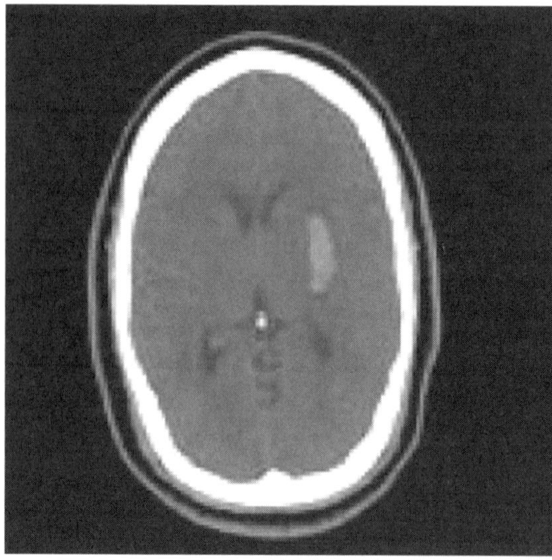

Figure 7.10 A hemorrhagic LHL in a 39-year-old, right-handed man who had neglect acutely, without aphasia.

constant sizes were lower than the 95 percent confidence limits for 6 of 12 continua and exceeded those of controls on one continuum.

These case studies are the first, to our knowledge, to show that left hemisphere injury can alter magnitude estimation in a manner similar, but not identical, to that observed following right hemisphere injury. In particular, values of the power function exponents were both increased and decreased following LHL, rather than decreasing, which is more typical following RHL. A similar pattern of results was observed in a group study of right and left hemisphere stroke patients that examined the relationship between perception of strength and stimulus intensity (Taylor-Cooke et al., 2006) (see next section).

MAGNITUDE ESTIMATES ARE OPPOSITE FOLLOWING LEFT AND RIGHT HEMISPHERE INJURIES

Falls by patients with neglect are commonly attributed to decreased awareness of weakness and to impulsivity (Webster et al., 1995; Rapport et al., 1993); however, the problem of altered strength perception after stroke has not been systematically studied. To examine this problem, we tested 13 patients with unilateral right hemisphere lesions and 6 with left hemisphere lesions while undergoing stroke rehabilitation. Only two patients in the RHL group had neglect; no patient had anosognosia. From these studies, we derived an index score of strength estimation accuracy (SEA) by comparing patients' ratings of contralesional limb strength to those of a physician and correlating them with power function exponents derived for length estimation on a bisection task. Line bisection was chosen because of previous experience with the test in stroke patients (Mennemeier et al., 2005). Strength perception of the contralateral limb was highly correlated with magnitude estimation for line length in both patient groups. Additionally, a subset of patients in the RHL group who had *decreased* power function exponents for length estimation *overestimated* contralateral limb strength, whereas a subset of patients in the LHL group who had *increased* exponents *underestimated* limb strength (Figure 7.11).

The results of this study suggest that altered strength perception may be quite common after a stroke, even in patients without frank neglect and anosognosia. Further, perception of strength and stimulus magnitude may be governed by a common neural mechanism. Finally, altered perception of strength after a stroke might help explain the abnormal reactions that patients sometimes have to stroke, such as a lack of concern shown by some patients with right hemisphere lesions (Starkstein, Federoff, Price, Leiguarda, & Robinson, 1992) and an over-concern or an extreme emotional response shown by some patients with left hemisphere lesions (Starkstein, Federoff, Price, Leiguarda, & Robinson, 1993). Together with functional imaging studies (Pinel, Piazza, LeBihan, & Dehaene, 2004), these patient studies indicate that both cerebral hemispheres generate magnitude estimates of stimulus intensity; however, lateralized brain injury may disrupt magnitude estimation in different ways. For example, left and right hemisphere lesions can have different affects on arousal (Heilman et al., 2003) which could alter magnitude estimation differently.

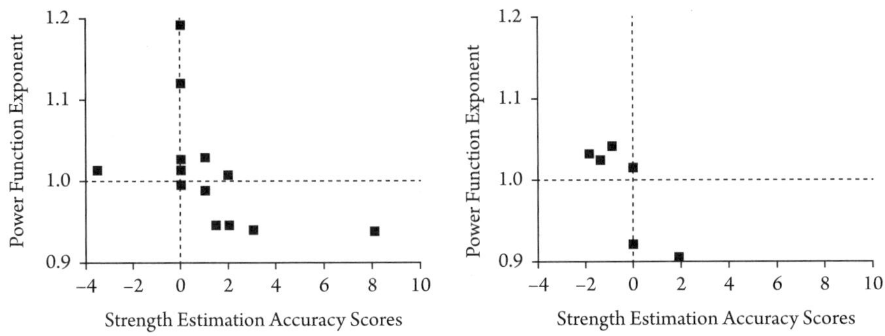

Figure 7.11 Strength estimation accuracy (SEA) scoring. A negative SEA score corresponded to underestimation of contralateral limb strength, and a positive score to overestimation, with a score of 0 indicating agreement between the estimations of patients and physician. The SEA score increased as the power function exponent for patients with right hemisphere stroke decreased (graph on **left**); in contrast, the SEA score decreased as the power function exponent increased in patients with left hemisphere stroke (graph on **right**: from Taylor-Cooke, et al 2006, figures 1 & 2, pages 1445 & 1446 respectively.

AROUSAL PROCESSES INFLUENCE MAGNITUDE ESTIMATION

Manipulations of arousal in patients with neglect, as described in the following case studies, demonstrates that arousal processes affect both stroke patients' estimation of the magnitude of stimulus intensity and behavioral symptoms of neglect.

Case 2 (Continued). In addition to deficits in magnitude estimation, patient J.W. was often drowsy during the day and even fell asleep during therapy when stimulation was minimal. He was given the psychostimulant modafinil (Provigil), 200 mg each morning, to increase arousal and alertness. Modafinil, with a half-life of 14–15 hours, is approved for the treatment of narcolepsy (McClellan & Spencer, 1998) and has been used experimentally to treat arousal deficits related to stroke (Sugden & Bourgeois, 2004; Smith, 2003). Both J.W.'s family and the rehabilitation staff reported a noticeable improvement in his alertness after he took modafinil. He was retested on tests of neglect and magnitude estimation 48 hours after taking his first dose (Woods et al., 2006). Figure 7.12 illustrates the positive effects of the drug on J.W.'s neglect on the cancellation test. His performance also normalized on all tests of magnitude estimation. These results suggest that medications designed to enhance arousal can improve neglect and related deficits in magnitude estimation.

Arousal can also be enhanced by nonpharmacological means. Irrigating the ear canal with either cold or warm water creates a temperature gradient across the tympanic membrane, precipitating caloric vestibular stimulation (CVS). CVS increases blood flow to heteromodal association areas, activates the striatum, thalamus, and midbrain (Chatterjee & Mennemeier, 1998), and thus can temporarily ameliorate neglect (Cappa, Sterzi, Vallar, & Bisiach, 1987; Storrie-Baker

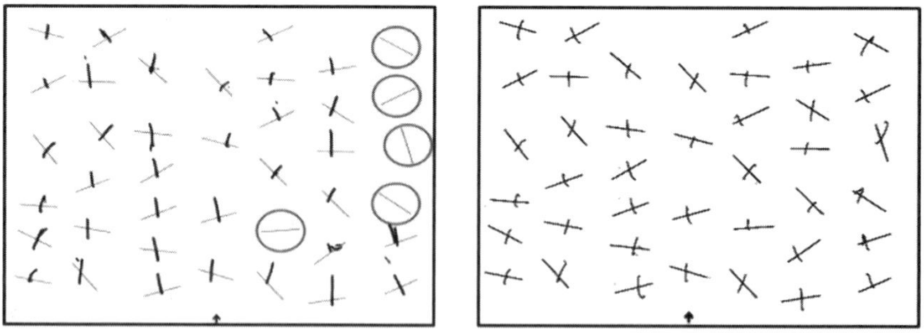

Figure 7.12 Effect of the psychostimulant modafinil on neglect in cancellation tests. **Left**, Before the start of modafinil therapy, patient J.W. neglected to cancel the circled lines. He performed normally on only 3 of 12 perceptual continua tests. **Right**, Forty-eight hours after taking his first dose, his performance on the cancellation text, as well as on 12 of 12 tests of magnitude estimation, normalized.

et al., 1997; Rubens, 1985). Although CVS is commonly thought to influence neglect via vestibular-mediated changes in spatial attention(Rubens, 1985), cold pressor stimulation (CPS) achieved by immersing a neglect patient's foot in ice water for 50 seconds can have the same ameliorating effect on magnitude estimation, neglect, alertness, and arousal. Both CVS and CPS may thus work by increasing arousal.

Case 3. Patient X was a 63-year-old woman with chronic left neglect 4 months after ischemic infarction of the frontotemporoparietal cortices of the right hemisphere (Woods et al. 2012). Magnitude estimation testing involved judgments of visual area and finger span of the right hand (see Table 7.1); a clock drawing test sought evidence for neglect, and a simple reaction time test examined alertness (Dinges, 1985). The amplitude of the P50 auditory evoked potential, a midlatency evoked response to a click sound recorded at the vertex (Robbins & Everitt, 1995; Kevanishivili & von Specht, 1979; Erwin & Buchwald, 1986b; Erwin & Buchwald, 1986a) was used to determine arousal. The amplitude is a measure of initial activation of reticular activating system (RAS) output.[11]

At baseline, exponents and constants of the power functions for visual area and finger span were altered on both tests of magnitude estimation; neglect was evident on the clock drawing test (Figure 7.13); and the patient's P50 amplitude was absent, and her reaction time slow (349 msec) (Figure 7.14). Immediately following CPS (immersion of her right foot in ice water for 50 sec), her P50 amplitude value normalized to 1.72 μV; her reaction time improved by 30 msec; her clock drawing became normal; and the power function parameters for finger span normalized: exponent, .38 vs. .64 (pre- vs. post-CPS; normal range, .69– .74); and constant, 5.88 vs. 3.5 (pre- vs. post-CPS; normal range, 3.3–4.3). Area judgment

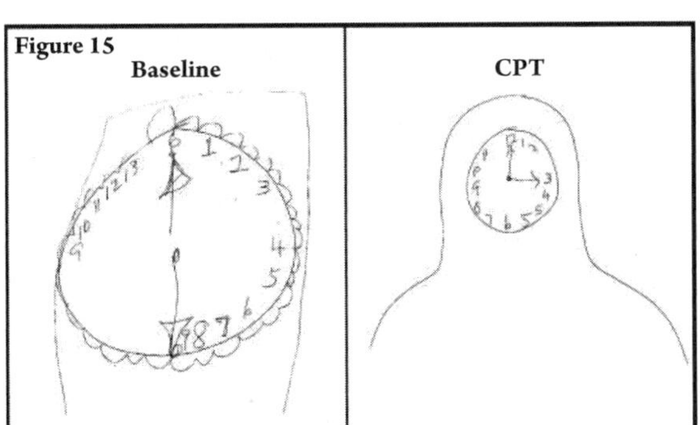

Figure 7.13 Clock drawing tests of patient X. **Left**, Neglect was evident at baseline. **Right**, A notable improvement followed the cold pressor stimulation (labeled CPT for cold pressor test) (from Woods, et al 2012, Figure 1, 5th page, reprinted by permission of the publisher (Taylor & Francis Ltd, http://www.tandf.co.uk/journals).

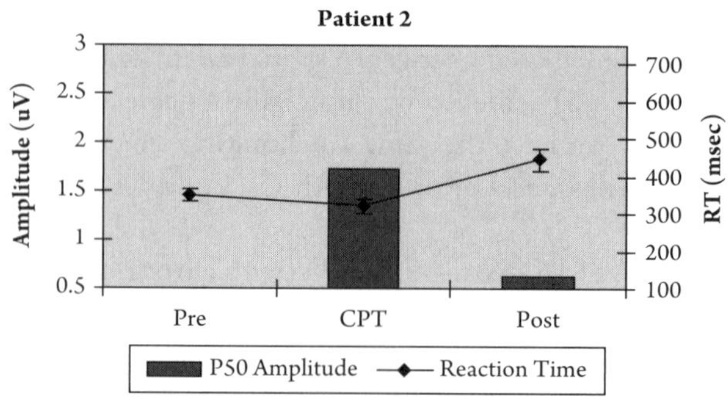

Figure 7.14 Arousal and alertness testing in patient X. The P50 amplitude was absent at baseline, and the patient's reaction time was slow (349 msec). Immediately following CPT, her P50 amplitude value normalized to a value of 1.72 μV, and her reaction time (RT) improved by 30 msec.

did not improve, possibly because this was the last test completed and the effect of CPS was waning. Twenty minutes after CPS, the P50 amplitude value was again below normal (.63 μV), and her reaction time increased by 100 msec over baseline (450 msec). Her fastest reaction time following CPS improved by only 4 percent from baseline, but the standard deviation improved 76 percent from baseline, indicating greater consistency. Variability is a significant contributor to the slow reaction times observed in patients with neglect (Anderson et al., 2000). These data converge to show improvement in neglect and magnitude estimation with improvement in arousal and alertness prompted by CPS. CPS also influences the P50 amplitude of normal subjects (Figure 7.15). Increasing arousal generally with CPS may "optimize" the P50 amplitude.

ALTERED PERCEPTION OF STIMULUS INTENSITY IS A TRANS-DISORDER PROCESS

Clinical studies show that neglect evident on the line bisection task predicts hospital falls during rehabilitation (Vlahov et al., 1990; Nyberg & Gustafson, 1997). The study of strength perception described above suggests a strong relationship between estimates of line length and strength perception. Further, patterns of length estimation that were opposite between patients with right and left hemisphere stroke were correlated with patterns of strength perception that were also opposite between patients with right and left hemisphere stroke. Deficits in magnitude estimation, therefore, may represent deficits common to both types of perception, but length estimation can manifest as a sign of neglect, whereas strength perception manifests as anosodiaphoria or anosognosia.

Symptoms of dysphagia may also be similar to those of neglect. For example, hemineglect in the pericutaneous buccal space (i.e., the mouth) has been described

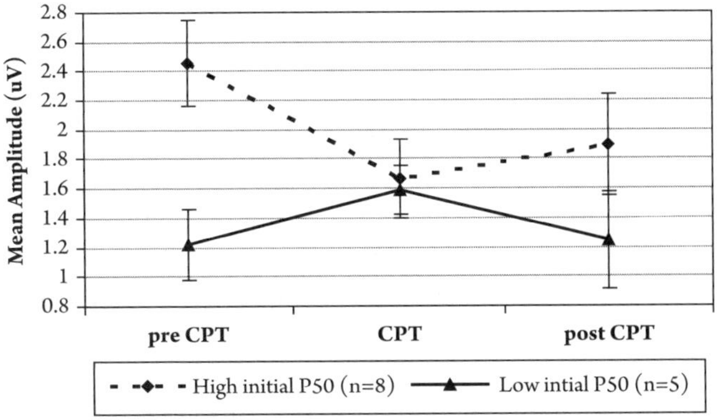

Figure 7.15 Effects of CPS on P50 amplitude in normal subjects. P50 amplitude and reaction times were obtained healthy, normal subjects, 10 men and 3 women, ranging in age from 20 to 28 years. The baseline range of P50 amplitude values was 1.0–3.5 μV, with a mean of 1.5 μV. Subjects were divided into two subsets according to whether their baseline P50 amplitude decreased or increased following CPS. Although one subgroup started with a high initial P50 amplitude and the other with a low initial amplitude, both groups exhibited the same P50 amplitude (1.6 μV) immediately following CPS. Twenty minutes after CPS, the P50 amplitude returned to its baseline level.

in monkeys following a contralateral lesions of area 6 corresponding to the post-arcuate cortex (Rizzolatti, Matelli, & Pavesi, 1983). Buccal hemineglect is also observed in humans in combination with the neglect syndrome, anosognosia, and parietal lesions (Andre et al., 2000), and is more common after right than left hemisphere injury. Clinical signs include impaired swallowing; failure to detect saliva or food in the hemibuccal cavity (usually the left); diminished taste sensation for salty, sweet, and acid tastes, with left-sided taste extinction; and impaired representation of the buccal cavity in drawings. In general, patients with right hemisphere stroke may have swallowing problems linked to a prolonged duration-of-stage transition (DST) (Robbins & Levine, 1998; John et al., 1998). One type of treatment, tactile thermal application (TTA), involves caloric stimulation, in which an ice stick or iced laryngeal mirror is rubbed on the anterior faucial pillars, to improve the onset of the pharyngeal swallow and temporarily reduce DST (Rosenbek, Roecker, Wood, & Robbins, 1996). TTA is similar to CVS, which temporarily improves neglect and magnitude estimation. Further, in a study of buccal hemineglect (Andre et al., 2000), CVS temporarily abolished all signs of buccal neglect in four subjects. Dysphagia, like altered perception of strength, is a common comorbidity of neglect. Altered perception of stimulus intensity in the buccal cavity may account for quantitative features of dysphagia, such as matching of the timing and strength of stage transitions to the volume of liquid and solid boluses in the buccal cavity, similarly to how it accounts for quantitative aspects of neglect.

Conclusions

Altered psychophysical function can manifest behaviorally as clinical symptoms of neglect, strength perception, and dysphagia. The strongest evidence for this conclusion can be found in patient studies of neglect. Whereas spatial theories are designed to explain where neglect occurs; altered psychophysical function can account for how much of something is neglected. Both explanations are necessary to account for the full range of neglect behavior. The psychophysical element of neglect has been emphasized in this chapter because it is not widely recognized as contributing to neglect behavior.

It is, admittedly, a peculiar proposal to ask readers to accept that altered psychophysical function can explain critical elements of neglect, and to then say, that this deficit is not specific to neglect, that it operates in parallel to spatial attention, representation and movement, and that the same deficit can manifest as elements of other clinical disorders which are commonly viewed as different from neglect. Where is the common ground? One basis for common ground is that perception of stimulus intensity explains quantitative elements of these other conditions as well as neglect. Another basis for common ground is that perception of stimulus intensity may be linked to changes in arousal following brain injury rather than to a specific clinical disorder. Arousal is a platform function that supports virtually all cognitive systems, so perceptual deficits related to fluctuations in arousal can conceivably influence behaviors as diverse as neglect on cancellation tests, swallowing and strength perception and perhaps many other functions. Consistent with this interpretation, we observed that psychophysical function is altered by stroke across multiple perceptual domains and in different clinical syndromes. Additionally, procedures designed to influence arousal can have ameliorative effects across multiple perceptual domains and behaviors including neglect, magnitude estimation and swallowing. One criticism of an explanation predicated on arousal is that it is not specific—increasing or optimizing arousal should improve cognitive function generally, and so, how can improvement in behaviors like neglect be attributed specifically to improvement in psychophysical function? No simple argument will dispel this criticism; rather, experiments are required to address the issue. The same criticism; however, can be made of the Yerkes-Dodson function that relates arousal and performance, yet somehow this criticism misses the point. It is probably more important to ask how fluctuations in arousal alter perception and how arousal deficits could be treated to improve neglect and related disorders.

Brain lesions that impair "arousal" presumably do so by disturbing the frequency, timing, or distribution of thalamocortical rhythms that facilitate conscious perception. Representations of sensory events formed under these abnormal circumstances may be more susceptible to bias, like contextual effects, which are normally present, but may alter the rate at which change in physical stimulus intensity is perceived. This change would alter the growth rate of power functions and presumably lead to behavioral abnormalities like under- or over-responding to stimulation. It is assumed here that perception of stimulus intensity is influenced by arousal in accordance with the Yerkes-Dodson function. Lateralized brain injury may have opposite effects on arousal, at least in some patients, that could alter perception of stimulus intensity in different ways and result in different behavioral abnormalities. So far, we have learned that lesions which affect the right cerebral hemisphere and cause hypoarousal are associated with a restricted range of perception such that greater stimulus intensities are underestimated and lesser intensities are overestimated. This pattern of bias is signaled by a decreased power function exponent and an increased constant and the associated behavioral manifestation is evident, for example, in the crossover effect on line bisection. In contrast, lesions of the left hemisphere might induce an opposite form of bias in some patients characterized by increased arousal and power function exponents that are elevated relative to normal. The behavior associated with this pattern of bias was underestimating limb strength. Finally, understanding the relationship between arousal, perception, and behavior may influence treatment. Caloric stimulation and arousal-enhancing medication, for example, can improve perception of stimulus intensity in hypoaroused patients. Caloric stimulation may impose fast oscillations on thalamocortical pathways via the peripheral sensory system that improves neglect, magnitude estimation, and dysphagia temporarily. Medications like modafanil might enhance thalamocortical activity chronically via intracortical mechanisms such as increasing gap junctions between cortical interneurons.

Notes

1. Hypersomnia is marked by excessive daytime sleepiness, inability to stay awake, and/or prolonged nighttime sleep due to decreased wakefulness, enhanced sleep mechanisms, or both.
2. The anterior cingulate gyrus may influence arousal systems in anticipation and preparation of responses; the dorsolateral frontal cortex may maintain and regulate cortical arousal over time by activating noradrenergic nuclei in the brainstem via the reticular nucleus of the thalamus; and the inferior parietal cortex may modulate arousal in response to stimulus processing via projections to the reticular nucleus(Sturm & Willmes, 2001).
3. Sensory perceptual deficits are most commonly evaluated for proprioception (with up to 52 percent of patients estimated to be affected), vibration (44 percent affected), light touch (37 percent affected), and loss of pinprick sensation (35 percent affected) (Hunter & Crome, 2002These deficits are as common, persistent, and debilitating (Fasoli & McKenna, 2007; Sullivan & Hedman, 208) as is motor impairment, with prevalence rates among stroke patients as high as 60 percent to 85 percent (Fasoli & McKenna, 2007) (Yekutiel, 2000) (Moskowitz, Lightbody F.E., & Freitag, 1972) (Kent, 1965) (Kim & Choi-Kwon, 1996).
4. In practice, it is debated whether the conditions for ratio scaling are ever satisfactorily achieved, so the term *magnitude estimation* will be used instead of ratio scaling after this introduction.

5. The term *perceptual continua* merely refers to the types of sensation under study, such as length, brightness, roughness, saltiness, etc.
6. Because lesser stimuli in the range of intensities, on average, are preceded by stimuli with higher intensities, and vice versa, contextual bias causes lesser stimuli to be overestimated and greater stimuli be underestimated (Cross, 1973).
7. Slow oscillations, which may have an intracortical origin, are present during sleep and anesthesia. Delta oscillations are slow rhythms which have cortical and thalamic origins and are believed to play a role in memory consolidation. Sleep spindles are slow rhythms which occur in intervals that may originate from an interaction between thalamic reticular and relay cells. Spindle oscillations are observed in association with early stage sleep and slow oscillations and play a role in memory formation.
8. Beta-gamma oscillations may have both extracortical origins, imposed by fast oscillations originating in peripheral motor and sensory systems, and intracortical mechanisms including intrinsic properties of fast rhythmic bursting neurons, activities of inhibitory interneurons, and gap junctions between axons of pyramidal cells.
9. The mechanism behind the 40 Hz rhythm appears to include layer IV cortical inhibitory interneurons which exhibit a sequential activation of a persistent low threshold sodium current followed by a subsequent potassium conductance. These cells can transmit the 40 Hz rhythm onto thalamic cells, allowing the entrainment of thalamocortical resonance.
10. Neglect is responsive to vestibular stimulation (Rubens, 1985), visual cues, and vibrotactile, optokinetic, and rotational stimulation(Pierce & Buxbaum, 2002). Amphetamine, methylphenidate, and bromocriptine have been used to improve arousal in neglect (Chatterjee & Mennemeier, 1998; Pierce & Buxbaum, 2002).
11. The P50 potential diminishes and disappears with progressively deeper stages of slow-wave sleep and is blocked by scopolamine. Its reappearance during REM sleep suggests that one generator is functionally related to states of arousal and modulated by cholinergic mesopontine cell groups (Buchwald, Rubenstein, Schwafel, & Strandburg, 1991; Erwin & Buchwald, 1986b; Garcia-Rill, 1997).

References

Adair, J. C., Na, D. L., Schwartz, R. L., & Heilman, K. M. (1998). Analysis of primary and secondary influences on spatial neglect. *Brain and Cognition, 37*, 351–367.

Adair, J. C., Schwartz, R. L., & Barrett, A. M. (2003). Anosognosia. In K. M. Heilman & E. Valenstein (eds.), *Clinical Neuropsychology* (4th ed., pp. 185–214). New York: Oxford University Press.

Albert, M. L. (1973). A simple test of visual neglect. *Neurology, 23*, 658–664.

Albert, M. L., Silverberg, R., Reches, A., & Berman, M. (1976). Cerebral Dominance for Consciousness. *Archives of Neurology, 33*, 453–454.

Algom, D., & Marks, L. E. (1990). Range and regression, loudness scales, and loudness processing. Toward a context-bound psychophysics. *Journal of Experimental Psychology Human Perception and Performance, 16*, 706–727.

Anderson, B., Mennemeier, M., & Chatterjee, A. (2000). Variability not ability: another basis for performance decrements in neglect. *Neuropsychologia, 38*, 785–796.

Andre, J. M., Beis, J. M., Morin, N., & Paysant, J. (2000). Buccal Hemineglect. *Archives of Neurology, 57*, 1734–1741.

Axelrod, B. N. (2002). Validity of the Wechsler Abbreviated Scale of Intelligence and Other Very Short Forms of Estimating Intellectual Functioning. *Assessment, 9*, 17–23.

Barer, D. H. (1989). The natural history and functional consequences of dysphagia after hemispheric stroke. *Journal of Neurology, Neurosurgy, & Psychiatry, 52*, 236–241.

Bassetti, C. (2001). Disturbances of consciousness and sleep-wake functions. In J. Bogousslavsky & L. R. Caplan (eds.), *Stroke Syndromes* (pp. 192–210). Cambridge: University Press.

Bazhenov, M., & Timofee, I. (2006). Thalamocortical oscillations. *Scholarpedia, 1*(6), 1319 [On-line at http://www.scholarpedia.org/article/Thalamocortical_oscillations, retrieved 9-24-2009].

Bisiach, E. (1993). Mental representation in unilateral neglect and related disorders: The twentieth Barlett Memorial Lecture. *Quarterly Journal of Experimental Psychology, 46A*, 435–461.

Bisiach, E., Bulgarelli, C., Sterzi, R., & Vallar, G. (1983). Line bisection and cognitive plasticity of unilateral neglect of space. *Brain and Cognition, 2*, 32–38.

Bisiach, E., Geminiani, G., Berti, A., & Rusconi, M. L. (1990). Perceptual and premotor factors of unilateral neglect. *Neurology, 40*, 1278.

Bisiach, E., & Luzzatti, C. (1978). Unilateral neglect of representational space. *Cortex, 14*, 129–133.

Bisiach, E., Rusconi, M. L., Peretti, V. A., & Vallar, G. (1994). Challenging current accounts of unilateral neglect. *Neuropsychologia, 32*, 1431–1434.

Buchwald, J. S., Rubenstein, E. H., Schwafel, J., & Strandburg, R. J. (1991). Midlatency auditory evoked responses: Differential effects of a cholinergic agonist and antagonist. *Electroencephalography and Clinical Neurophysiology, 80*, 303–309.

Cappa, S., Sterzi, R., Vallar, G., & Bisiach, E. (1987). Remission of hemineglect and anosognosia during vestibular stimulation. *Neuropsychologia, 25*, 775–782.

Cappelletti, M., Barth, H., Fregni, F., Spelke, E., & Pascual-Leone, A. (2007). rTMS over the intraparietal sulcus disrupts numerosity processing. *Experimental Brain Research, 179*, 631–642.

Carey, L. (1995). Somatosensory loss after stroke. *Critical Reviews in Physical and Rehabilitation Medicine, 7*, 51–91.

Carpenter, M. B. (1976). *Human Neuroanatomy*. (7th ed.) Baltimore: Waverly Press.

Chatterjee, A. (1995). Cross-over, completion and confabulation in unilateral spatial neglect. *Brain, 118*, 455–465.

Chatterjee, A., & Mennemeier, M. (1998). Diagnosis and treatment of spatial neglect. In R. B. Lazar (ed.), *Principles of neurologic rehabilitation* (pp. 597–612). New York: McGraw-Hill.

Chatterjee, A., Mennemeier, M., & Heilman, K. M. (1992a). A stimulus-response relationship in unilateral negelct: the power function. *Neuropsychologia, 30*, 1101–1108.

Chatterjee, A., Mennemeier, M., & Heilman, K. M. (1992b). Search patterns and neglect: a case study. *Neuropsychologia, 30*, 657–672.

Chatterjee, A., Thompson, K. A., & Ricci, R. (1998). Weigh(t)ing for awareness. *Brain and Cognition, 37*, 477–409.

Coslett, H. B., Bowers, D., Fitzpatrick, E., Haws, B., & Heilman, K. M. (1990). Directional hypokinesia and hemispatial inattention in neglect. *Brain, 113*, 475–486.

Coslett, H. B., Bowers, D., & Heilman, K. M. (1987). Reduction in cerebral activation after right hemisphere stroke. *Neurology, 37*, 957–962.

Cross, D. V. (1973). Sequential dependencies and regression in psychophysical judgments. *Perception and Psychophysics, 14*, 547–552.

Cucchiara, B., Kasner, S. E., Wolk, D. A., Lyden, P. D., Knappertz, V. A., Ashwood, T. et al. (2003). Lack of hemispheric dominance for consciousness in acute ischaemic stroke. *Journal of Neurology, Neurosurgery, and Psychiatry, 74*, 889–892.

Dinges, P. (1985). Microcomputer analyses of performance on a portable, simple visual RT task during sustained operations. *Behavior Research Methods, 17*, 652–655.

Erwin, R. J., & Buchwald, J. S. (1986a). Midlatency auditory evoked responses: differential effects of sleep in the human. *Electroencephalography and Clinical Neurophysiology, 65*, 383–392.

Erwin, R. J., & Buchwald, J. S. (1986b). Midlatency auditory evoked responses: Differential recovery cycle characteristics. *Electroencephalography and Clinical Neurophysiology, 64*, 417–423.

Farne, A., Buxbaum, L. J., Ferraro, M., Frassinetti, F., Whyte, J., Veramonti, T. et al. (2004). Patterns of spontaneous recovery of neglect and associated disorders in acute right brain-damaged patients. *Journal of Neurology, Neurosurgery, and Psychiatry, 75*, 1401–1410.

Fasoli, D. S., & McKenna, K. T. (2007). Interventions for sensory impairment in the upper limb after stroke (protocol). *Cochrane Database of Systematic Reviews*, 1–8.

Fuller, P. M., Gooley, J. J., & Saper, C. B. (2006). Neurobiology of the Sleep-Wake Cycle: Sleep Architecture, Circadian Regulation, and Regulatory Feedback. *Journal of Biological Rhythms, 21*, 482–493.

Gainotti, G., & Tiacci, C. (1971). The relationships between disorders of visual perception and unilateral spatial neglect. *Neuropsychologia, 9*, 451–458.

Garcia-Rill, E. (1997). Disorders of the reticular activating system. *Med Hypoth, 49*, 379–387.

Garcia-Rill, E. (2009a). Reticular Activating System. In L. R. Squire (ed.), *Encyclopedia of Neuroscience* (pp. 137–143). Oxford: Academic Press.

Garcia-Rill, E. (2009b). Sleep and arousal states: reticular activating system. In L. R. Squire, F. E. Bloom, N. Spitzer, F. Gage, & Albright, T. (eds.), *New Encyclopedia of Neuroscience* (pp. 137–143). Oxford: Elsevier.

Gescheider, G. A. (1997a). Psychophysical ratio scaling. In G. A. Gescheider (ed.), *Psychophysics: the fundamentals* (3 ed., pp. 231–263). Mahwah: Lawrence Erlbaum Associates.

Gescheider, G. A. (1997b). *Psychophysics: the fundamentals.* London: Lawrence Erlbaum Associates.

Golay, L., Schnider, A., & Ptak, R. (2008). Cortical and subcortical anatomy of chronic spatial neglect following vascular damage. *Behavioral and Brain Functions, 4*, 43.

Gordon, C., Hewer, R. L., & Wade, D. T. (1987). Dysphagia in acute stroke. *British Medical Jounral (Clinical Research Edition)., 295*, 411–414.

Halligan, P. W., & Marshall, J. C. (1991). Figural modulation of visuo-spatial neglect: a case study. *Neuropsychologia, 29*, 619–628.

Halligan, P. W., & Marshall, J. C. (1988). How long is a piece of string? A study of line bisection in a case of visual neglect. *Cortex, 24*, 321–328.

Heilman, K. M., Blonder, L. X., Bowers, D., & Valenstein, E. (2003). Emotional disorders associated with neurological diseases. In K. M. Heilman & E. Valenstein (eds.), *Clinical Neuropsychology* (4 ed., pp. 447–478). New York: Oxford University Press.

Heilman, K. M., Schwartz, H. D., & Watson RT (1978). Hypoarousal in patients with the neglect syndrome and emotional indifference. *Neurology, 28*, 229–232.

Heilman, K. M., & Valenstein, E. (1972). Frontal lobe negelect in man. *Neurology, 22*, 660–664.

Heilman, K. M., & Van Den Able, T. (1980). Right hemisphere dominance for attention: the mechanism underlying hemispheric asymmetries of inattention. *Neurology, 30*, 327–330.

Heilman, K. M., Watson, R. T., & Valenstein, E. (1985). Neglect and related disorders. In K. M. Heilman & E. Valenstein (eds.), *Clinical Neuropsychology* (2 ed., pp. 243–293). New York: Oxford University Press.

Hollingworth, H. L. (1909). The indifference point. In H. L. Hollingworth (ed.), *The inaccuracy of movement* (pp. 21–39). New York: The Science Press.

Hunter, S. M., & Crome, P. (2002). Hand function and stroke. *Reviews in Clinical Gerontology, 12*, 66–81.

Husain, M., & Rorden, C. (2003). Non-spatially lateralized mechanisms in hemispatial neglect. *Nature Reviews Neuroscience, 4*, 26–36.

Jewell, G. (2003). *Psychophysical scaling of prothetic and metathetic continua in lateralized brain injury and neglect: where and how much?* Dissertation for the Doctor of Philosophy Degree in the Department of Psychology University of Alabama at Birmingham. Graduate School, University of Alabama at Birmingham.

Rosenbek, J. C., Robbins, J., Willford, W. O., Kirk, G., Schiltz, A., Sowell, T. W.,…, Hansen, J. E. (1998). Comparing Treatment Intensities of Tactile-Thermal Application. *Dysphagia, 13*, 1–9.

Karnath, H. O., Ferber, S., & Himmelbach, M. (2001). Spatial awareness is a function of the temporal not the posterior parietal lobe. *Nature,411 (6840)*, 950–953.

Karnath, H. O., Fruhmann Berger, M., Kuker, W., & Rorden, C. (2004). The anatomy of spatial neglect based on voxelwise statistical analysis: A study of 140 patients. *Cerebral Cortex, 14,* 1164–1172.

Karnath, H. O., Himmelbach, M., & Rorden, M. (2002a). The subcortical anatomy of human spatial neglect; putamen, caudate nucleus and pulvinar. *Brain, 125,* 350–360.

Karnath, H. O., Himmelbach, M., & Rorden, C. (2002b). The subcortical anatomy of human spatial neglect: putamen, caudate nucleus and pulvinar. *Brain, 125,* 350–360.

Kent, B. (1965). Sensory-motor testing: the upper limb of adult patients with hemiplegia. *Physical Therapy, 45,* 550–561.

Kerkhoff, G. (2001). Spatial hemineglect. *Progress in Neurobiology, 63,* 1–27.

Kevanishivili, Z., & von Specht, H. (1979). Human auditory evoked potentials during natural and drug-induced sleep. *Electroencephalography and Clinical Neurophysioly, 47,* 280–288.

Kim, J. S., & Choi-Kwon, S. (1996). Discriminative sensory dysfunction after unilateral stroke. *Stroke, 27,* 677–682.

Kim, M., Schwartz, R. L., & Heilman, K. M. (1999). Pupillographic findings in neglect. *Journal of Neurology, Neurosurgery, and Psychiatry, 67,* 82–85.

Kinsbourne, M. (1970). The cerebral basis of lateral asymmetries in attention. *Acta Psychologica, 33,* 193–201.

Kinsbourne, M. (1993). Orientation bias model of unilateral neglect: evidence from attentional gradients within hemispace. In I. H. Robertson & J. C. Marshal (eds.), *Unilateral neglect: clincal and experimental studies.* (pp. 63–86). UK: Hove.

Ladavas, E. (1987). Is the hemispatial deficit produced by right parietal lobe damage associated with retinal or gravitational co-ordinates? *Brain, 110,* 167–180.

Llinas, R. (2001). *The I of the vortex, from neurons to self.* Cambridge: MIT Press.

Llinas, R., Ribary, U., Contreras, D., & Pedroarena, C. (1998). The neuronal basis for consciousness. *Philosophical Transactions of the Royal Society of London,* 1841–1849.

Marshall, J. C., & Halligan, P. W. (1989). When right goes left: an investigation of line bisection in a case of visual neglect. *Cortex, 25,* 503–515.

Marshall, R. S., Lazar, R. M., Krakauer, J. W., & Sharma, R. (1998). Stimulus contex in hemineglect. *Brain, 121,* 2003–2010.

McClellan, K. C., & Spencer, C. M. (1998). Modafinil: a review of its pharmacology and clinical efficacy in the management of narcolepsy. *CNS Drugs, 9,* 311–324.

Meador, K. J., Ray, P. G., Day, L. J., & Loring, D. W. (2000). Train Duration Effects on Perception: Sensory Deficit, Neglect, and Cerebral Lateralization. *Journal of Clinical Neurophysiology, 17,* 406–413.

Mennemeier, M., Pierce, C. A., Chatterjee, A., Anderson, B., Jewell, G., Dowler, R. et al. (2005). Bias in attentional orientation and magnitude estimation explain crossover: neglect is a disorder of both. *Journal of Cognitive Neuroscience, 17,* 1194–1211.

Mennemeier, M., Rapcsak, S. Z., Dillon, M., & Vezey, E. (1998). A search for the optimal stimulus. *Brain and Cognition, 37,* 439–459.

Mennemeier, M., Vezey, E., Lamar, M., & Jewell, G. (2002). Crossover is not a consequence of neglect. *Journal of the International Neuropsychological Society, 8,* 107–114.

Mesulam, M. (1981). A cortical network for directed attention and unilateral neglect. *Annals of Neurology, 10,* 309–325.

Milner, A. D., Harvey, M., Roberts, R. C., & Forster, S. V. (1993). Line bisection errors in visual neglect: misguided action or size distortion? *Neuropsychologia, 31,* 39–49.

Mohr, J. P., & Barnett, J. M. (1986). Classification of ischemic strokes. In H. J. M. Barnett, J. P. Mohr, B. M. Stein, & F. M. Yatsu (eds.), *Stroke, pathophysiology, diagnosis, and management* (pp. 281–291). New York: Churchill Livingstone.

Monaghan, P., & Shillcock, R. (1998). The cross-over effect in unilateral neglect. Modelling detailed data in the line-bisection task. *Brain, 121,* 907–921.

Morrow, L., Vrtunski, K., Kim, Y., & Boller, F. (1981). Arousal responses to emotional stimuli and laterality of lesion. *Neuropsychologia, 19,* 65–71.

Moskowitz, E., Lightbody, F. E., & Freitag, N. S. (1972). Long-term follow-up of the poststroke patient. *Archives of Physical Medicine and Rehabilitation, 53*, 167–172.

Na, D. L., Adair, J. C., Williamson, D. J. G., Schwartz, R. L., Haws, B., & Heilman, K. M. (1998). Dissociation of sensory-attentional from motor-intentional neglect. *Journal of Neurology, Neurosurgery, and Psychiatry, 64*, 331–338.

Nolte, J. (2009). *The Human Brain: an introduction to its functional anatomy.* (6th ed.) Philadelphia: Mosby Elsevier.

Nyberg, L., & Gustafson, Y. (1997). Fall Prediction Index for Patients in Stroke Rehabilitation. *Stroke, 28*, 716–721.

Ogden, J. A. (1987). The neglected left hemisphere and its contribution to visuo-spatial neglect. In M. Jeannerod (ed.), *Neurophysiological and neuropsychological aspects of spatial neglect* (1st ed., pp. 215–234). Amsterdam: North-Holland.

Pare Denis & Llinas, R. (1995). Conscious and pre-conscious processes as seen from the standpoint of sleep-waking cycle neurophysiology. *Neuropsychologia, 33*, 1155–1168.

Pierce, S. R., & Buxbaum, L. J. (2002). Treatments of unilateral neglect: a review. *Archives of Physical Medicine and Rehabilitation, 83*, 256–268.

Pinel, P., Piazza, M., Biham, D. L., & Dehaene, S. (2004). Distributed and overlapping cerebral representations of number, size and luminance during comparative judgments. *Neuron, 41*, 983–993.

Pinel, P., Piazza, M., LeBihan, D. L., & Dehaene, S. (2004). Distributed and overlapping cerebral representations of number, size and luminance during comparative judgments. *Neuron, 41*, 983–993.

Posner, M. I., & Boies, S. J. (1971). Components of attention. *Psychological Review, 78*, 391–408.

Posner, M. I., & Dehaene, S. (1994). Attentional networks. *Trends in Neuroscience, 17*, 75–79.

Posner, M. I., & Rafal, R. D. (1987). Cognitive theories of attention and the rehabilitation of attentional deficits. In M. J. Meier, A. L. Benton, & L. Diller (eds.), *Neuropsychological Rehabilitation* (pp. 182–201). Edinburgh: Churchhill Livingstone.

Poulton, E. C. (1979). Models for biases in judging sensory magnitude. *Psychological Bulletin, 86*, 777–803.

Poulton, E. C. (1968). The new psychophysics: six models for magnitude estimation. *Psychological Bulletin, 69*, 1–19.

Rand, D., Gottlieb, D., & Weiss, P. (2001). Recovery of patients with a combined motor and proprioception deficit during the first six weeks of post stroke rehabilitation. *Physical and Occupational Therapy in Geriatrics, 18*, 69–87.

Rapport, L. J., Webster, J. S., Flemming, K. L., Lindberg, J. W., Godlewski, M. C., Brees, J. E. et al. (1993). Predictors of falls among right-hemisphere stroke patients in the rehabilitation setting. *Archives of Physical Medicine and Rehabilitation, 74*, 621–626.

Ringman, J. M., Saver, J. L., Woolson, R. F., Clarke, W. R., & Adams, H. P. (2004). Frequency, risk factors, anatomy, and course of unilateral neglect in an acute stroke cohort. *Neurology, 63*, 468–474.

Rizzolatti, G., & Berti, A. (1993). Neural mechanisms of spatial neglect. In I. H. Robertson & J. C. Marshal (eds.), *Unilateral neglect: clinical and experimental studies* (1 ed., Hove-UK: Lawrence Erlbaum Associates.

Rizzolatti, G., Matelli, M., & Pavesi, G. (1983). Deficits in Attention and Movement Following the Removal of Postarcuate (Area 6) And Prearcuate (Area 8) Cortex in Macaque Monkeys. *Brain, 106*, 655–673.

Robbins, J. A., & Levine, R. L. (1998). Swallowing after unilateral stroke of the cerebral cortex: preliminary experience. *Dysphagia, 3*, 11–17.

Robbins, T. W., & Everitt, B. J. (1995). Arousal systems and attention. In M. Gazzaniga (ed.), *The cognitive neurosciences* (pp. 703–720). Cambridge: MIT Press.

Robertson, I. H. (1993). The relationship between lateralized and non-lateralized attentional deficits in unilateral neglect. In I. H. Robertson & J. C. Marshall (eds.), *Unilateral neglect: clinical and experimental studies.* (pp. 257–275). Hove: Lawrence Erlbaum.

Robertson, I. H. (2001). Do we need the "lateral" in unilateral neglect? Spatially nonselective attention deficits in unilateral negelct and their implications for rehabilitation. *Neuroimage, 14*, S85–S90.

Robertson, I. H., & Garavan, H. (2004). Vigilant Attention. In M. S. Gazzaniga (ed.), *The Cognitive Neurosciences III* (3 ed., pp. 631–640). Cambridge: MIT Press.

Robertson, S. L., & Jones, L. A. (1994). Tactile sensory impairment and prehensile function in subjects with left hemisphere cerebral lesions. *Archives of Physical Medicine and Rehabilitation, 75*, 1108–1117.

Rosenbek, J. C., Roecker, E. B., Wood, J. L., & Robbins, J. (1996). Thermal application reduces the duration of stage transition in dysphagia after stroke. *Dysphagia, 11*, 225–233.

Rubens, A. B. (1985). Caloric stimulation and unilateral visual neglect. *Neurology, 35*, 1019–1024.

Samuelsson, H., Hjelmquist, E. K., Jenson, C., Ekholm, S., & Blomstrand, C. (1998). Nonlateralized attention deficits; an important component behind persisting visuospatial neglect. *Journal of Clinical & Experimental Neuropsychology, 20*, 73–88.

Smith, B. (2003). Modafinil for treatment of cognitive side effects of antiepileptic drugs in a patient with seizures and stroke. *Eplilepsy & Behavior, 4*, 352–353.

Starkstein, S. E., Federoff, J. P., Price, T. R., Leiguarda, R., & Robinson, R. G. (1992). Anosogosia in patients with cerebrovascular lesions. A study of causative factors. *Stroke, 23*, 1446–1453.

Starkstein, S. E., Federoff, J. P., Price, T. R., Leiguarda, R., & Robinson, R. G. (1993). Catastrophic reaction after cerebrovascular lesions: frequency, correlates, and validation of a scale. *Journal of Neuropsychiatry and Clinical Neurosciences, 5*, 189–194.

Steriade, M., Curro, D. R., Pare, D., & Oakson, G. (1991). Fast oscillations (20–40 Hz) in thalamocortical systems and their potentiation by mesopontine cholingergic nuclei in the cat. *Proceedings of the National Academy of Sciences U S A, 88*, 4396–4400.

Steriade, M., McCormick, D. A., & Sejnowski, T. J. (1993). Thalamocortical oscillations in the sleeping and aroused brain. *Science, 262*, 679–685.

Stevens, S. S. (1971). Issues in psychophysical measurement. *Psychological Review, 78*, 426–450.

Stevens, S. S. (1975a). *Psychophysics: introduction to its perceptual, neural, and social prospects*. New York: John Wiley & Sons.

Stevens, S. S. (1975b). The psychophysical law. In G. Stevens (Ed.), *Psychophysics: introduction to its perceptual neural and social prospects* (pp. 1–36). Toronto: John Wiley & Sons.

Stevens, S. S., & Galanter, E. H. (1957). Ratio scales and category scales for a dozen perceptual continua. *Journal of Experimental Psychology, 54*, 377–411.

Stone, S. P., Wilson, B., Wroot, A., Halligan, P. W., Lange, L. S., Marshall, J. C. et al. (1991). The assessment of visuo-spatial neglect after acute stroke. *Journal of Neurology, Neurosurgery, and Psychiatry, 54*, 345–350.

Storrie-Baker, H. J., Segalowitz, S. J., Black, S. E., McLean, J. A., & Sullivan, N. (1997). Improvement of hemispatial neglect with cold-water calorics: an electrophysiological test of the arousal hypothesis of neglect. *Journal of the International Neuropsychological Society, 3*, 394–402.

Sturm, W., & Willmes, K. (2001). On the Functional Neuroanatomy of Intrinsic and Phasic Alertness. *NeuroImage, 14*, S76–S84.

Sugden, S. G., & Bourgeois, J. A. (2004). Modafinil Monotherapy in Poststroke Depression. *Psychosomatics, 45*, 80–81.

Sullivan, J. E., & Hedman, L. D. (2008). Sensory dysfunction following stroke: incidence, significance, examination, and intervention. *Topics in Stroke Rehabilitation, 15*, 200–217.

Tartaglione, G., Bino, L., Spadavecchia, L., & Favale, E. (1986). Simple reaction time changes in patients with unilateral brain injury. *Neuropsychologia, 24*, 649–658.

Taylor-Cooke, P. A., Ricci, R., Banos, J. H., Zhou, X., Woods, A. J., & Mennemeier, M. S. (2006). Perception of motor strength and stimulus magnitude are correlated in stroke patients. *Neurology, 66*, 1444–1456.

Tegner, R., & Levander, M. (1991a). The influence of stimulus properties on visual neglect. *Journal of Neurology, Neurosurgery, and Psychiatry, 54*, 882–886.

Tegner, R., & Levander, M. (1991b). Through the looking glass. A new technique to demonstrate directional hypokinesia in unilateral neglect. *Brain, 114*, 1943–1951.

Vallar, G., & Perani, D. (1987). The anatomy of spatial neglect in humans. In M. Jeannerod (ed.), *Neurophysiological and neuropsychological aspects of spatial neglect* (pp. 235–258). North Holland: Elsevier.

Veis, S. L., & Logemann, J. A. (1985). Swallowing disorders in persons with cerebrovascular accident. *Archive of Physical Medicine and Rehabilitation, 66*, 372–375.

Vlahov, D., Myers, A. H., & Al-Ibrahim, M. S. (1990). Epidemiology of falls among patients in a rehabilitation hospital. *Archives of Physical Medicine and Rehabilitation, 71*, 8–12.

Volpe, B. T., Ledoux, J. E., & Gazzaniga, M. S. (1979). Information processing of visual stimuli in an "extinguished" field. *Nature, 282*, 722–724.

Walsh, V. (2003). A theory of magnitude; common cortical metrics of time, space and quantity. *Trends in Cognitive Neuroscience, 7*, 483–488.

Watson, R. T., Heilman, K. M., Miller, B. D., & King, F. A. (1974). Neglect after mesencephalic reticular formation lesions. *Neurology, 24*, 294–298.

Watson, R. T., Valenstein, E., & Heilman, K. M. (1978). Nonsensory neglect. *Annals of Neurology, 3*, 505–508.

Watson, R. T., Valenstein, E., & Heilman, K. M. (1981). Thalamic neglect. Possible role of the medial thalamus and nucleus reticularis in behavior. *Archives of Neurology, 38*, 501–506.

Webster, J. S., Roades, L. A., Morrill, B., Rapport, L. J., Abadee, P. S., Sowa, M. V. et al. (1995). Rightward orienting bias, wheelchair maneuvering, and fall risk. *Archives of Physical Medicine and Rehabilitation, 76*, 924–928.

Wilson, B., Cockburn, J., & Halligan, P. W. (1987). Behavioral Inattention Test. *Titchfield, Tants, Thames Valley Test Co.*

Woods, A., Mennemeier, M., Garcia-Rill, E., Huitt, T., Chelette, K. C., McCullough, G., Munn, T., Brown, G., & Kiser, T. S. (2012). Improvement in arousal, visual neglect, and perception of stimulus intensity following cold pressor stimulation. *Neurocase, 18*(2), 115–122.

Woods, A. J., Mennemeier, M., Garcia-Rill, E., Meythaler, J., Mark, V. W., Jewel, G. R., et al. (2006). Bias in magnitude estimation following left hemisphere injury. *Neuropsychologia, 44*, 1406–1412.

Yekutiel, M. (2000). *Sensory re-education of the hand after stroke*. Philadelphia: Whurr.

Yerkes, R. M., & Dodson, J. D. (1908). The relation of strength of stimulus to rapidity of habit-formation. *Journal of Comparative Neurology and Psychology, 18*, 459–482.

CHAPTER 8

Perceptual-Attentional "Where" and Motor-Intentional "Aiming" Spatial Systems

A.M. Barrett

Introduction

Dedicated brain-behavior networks continuously compute the relationships between our bodies and the world around us: when we are at rest, when we move, and when both we and the environment are in motion. These *spatial cognitive* systems are akin to, but not synonymous with, visual cognitive systems. Patient-based work has strong theoretical relevance, and is also *translational,* in that it directly informs the distinction between spatial and visual cognition. In this chapter, I will suggest that patient-based studies provide an essential basis to understand spatial information processing in human and also animal models.

Spatial cognitive systems in patients who have neurological conditions or brain injury can be studied using precise experimental psychological methods. Since brain-injured subjects can have difficulty responding reliably in rigidly timed protocols; may only be able to complete relatively few task trials; may be heterogeneous with respect to physical health, the researcher needs to use imaginative methods to obtain reliability and internal validity of these experiments.

The reward of performing spatial cognitive experiments in brain-injured people lies in the very large magnitude effects which patient-centered research may yield, eloquently demonstrated in experiments by Kenneth Heilman, Edward Valenstein, Robert Watson, and their collaborators. Certainly, their magnitude far exceeds that of confounding influences we work so hard to avoid inducing in the experimental psychology laboratory when we test healthy young subjects. There is a second surprise from this work: dissociated effects demonstrated in these patients are not consistent with the visual cognitive, perceptual psychological approaches we are used to using to explain spatial behavior.

The distinctive behavioral dissociations observed in spatial dysfunction produce strong evidence to separate spatial and visual thinking. They suggest spatial cognition is distinct from processing in the dorsal visual stream in at least three ways. Dedicated spatial cognitive networks may include information processing beyond initial attentional, and perceptual stages. Patients with spatial disorders show problems with asymmetrically disorganized, degraded, or distorted body and environmental *knowledge*, or *representations*. Further, perceptual and representational stages of spatial processing are convincingly demonstrated in patient-based experiments to be *multimodal*. These stages integrate spatial properties of tactile and auditory perceptual processing; they also integrate spatial visual, auditory, and somesthetic representations, maps, or imagery.

Perhaps most interesting, patient-based research extends the spatial cognitive model beyond traditional perceptual, integrative, and representative processing stages. Patient-based studies suggest that spatial cognition may involve processes previously associated with motor planning, control, and learning. A spatial cognitive model with perceptual, representational, and motor-intentional components can be investigated by patient-based studies conducted in parallel with experiments investigating similar systems and processes in the healthy brain, resulting in converging information of exceptional internal validity.

In summary, we will discuss translational, patient-based data in this chapter that is consistent with animal spatial literature. These systematic, "n = 1" single-case analyses, prospective case series, or larger group designs, may bring us to understand spatial cognition as an embodied function, having not only perceptual attentional capacity, but both representational and motor-execution "aiming" stages, function and ability.

General Description

WHY IS SPATIAL PROCESSING COGNITIVE?

We will discuss an information processing model for spatial function, stressing three processing stages: dedicated perceptual-attentional, representational, and motor-intentional operations. This kind of an engineering input-output components model is part of what defines a mental function as *cognitive*.[1]

Spatial cognitive representations are also multimodal. They can reference the body from an inherently invisible perspective—that of the person living within (body schema).[2] However, internal reference systems (spatial maps or profiles) are not only referenced by visual parameters but also reference auditory or vestibular parameters.[3,4]

Thirdly, spatial neglect, as one of the few *class-common* mammalian cognitive disorders, apparently employs specialized output information processing. Early reports of spatial neglect in animals[5,6] clearly associated this syndrome with asymmetric movements (e.g. rotatory behaviors), and head/eye/postural turning. Although cortical ablation leads to spatial neglect in rodents, cats, dogs and monkeys,[7-10] subcortical dopamine depletion with 6-hydroxydopamine is a well-known paradigm for spatial neglect induction.[11] In these animals, body-centered biases accompanied systematic changes in response to contralesional tactile/somesthetic and visual stimulation, and symptoms were pharmacologically manipulable. Thus, a paradigm designed to study a movement disorder ("hemi-parkinsonism"), in fact produces a model of spatial cognitive dysfunction. The animal and human spatial neglect literature suggests that spatial *movement* could be cognitive.

The idea of visual systems dedicated to movement-related processing is not new. In a classic chapter, Ungerleider and Mishkin[12] suggested visual input processing determining "where" stimuli (a dorsal visual stream) is topologically segregated from cortical object recognition, which determines "what" stimuli are being processed (a ventral visual stream). However, the dorsal visual stream is a distinct system from that dedicated to spatial cognitive processing in at least two ways. First, dorsal systems may process many kinds of action- and movement-related information, and not exclusively spatial information (for example, images of grasping hands[13]). Dorsal visual stream, or streams[14,15] also inherently focus on input and representation stages of information processing. In contrast, an information processing spatial cognitive model describing a continuum of input, representational, and *also* output function[16-18] was proposed by Heilman, Valenstein,Watson and their colleagues starting in the 1970s. In this system, dedicated spatial attention directs spatial perceptual, representational, and eventually spatial motor-intentional "aiming" response execution.

MODULAR SPATIAL COGNITION AS EXPLAINED BY HEILMAN AND COLLEAGUES

In three manuscripts exploring spatial deficits in humans and monkeys,[16-18] three subsequent monkey studies,[19,25,26] and several chapters,[20-22] Heilman, Watson, Valenstein and their colleagues described the behavioral and neuroanatomic basis for input and output information processing modules dedicated to spatial cognition. Critically, these studies allowed for fractionation of potential input, representational and output spatial cognitive information processing stages by using novel training and performance testing.

The investigators designed a stimulus-response method of testing monkeys,[16] allowing them to separate perceptual-attentional "where" input-related response failure from motor-intentional "aiming" output-related response failures. Monkeys were trained to respond to a tactile stimulus (a brush touching one of their legs, out of view) by using one arm to open a door. The investigators cleverly designed a paradigm in which the monkeys responded with the *opposite* arm to a leg being touched (left leg brushed by experimenter → use right arm to open a door on the right side, and vice versa). In this way, they dissociated the body-referenced space of the stimulus (left leg, right leg) and the response (left arm, right arm). After the monkeys were trained, the investigators ablated frontal cortical and subcortical reticular formation regions in the intralaminar region of the thalamus and bordering the dorsal reticular formation. Five animals were trained, operated, and tested post-ablation. The experimenters observed that, although none of the monkeys had a weak arm (no motor deficits), all failed to open the contralesional door after stimulation of the ipsilesional leg. Impaired perceptual-attentional "where" input should not have occurred on the ipsilesional side of the body after the induced brain lesion—this should only occur on the contralesional side of the body. Because sensory input on the ipsilesional leg should have been correctly attended and perceived, and because monkeys apparently consistently reacted appropriately to contralesional leg stimulation, opening the ipsilesional door, the authors concluded that there was no major deficit of spatial-related perceptual-attentional processing. Rather, they concluded that the responsible deficit was at the stage of spatial-related action. Spatial input was being processed from the contralesional leg, but the contralesional arm action system was not prepared to respond (see the portion of the flowchart in Figure 8.1 labeled "Movement"). Postmortem examination of the lesions the examiners

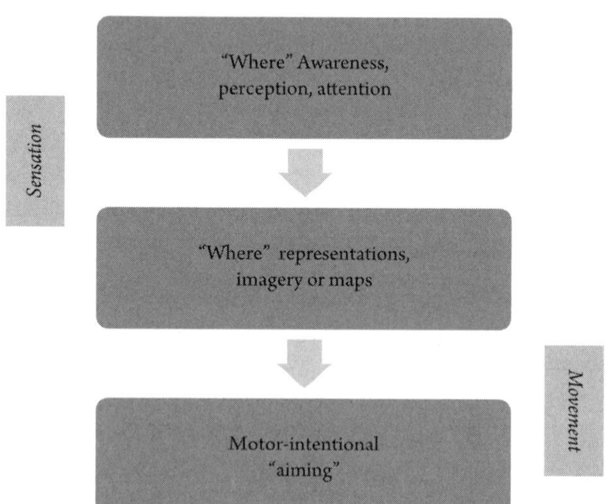

Figure 8.1 A schematic drawing of processes involved in the translation of sensory input to action.

made in the animals' brains revealed, of six lesions, that two affected the frontal arcuate gyrus, three affected the intralaminar nucleus of the thalamus, and two appeared to affect the dorsal reticular formation.

Initially,[16, 17] the authors labeled this phenomenon anatomically as "frontal neglect." They also labeled the syndrome based on unaffected primary sensory and perceptual stages of information processing: "nonsensory neglect". However, in subsequent studies, the authors clarified their construct by defining the affected and abnormal spatial cognitive processing stages, which were deemed motor output-related.[18-20] Their reports specified abnormal aspects of motor preparatory functions that they observed, such as unilateral hypokinesia (decreased movement specific to one side of the body, not due to weakness) and motor extinction (inability to activate the affected body side, but only when motor-activation resources must be allocated to both sides of the body simultaneously).[18] They directly compared this phenomenon to previous reports of "motor" output-related spatial dysfunction.[23, 24] They further demonstrated that dysfunction affecting specific spatial cognitive processing stages is not synonymous with dysfunction affecting a specific brain anatomic region, as they reported that "aiming" motor-intentional dysfunction could occur after both anterior cortical lesions and posterior association cortex lesion in monkeys.[25,26]

Relevant Experimental Work

In this section, I will review selected reports of spatial cognitive disorders in humans. These manuscripts suggested that input spatial cognitive information processing stages may be dissociable and distinct from output spatial cognitive information processing stages, because they may be independently impaired. We will consider in the following sections 1) spatial perceptual-attentional awareness, 2) spatial representations or internal images and 3) spatial motor-intentional action.

SPATIAL COGNITION: "WHERE" PERCEPTUAL ATTENTION

Multimodal perception. Spatial perception mandates a continuous computation not required by visual attentional or visual perceptual processing: the "where" inter-relationship between the body and space, in which both are assigned three-dimensional coordinates. Because spatial perceptual attention provides information dedicated to systems representing both the body and the external environment, it triages multimodal inputs, and is highly specialized to make predictions about 3-D stimulus-response associations. This system also provides inputs which are representationally integrated (see next section), so as to project the impact of self-movement on body position and thus on the body-environment spatial coordinate system. Spatial stimulus detection and perception of the external world thus may require tactile-somesthetic, haptic, vestibular, and motor efferent input as well as visual information.

Heilman and Valenstein [27, 28] provided some of the first information about stimulus unawareness in the auditory modality. In nine of their patients consistently able to identify ipsilesional auditory stimuli but unable to identify the contralesional stimulus with bilateral presentation (auditory neglect), who also had brain scans (technicium-99 uptake studies), the responsible lesion was in the inferior parietal lobe; one patient in their series had a frontal lobe lesion.[27] This finding was consistent with earlier work in monkeys, in which auditory inattention (unawareness), accompanied by visual and somesthetic inattention, was produced by lesions to caudal inferior parietal lobe and causal superior temporal sulcus, but not to temporal cortex.[29] Interestingly, another study demonstrated that patients with temporal lobe dysfunction (who had either undergone anterior temporal lobectomy for intractable seizures, or had EEG-confirmed seizure foci in the temporal lobe) had auditory discrimination deficits in the contralateral ear (although hearing threshold was unaffected).[30] Spatial neglect was not reported in association with this phenomenon, and patients with both left and right temporal surgery were among the 18 subjects tested. However, the "selective hearing" advantage on the ipsilesional side might represent a perceptual-attentional "where" bias selective to the auditory modality.

Visual unawareness. Kooistra and Heilman[31] and Nadeau and Heilman[32] pointed out that unlike a primary visual disorder (hemianopsia), unawareness of contralesional visual stimuli is relatively sensitive to the body space in which the relevant stimulus appears. This means that a stimulus which falls at the same place on the retina (and thus in the visual field) may be perceived when it falls to the right of the body midline (with rightward gaze), but may fail to be processed and perceived when it falls to the left of body midline, with leftward gaze. This may occur because the problem with stimulus detection is a *spatial* processing problem rather than a *visual* processing problem—spatial systems overweight the body reference system (egocentric system) relative to the retinotopic reference system.

Their patient's deficit is consistent with spatial perceptual-attentional neglect, because he manifested an isolated failure to detect left-sided visual stimuli when he looked straight ahead with his head in midposition facing forward. The phenomenon was demonstrated to be body-space dependent (consistent with spatial processing) rather than retinal hemifield-dependent (consistent with hemianopsia). Unawareness of left-sided stimuli worsened with his head turned into left (contralesional) space, even though stimuli maintained the same retinotopic position. The phenomenon also improved when the head was turned into right (ipsilesional) space.

Abnormalities of Habituation and Distraction

An important ability of the visual perceptual-attentional system is to manage bottom-up (stimulus-driven) and top-down (goal-driven) processing. "Visual persistence" allows us to focus and orient to visual stimuli without intrinsic environmental relevance, which are important to a top-down cognitive goal. Healthy subjects experience the Troxler effect, fading of a peripheral visual stimulus when one fixates centrally.[33] In a study of six patients with cortical lesions, Mennemeier and colleagues[34] observed that peripheral stimuli faded faster, in particular those lesions involving Brodmann's area 19, and peripheral moving stimuli, which did not fade in healthy controls, faded abnormally in these patients. Interestingly, absence of contralesional Troxler fading (abnormal persistence of a stationery visual peripheral stimulus) was associated with frontal lobe lesions. In one patient with both a parietal and frontal lesion, on opposite sides of the brain, abnormal fading occurred opposite the parietal lesion, and abnormal persistence, opposite the frontal lesion.

A triage system allows for novel or potentially environmentally relevant stimuli to be processed even when orienting to these stimuli would interfere with top-down, goal-driven stimulus processing. Conversely, novel stimuli without survival or ecological importance are rapidly triaged out of processing, such that after a certain amount of time, or a certain stimulus persistence, these stimuli no longer prompt orientation. Barrett and colleagues[35] reported that after an anteromedial thalamic stroke, a patient veered uncontrollably toward peripheral stimuli in far space while driving, on one occasion running off the road. They demonstrated that this patient erred significantly contralesionally when bisecting lines in far space in the presence of a contralesional distractor; she was not distracted in near space, nor did she make errors in the presence of an ipsilesional distractor. The authors interpreted this as potential evidence of an inhibitory-avoidance network in which dorsolateral frontal cortex, anterior thalamus, and retrosplenial cortex participate, since Heilman et al. [36] had previously reported veering while driving occurred in a man with a retrosplenial lesion. Such an inhibitory-avoidance network may modulate approach-orienting behaviors mediated by the superior colliculus and parietal lobe.

Other Problems: Avoidance

Just as perceptual-attentional "where" systems may abnormally engage to stimuli in a neglected spatial region (distraction), these systems might abnormally fail to engage to, or engage away from stimuli in a neglected spatial region (avoidance). Kodsi and Heilman [37] demonstrated that a single subject made more rightward errors in a workspace when she viewed her hand in left space on a video apparatus. They pointed out that this disorder was not likely to be related to asymmetric motor-intention based on results when they used a digital editor to rotate the axis of horizontal lines so that they appeared vertical. Under these testing conditions, the subject made mean leftward, contralesional direction in the workspace (apparently, not significantly different from accurate performance), rather than making rightward errors in the workspace, as would be expected with a pure directional hypokinesia. Since the direction of the subjects' errors was away from her viewed hand on the screen, the investigators suggested that seeing her hand on the video screen in contralateral space might provoke rightward avoidance errors. However, because the investigators did not compare an avoidance response to her own viewed hand, with avoidance that might be provoked by other kinds of stimuli that might increase the salience of the left, neglected space, it was unclear whether avoidance in this case was hand-specific. Indeed, if other stimuli in left space such as the left side of a line to be bisected had also provoked an avoidance response, secondary contralesional "where" perceptual-attentional errors reported by others using similar video technique [38-40] might be mechanistically related to an avoidance phenomenon.

SPATIAL COGNITION: INTERNAL "WHERE" REPRESENTATIONS

Multimodal internal representations and internal reference frames. Heilman et al. [41] presented eight patients with spatial neglect after right stroke with random auditory letter strings (auditory consonant trigrams) to one ear. Although participants' repetition was comparable when letters were presented to their right versus left ear, subjects repeated more letters presented to the non-neglected ear after a delay. This was interpreted as evidence of asymmetric auditory internal representations, or memory, since the asymmetry was present only after a delay. Heilman et al.[42] also reported that right brain stroke survivors with left neglect performed differently from left stroke survivors without neglect when they were asked to point to an imaginary point directly in front of them, corresponding to the midline of their chest. On average, the patients with right brain stroke and neglect pointed to the right of midline (8.8 cm rightward); patients with left brain stroke, aphasia and no neglect performed similarly to healthy controls (left brain stroke survivors: 1.2 cm to the left; controls: 1.1 cm to the left). Patients did not process any visual input during this task, and thus results support a bias related either to multimodal internal representations of the body (vestibular /tactile/ proprioceptive), or to biased motor-intentional "aiming" based upon those representations (hemispatial or directional akinesia). Both deficits could also have been present in the subjects reported.

Vestibular and somatic input may alter internal spatial representations based on the critical role of this input on the egocentric, body-centered reference. People with neglect may preferably report the body-centered right side of an imagined scene.[43] However, Meador and colleagues[44] replicated that study and, further, demonstrated that shifting the eyes and head into right body space increased access to left-sided environmental memories in one subject by 26 percent.

Other Representational Deficits: Spatial Syntactic Deficit

A complete review of deficits affecting spatial representational processing, which include body representations and magnitude estimation (working with a mental number line, estimating size, extent, weight, or other parameters; see Table 1), is beyond the scope of this chapter. These topics are taken up elsewhere[20,21,70] and in this volume (Mennemeier, Chapter 7; Coslett, Chapter 10). However, Heilman and his colleagues[45,46] also reported an unusual deficit affecting spatial representations relevant to syntactic thematic expression. In these studies, the authors demonstrated that a fundamental or primitive syntactic representation of agent and action, versus object, may be critically supported by the right hemisphere. Healthy controls may be biased to place the actor or agent of a sentence on the left side of a piece of paper, or leftward, when drawing the action of a sentence. This leftward spatial-syntactic bias can be dysfunctionally lost in association with spatial neglect after right hemisphere injury.

SPATIAL COGNITION: MOTOR-INTENTIONAL "AIMING"

Different Motor-Intentional Activities

Types of spatial motor response errors demonstrated in patient-based experiments are summarized in Table 1. Perceptual-attentional or representational systems may define the three-dimensional spatial trajectory of a movement. However, "when" to move and "when" to stop moving—which complete the definition of

Table 8.1 **Types of Spatial Dysfunction, by Spatial Processing Stages, as Described in Articles by Heilman and Colleagues. See text for full details.**

Perceptual-attentional "where"	*Representational "where"*	*Motor-intentional "aiming"*
Asymmetric unawareness	Asymmetrically degraded internally-stored information (asymmetrically reduced spatial magnitude)	Asymmetric hypokinesia, bradykinesia or hypometria(may be directional, hemispatial, or affect only left/right body)
Asymmetrically abnormal habituation	Asymmetrically activated internally-stored information	Asymmetric perseveration
Asymmetric decreased vigilance	Abnormally asymmetric mental manipulation of a number line	Asymmetric (or hemispatial) motor impersistence
Asymmetric distraction (Avoidance?)	Abnormal spatial-syntactic asymmetry	Asymmetric abnormal motor response inhibition

a movement by adding its parameters over time—may be primarily managed by “”motor-intentional systems “”[21, 47]. If the threshold for “when” to move into one body space, in one direction, or with one side of the body is too high, the organism manifests asymmetric hypokinesia /akinesia. If the threshold for “when” to move is too low, the organism manifests asymmetric disinhibited motor responses. Movement components also need to be timed: their start, speed, and termination, including repetitions. If timing of motor responses is too strictly limited, asymmetric hypometria or bradykinesia may occur. If the speed, gain, or number of motor responses is excessive, we may observe asymmetric perseveration.

Asymmetric Kinesis

Heilman and colleagues [48-50, 38] demonstrated directional and hemispatial abnormalities of kinesis in several clever patient studies. A common theme in these experiments was an effort to ensure that patients demonstrated evidence that they were aware of and attended to leftward space, left space, or left body, but still responded asymmetrically. Asymmetric performance was then attributed to spatial motor processing bias. A lesser capacity for contralesional, leftward movement, especially in left space, [20] a greater delay initiating contralesional movements than those in an ipsilesional direction,[48] slower movements in contralesional than in ipsilesional body space[49] and failure to move leftward when the hemispace of movement and action are dissociated[50,38] all support a spatial neglect-associated movement abnormality. The bias pertains for both continuously-monitored and rapid, ballistic movements. For example, as above, a systematic rightward bias in pointing to a spot opposite the body center, associated with spatial neglect [42], may have been related directional hypokinesia—a failure to move leftward. In all of these experiments, spatially asymmetric movements may be analogous to circling behavior in animal neglect models. [51]

Although dopamine-depletion models referred to “sensory neglect” in animals such as rats, some investigators used a crossed-response paradigm similar to those used by Watson, Valenstein, Heilman and colleagues. [17, 19, 26] Rats were conditioned to respond to sensory stimulation by turning to the side *opposite* the stimulus, instead of turning toward the stimulus. In these animals, lateral hypothalamic ablation produced no abnormality of ipsilesional turning to contralesional stimulation; rather, the rats manifested inability to turn contralesionally when stimulated on the good side. [53]

Other Problems

Stroke survivors may manifest defective inhibition of motor responses toward the neglected space.[53-55] This is comparable to the “allokinesia” and “disinhibition hyperkinesias” Heilman and colleagues[19] observed in monkeys with spatial neglect, whose contralesional limb made many errors of commission.

Motor output abnormalities can occur in both the neglected and the "normal" hemispace. Mizuno et al.[56] demonstrated progressive hypometria in eleven right hemisphere-damaged patients with spatial neglect who drew successive horizontal lines, end-to-end. Although leftward hypokinesia might have contributed to this phenomenon (shorter lines were drawn leftward and the workspace shifted progressively rightward), lines drawn rightward and in right space also became progressively smaller in gain.

Relevance to Functional and Anatomic Theory

Distinction between dorsal visual processing and spatial processing. Some modern cognitive neuroscience theorists treat spatial cognitive networks as greatly overlapping with dorsal visual cognitive networks. [57] However, as summarized above, the dorsal visual processing model is spatially incomplete. It does not include the integrative, *multimodal* nature of spatial cognition at input and output processing stages. Specifying the underlying system as spatial allows for a more parsimonious unified, multimodal spatial reference system instead of multiple, integrated auditory, haptic, tactile, somesthetic, and vestibular as well as dorsal visual maps. It is logical that this reference system may be critically supported by the tertiary sensory association cortex, but subcortical regions may also participate [58, 59], and more work is needed to define how primate cortical systems contribute to and support multimodal sensory and sensorimotor spatial mapping.

The dorsal perceptual system also has non-spatial functions, such as processing emotional facial movements.[60] Lastly, Heilman [21,47] points out that a major strength of including motor output in the spatial cognitive model is that this allows it to include both abnormal motor cortical system activation and "uncovered" primitive motor response. Although the superior colliculus plays an important role in the dorsal visual system, the lateral hypothalamus and striatum, to which the midbrain projects dopaminergic output, are not critical to the dorsal visual stream.[51,67]

Bidirectional networks. A conceptual challenge of the spatial cognitive information processing model is that methodological fractionation of "where" perceptual-attention and "aiming" motor-intention may be incomplete. For example, experimental tasks may dissociate one task primarily reliant on perceptual-attention (viewing a line), from another primarily reliant on motor-intention (moving in one direction).[38] However, the dissociation may not be pure: viewing a line is accompanied by motor-intentional eye movements, even when the head is fixed or exposure time very limited. Similarly, interventions primarily affecting one information processing stage (e.g. prism adaptation primarily altering directional hypokinesia[61] and hemispatial motor learning[62]) may also affect other stages of spatial information processing[63]. Lastly, neuroanatomic regions primarily associated input or output spatial processing. For example, injury to parietal association cortex supporting "where" perceptual-attentional processing may still adversely affect "aiming" motor-intention[64].

We might consider that spatial cognitive information processing can proceed bidirectionally. Motor-intention may "back-activate" representations and perceptual-attention. This is intuitively appealing: ecologically, "where" perceptual-attention and "aiming" motor-intention should be intimately coordinated and difficult to separate.

Back-activation could still be systematic. Its organization could thus be inquired in future research. For example, "aiming" motor-intention may primarily register on body-centered reference frames (multimodal internal spatial representations). Thus, spatial representations facilitated by motor-intentional "aiming" processing might primarily be those relevant to the body (i.e., tactile-somesthetic).

Heilman[65] proposed "substreams" within the spatial cognitive processing model, with preferential communication and correspondence between some perceptual-attentional and motor-intentional processes. For example, perceptual-attentional systems supporting inhibition-avoidance of attention to distractors may communicate closely with motor-intentional systems supporting inhibition of inappropriate motor responses.

Opportunities for Translation

Lastly, dissociated information processing in the spatial cognitive model proposed by Heilman, Watson, Valenstein and their collaborators is translationally important. First, it allows for theoretical stratification of between-subject heterogeneity in group studies of patients with spatial neglect—different subjects, with impairments affecting different stages of processing, would be expected to respond differently to interventions[20-22]. This is highly relevant to how we interpret intervention studies performed using linear regression-based analytic techniques. Such approaches underestimate treatment effects when data collected from the same subject (nested data) is highly inter-correlated, and subgroup differences are not analyzed. Thus, subgroups of patients with deficits primarily at one information processing stage (e.g. "where" perceptual attention) may experience robust treatment benefit. However, if the treatment does not affect patients with deficits at later processing stages, or adversely affects deficits at "aiming" processing stages[66], a group treatment effect may be lost.

The spatial cognitive model also allows the scholar to consider animal literature on subcortical-cortical interactions. Separating perceptual-attentional and representational "where" spatial processing and motor-intentional "aiming" allows us to consider the relevance of several "motor" primitive systems to spatial behavior, especially in the midbrain. These include, as above, the substantia nigra [67], the superior colliculi, and the midbrain reticular activating system[69] (which neurons may overlap with the deep motor colliculus). Interhemispheric interaction relevant to spatial cognition[70] and other high-order functions[71] may critically involve relay and modulation via these subcortical systems. Spatial cognitive behaviors are, like communicative behaviors, very complex. Thus, the modular theory of spatial cognition proposed by Heilman and colleagues may not only benefit our understanding of human-environmental interaction: this model may also improve the validity of our hypotheses of interactions between cognitive systems, whether localized in the same or different cerebral hemispheres.

References

Adair, J.C., Na, D.L., Schwartz, R.L., & Heilman, K.M. (1998). Analysis of primary and secondary influences on spatial neglect. *Brain and Cognition* 37(3), 351–367.

Barrett, A. M. & Burkholder, S. (2006). Monocular patching in subjects with right hemisphere stroke affects perceptual-attentional bias. *Journal of Rehabilitation Research and Development* 43(3), 337–346.

Barrett, A. M., Schwartz, R. L., Crucian, G. P., & Heilman, K. M. (1999). Adverse Effect of Dopamine Agonist Therapy in a Patient With Motor-Intentional Neglect. *Archives of Physical Medicine and Rehabilitation 80*, 600–603.

Barrett, A.M., Crucian, G.P., Kim, M.H., and Heilman, K.M. (2000). Attentional grasp in far extrapersonal space after thalamic infarction. *Neuropsychologia 38*, 778–784.

Barrett, A.M., Kim, M.H., & Heilman, K.M. (2002a) Spatial bias in Korean right-left, vertical readers. *Neuropsychologia 40*, 1003–1012.

Berthoz, A., Israël, I., Georges-François, P., Grasso, R., & Tsuzuku, T. (1995) Spatial memory of body linear displacement: what is being stored? *Science 269*, 95–98.

Bianchi, L.(1895). The function of the frontal lobes. *Brain 18*, 497–522.

Bisiach, E. & Luzzatti, C. (1978). Unilateral neglect of representational space. *Cortex 14*, 129–133.

Brown, V.J. (2002). The neurobehavioral analysis of visuospatial attention in the rat. In: (Eds. Karnath, H-O., Milner, D., & Vallar, G.) *The Cognitive and Neural Basis of Spatial Neglect* (pp. 233–242). New York, NY: Oxford University Press.

Burnett, L.R., Stein, B.E., Chaponis, D., & Wallace, M.T. (2004). Superior colliculus lesions preferentially disrupt multisensory orientation. *Neuroscience 124* (3), 535–547.

Butter, C.M., Rapcsak, S.Z., Watson, R.T., & Heilman, K.M. (1988). Changes in sensory inattention, direction hypokinesia, and release of the fixation reflex following a unilateral frontal lesion: a case report. *Neuropsychologia 26*, 533–545.

Castaigne, P., Laplane, D., & Degos, J-D.(1972). Trois cas de negligence motrice par Ibion frontale pre-rolandique. *Revue Neurologique* (Paris) *126*, 5–15.

Chatterjee, A., Maher, L.M, & Heilman, K.M. (1995). Spatial characteristics of thematic role representation. *Neuropsychologia* 33(5),643–648.

Coslett, H.B., Bowers, D., Fitzpatrick, E., Haws, B., & Heilman, K.M. (1990). Directional hypokinesia and hemispatial inattention in neglect. *Brain 113*, 475–486.

Critchley, M: (1969). *The Parietal Lobes*. New York: Hafner, p. 227.

Fortis, P., Kornitzer, J., Goedert, K.M., & Barrett, A.M. (2009, April). Effect of prism adaptation on "aiming" spatial bias and functional abilities [abstract]. *Neurology, 72,11(S1)*, A332.

Heilman, K.M. (1979). Neglect and related disorders. In: Eds. Heilman, K.M. & Valenstein, E., *Clinical Neuropsychology* (pp. 269–307). New York: Oxford University Press.

Heilman, K.M. (2004). Intentional neglect. *Frontiers in Bioscience 9*, 694–705.

Heilman, K.M. & Valenstein, E. (1972). Auditory Neglect in Man. *Archives of Neurology* 26(1), 32–35.

Heilman, K.M. & Valenstein, E. (1972). Frontal lobe neglect in man. *Neurology 22*, 660–664.

Heilman, K.M. and Watson, R.T.(1991) Intentional motor disorders. In: Eds. Levin, H.S., Eisenberg, H.M., & Benton, A.L., *Frontal lobe function and dysfunction* (pp. 199–213). New York: Oxford University Press.

Heilman, K.M. (2003) Motor neglect. Neurology Department Grand Rounds Lecture, Penn State College of Medicine.

Heilman, K.M., Bowers, D., & Watson, R.T. (1983). Performance on hemispatial pointing task by patients with neglect syndrome. *Neurology 33*, 661–664.

Heilman, K.M., Bowers, D., Coslett, H.B., Whelan, H., & Watson, R.T. (1985). Directional hypokinesia: prolonged reaction times for leftward movements in patients with right hemisphere lesions and neglect. *Neurology 35*, 855–860.

Heilman, K.M., Bowers, D., Watson, R.T., Day, A., Valenstein, E., Hammon, E., & Duara, R.R (1990). Frontal hypermetabolism and thalamic hypometabolism in a patient with abnormal orienting and retrosplenial amnesia. *Neuropsychologia 28*, 161–169.

Heilman, K.M., Hammer, L.C., and Wilder, B.J. (1973). An audiometric defect in temporal lobe dysfunction. *Neurology 23*, 384–386.

Heilman, K.M., Pandya, D.N., & Geschwind, N. (1970). Trimodal inattention following parietal lobe ablations. *Transactions of the American Neurological Association 95*, 259–261.

Heilman, K.M., Pandya, D.N., Karol, E.A., & Geschwind, N. (1971). Auditory Inattention. *Archives of Neurology 24*(4), 323–325.

Heilman, K.M., Valenstein, E., Day, A. & Watson, R.T. (1995). Frontal lobe neglect in monkeys. *Neurology 45*, 1205–1210.

Heilman, K.M., Watson, R.T. &Valenstein, E. (2002). Spatial neglect. In: Eds. Karnath, H-O., Milner, D., & Vallar, G.). *The Cognitive and Neural Bases of Spatial Neglect* (pp. 3–30). New York: Oxford University Press.

Heilman, K.M., Watson, R.T., & Schulman, H,M. A unilateral memory defect. *Journal of Neurology, Neurosurgery and Psychiatry* 37(7): 790–793.

Hoyman, L., Weese, G.D., Frommer, G.P. (1979). Tactile discrimination performance deficits following neglect-producing unilateral lateral hypothalamic lesions in the rat. *Physiology and Behavior 22*, 139–147.

Jacquin-Courtois, S., Rode, G.,Pavani, F.,O'Shea, J.,Giard, M. H.,Boisson, D.,& Rossetti, Y. (2010). Effect of prism adaptation on left dichotic listening deficit in neglect patients: glasses to hear better? *Brain 133*(3), 895–908.

Kayser, C., Petkov, C., Lippert, M., & Logothetis, M.K. (2005). Mechanisms for allocating auditory attention: an auditory saliency map. *Current Biology 15*(21), 1943–1947.

Kodsi, M.H. & Heilman, K.M. (2002). The contribution of an avoidance response to contralateral neglect. *Neurology 58(11)*,1692–1694.

Kooistra, C.A. & Heilman, K.M. (1989). Hemispatial visual inattention masquerading as hemianopsia. *Neurology 39*, 1125–1127.

Kosslyn,S.M, Koenig, O., Barrett, A., Cave, C.B., Tang, J. & Gabrieli, J.D.E. (1989). Evidence for two types of spatial representations: hemispheric specialization for categorical and coordinate relations. *Journal of Experimental Psychology: Human Perception and Performance 15*, 723–735.

Kwon, S.E. & Heilman, K.M. (1991). Ipsilateral neglect in a patient following a unilateral frontal lesion. *Neurology 41*, 2001–2004 .

Lunenburger, L., Kleiser, R., Stuphorn, V., Miller, L.E. & Hoffmann, K.P. (2001) A possible role of the superior colliculus in eye-hand coordination. *Progress in Brain Research134*, 109–125.

Marshall, J. F. (1979). Somatosensory inattention after dopamine depleting intracerebral 6-OHDA injections: spontaneous recovery and pharmacological control. *Brain Research 177*, 311–324.

Marshall, J.F., Richardson, J.S, & Teitelbaum, P.(1971). Sensory neglect produced by lateral hypothalamic damage. *Science 174*, 523–525.

Meador, K., Watson R. T., Bowers, D., & Heilman, K.M. (1986). Hypometria with hemispatial and limb motor neglect. *Brain 109*, 293–305 .

Meador, K.J., Loring, D.W., & Heilman, K.M. (1987). Remote memory and neglect syndrome. *Neurology* 37 (3), 522–526.
Mennemeier, M.S., Chatterjee, A., Watson, R.T., Wertman, E., Carter, L.P. & Heilman, K.M. (1994). Contributions of the parietal and frontal lobes to sustained attention and habituation. *Neuropsychologia* 32(6), 703–716.
Mizuno, T., Crucian, G.P., Finney, G.R., Jeong, Y., Drago, V.,& Heilman, K.M. (2006). Incremental limb hypometria. *Journal of Neurology, Neurosurgery and Psychiatry* 77(6), 793–795.
Na, D. L., Adair, J. C., Williamson, D. J., Schwartz, R. L., Haws, B., Heilman, K. M. (1998). Dissociation of sensory-attentional from motor-intentional neglect. *Journal of Neurology, Neurosurger y, and Psychiatry 64*, 331–338.
Nadeau, S.E. & Heilman, K.M. (1991). Gaze-dependent hemianopia without hemispatial neglect. *Neurology 41*, 1244–1250.
Neisser, U. The Cognitive Approach. In: *Cognitive Psychology*. (p. 3). New York, NY: Prentice Hall.
Parkinson, R. B., Raymer, A.,Chang, Y.-L., FitzGerald, D. B., & Crosson, B. (2009). Lesion characteristics related to treatment improvement in object and action naming for patients with chronic aphasia. *Brain and Language,110*, 75–84.
Payne, B.R. & Rushmore, R.J. (2003). Animal models of cerebral neglect and its cancellation. *The Neuroscientist* 9(6), 446–454.
Payne, B.R. & Rushmore, R.J. (2003). Animal models of cerebral neglect and its cancellation. *Neuroscientist* 9(6), 446–454.
Pisella, L., Binkofski, F., Lasek, K., Toni, I. & Rossetti, Y. (2006). No double-dissociation between optic ataxia and visual agnosia: Multiple sub-streams for multiple visuo-manual integrations. *Neuropsychologia 44 (13)*, 2734–2748.
Rode, G., Rossetti, Y., Farnè, A., Boisson, D. & Bisiach, E. (2000). The motor control of a movement sequence ending to the left is altered in unilateral neglect. European Conference on Cognitive and Neural Bases of Spatial Neglect. Cuomo, Italy; Sept. 2000.
Schwarting, R. K. & Huston, J.P. (1996). The unilateral 6-hydroxydopamine lesion model in behavioral brain research. Analysis of functional deficits, recovery and treatments. *Progress in Neurobiology* 50(2–3), 275–331.
Schwartz, R. L., Barrett, A. M., Crucian, G. & Heilman, K. M. (1998). Dissociation of Gesture and Object Recognition. *Neurology, 50(4)*, 1186–1188.
Schwoebel, J. & Coslett, H.B. (2007). Evidence for multiple, distinct representations of the human body. *Journal of Cognitive Neuroscience* 17(4), 543–553.
Shmuelof, L. & Zohary, E. (2005). Dissociation between ventral and dorsal fMRI activation during object and action recognition. *Neuron* 47(3), 457–470.
Sprague, J. M. (1966). Interaction of cortex and superior colliculus in mediation of visually guided behavior in the cat. *Science 153*, 1544–1547.
Stein, B.E. (1998). Neural mechanisms for synthesizing sensory information and producing adaptive behaviors. *Experimental Brain Research 123*, 124–135.
Striemer, C.L. & Danckert, J.A. (2010).Through a prism darkly: re-evaluating prisms and neglect. *Trends in Cognitive Science* 14(7), 308–316.
Triggs, W.J., Gold, M., Gerstle, G., Adair, J. & Heilman, K.M. (1994). Motor neglect associated with a discrete parietal lesion. *Neurology, 44*, 1164–1166.
Troxler, D. (1804). Ueber das Verschwindern gegebener Gegenstaende innerhalb unsers Gesichtskreises. In: Eds. Himly, K & Schmidt, J.A. *Ophtalmologisches Bibliothek* 2, 51–53.
Ungerleider, L.G. & Mishkin. M. (1982). Two cortical visual systems. In: Eds. Ingle, D.J., Goodale, M.A., & Mansfield, R.J.W. *Analysis of visual behavior* (pp. 263–299). Cambridge, MA: MIT Press.
Ungerstedt, U. (1973). Sensory neglect following removal of the nigrostriatal DA system. In: (Eds.) Ehrenrpreis, S.& Kopin, I. *Neuroscience Research*, vol. 5. Orlando, FL: Academic Press.
Ungerstedt, U. (1976). 6-hydroxydopamine-induced degeneration of the nigrostriatal dopamine pathway: the turning syndrome. *Pharmacology and Therapeutics: Part B—General and Systematic Pharmacology* 2(1): 37–40.

Valenstein, E. & Heilman, K.M. (1981). Unilateral hypokinesia and motor extinction. *Neurology 31*: 445–448.

Valenstein, E., Heilman, K.M., Watson, R.T., &Van Den Abell, T. (1982). Nonsensory neglect from parietotemporal lesions in monkeys. *Neurology 32,* 1198–1201.

Verfaellie, M., Heilman, K.M. (1987). Response preparation and response inhibition after lesions of the medial frontal lobe. *Archives of Neurology 44,* 1265–1271.

Watson, R. T., Heilman, K. M., Miller, B. D., & King, F. A. Neglect After Mesencephalic Reticular Formation Lesions. *Neurology 24,* 294–298.

Watson, R.T., Miller, B.D., & Heilman, K.M. (1978). Nonsensory neglect. *Annals of Neurology 3,* 505–508.

Watson, R.T., Valenstein, E., Day, A. & Heilman, K.M. (1986). Normal tactile threshold in monkeys with neglect. *Neurology 36*(5): 636–640.

CHAPTER 9

Limb Apraxia: A Disorder of Goal-Directed Actions

Anne L. Foundas

Apraxia is a disturbance in goal-directed behavior defined as a cognitive-motor disorder specific to learned skilled movements (e.g., tool use). Goal-directed behaviors, like the ability to use a toothbrush, require the acquisition of the knowledge and the motor representations to perform the purposeful skilled movements associated with an action. Apraxia (dyspraxia) is found in many acquired and developmental brain disorders, and is often diagnosed based on difficulty in pantomiming tool-gestures to command. The disordered movement can manifest as the imprecise orientation (spatial disturbance) of the object (e.g., toothbrush not oriented correctly to the teeth) or as the incorrect sequencing (temporal disturbance) of an action at a proximal rather than a distal limb joint (e.g., rotating at the shoulder rather than moving at the wrist to brush your teeth). This is an operational definition based on behavioral observations consistent with the fact that limb apraxia, which is the topic of this chapter, is a clinical diagnosis that requires the direct observation of a patient performing a variety of upper limb movements. In this chapter, several cognitive-process models of limb apraxia will be discussed including a brief reference to Liepmann's early model (presented in detail in the "History of Cognitive Neurology" chapter); Geschwind's disconnection model; De Renzi's multi-modal model; and the Heilman-Rothi dual-component model of limb apraxia. Lesion localization studies and converging evidence from functional imaging studies will be reviewed to present an updated anatomical model of limb praxis with an emphasis on the praxis production system.

Cognitive-Process Models of Limb Apraxia

The term apraxia is commonly ascribed to Gogol (1873), although Steinthal used the term in 1871 and is credited with the original definition that included "the movement of the limb is restricted, particularly the relation of the movement to the object to be handled; the relation of the movement to the purpose is disturbed." Hugo Karl Liepmann (1863–1925) is credited with the first description of the neuropsychological mechanisms that mediate learned, skilled movements (Figure 9.1).

Liepmann (Liepmann, 1920) described three types of apraxia: (1) limb kinetic apraxia, (2) ideokinetic (ideomotor) apraxia, and (3) ideational (conceptual) apraxia. The regions that Liepmann considered to be especially important for the acquisition of these "movement formulae" included the: (1) left parietal lobe, (2) precentral gyrus, (3) parieto-occipital region, and (4) corpus callosum. Liepmann's original concept was that the right precentral gyrus was not subject to the person's will without guidance through the left precentral gyrus. Liepmann viewed the supramarginal gyrus (SMG) as the region that integrates sensory impulses necessary for the formulation of the movement representation. These movement formulae must then pass through this area to the physiological center for hand movement. Thus, a lesion to the SMG interrupts these impulses that are on the way to the frontal motor regions for the planning and production of the movement sequence. For this reason, Liepmann speculated that a lesion near the SMG would cause ideomotor apraxia in both hands. Consistent with this model,

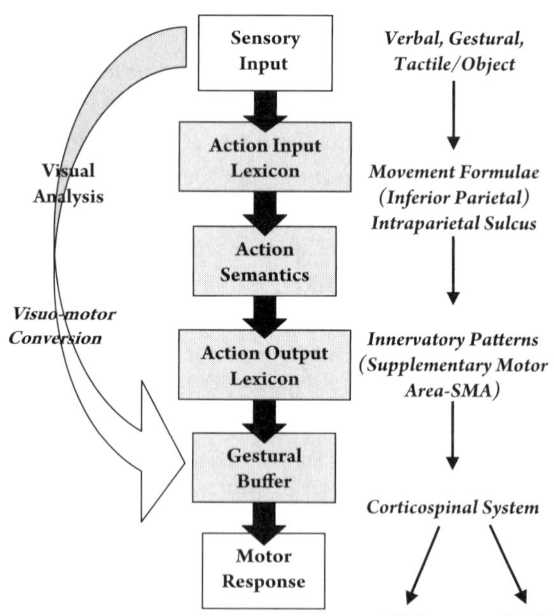

Figure 9.1 Liepmann's Praxis Process Model. This modified "box diagram" depicts Liepmann's model that supports the idea that the left hemisphere controls the movement formulae and kinematic representations for learned skilled movements.

Liepmann also proposed that a lesion to the dominant left precentral gyrus would cause ideomotor apraxia of both sides. Liepmann also postulated that a more general cortical dysfunction was necessary to disrupt the ideation of motor function that would produce ideational (conceptual) apraxia. Limb kinetic apraxia, in contrast, was defined as a deficit in the deftness of a limb movement rather than a higher-order problem associated with cognitive-motor aspects of goal directed movements. Thus, in contrast to ideomotor or ideational apraxia, Liepmann thought that limb kinetic apraxia was more directly linked to elemental motor systems associated with a paralysis or problem with deftness of the hand or arm movement.

GESCHWIND'S DISCONNECTION MODEL OF APRAXIA

Geschwind, like Liepmann, believed that the left hemisphere was specialized for the performance of learned skilled movements. Geschwind elaborated on Liepmann's model by defining a neural network aligned with Wernicke's model of speech (Geschwind, 1965). He postulated that the stored movement representations are localized to the left parietal cortex and the gesture production components are located in frontal motor regions interconnected by white matter pathways specific to this neural network. He used a disconnection model of apraxia to reconcile the observations of Liepmann & Maas (1907) with the additional observations seen in a patient that he evaluated with Edith Kaplan (Geschwind & Kaplan, 1962).

Liepmann & Mass (1907) reported on a patient with a right hemiplegia who performed poorly when gesturing-to-command and to imitation with the left hand. This patient also had difficulty manipulating actual tools. On postmortem examination, one small lesion was found in the left basis pontis that probably accounted for the contralateral hemiparesis. Another lesion was found in the anterior and mid-corpus callosum. The authors postulated that the disordered behavior in this patient resulted from the inability of the right hemisphere to gain access to the time-space-form picture of the movement located in the left hemisphere (Liepmann & Mass, 1907). Liepmann (1920) used this case to support his idea that the left hemisphere contains the "movement formulae" that control purposeful skilled movements (Figure 9.1).

The patient reported by Geschwind & Kaplan (1962) was examined following a left-hemisphere tumor resection and a post-operative anterior cerebral artery stroke with a residual lesion to the anterior two-thirds of the corpus callosum. This patient had difficulty performing gestures to command with the left hand. Unlike the patient described by Liepmann, he was able to perform gestures to imitation, and to manipulate and use tools with his left hand. This patient was able to gesture and write with his right hand, but he was not able to write or type with his left hand. Geschwind and Kaplan explained this pattern of behavior as a *disconnection* of motor representations from the language representations stored in the left hemisphere. This case and the case reported by Liepmann & Mass (1907) had common lesions to the anterior corpus callosum, although the extent of the lesion and other brain injury differed in these two patients. Thus, lesion localization differences and compensatory mechanisms may contribute to performance differences in these two cases of patients who were examined many months following initial brain injury. It may be that the patient described by Geschwind & Kaplan (1962) had language lateralized to the left with bilateral praxis representations.

Geschwind postulated that left brain damage to parietal and frontal motor regions or to the interconnecting pathways induces limb apraxia because the left hemisphere that comprehends the verbal command is disconnected from the right premotor and motor areas which control the left hand (Geschwind, 1965). He stressed that apraxia is common, especially following acute lesions to the left frontal association areas. Geschwind also noted that many neurologists fail to diagnose apraxia because a large number of apraxic patients can actually manipulate and use familiar objects in their environment, but fail with more specific testing. He recognized four settings in which apraxia could be demonstrated: (1) failure to produce a correct movement in response to a verbal command; (2) failure to produce a correct response to imitation; (3) failure to produce a movement in response to seeing the actual object; and (4) failure to handle and use an object correctly. Geschwind emphasized the importance of examining gestures in all of these settings.

MULTI-MODAL MODEL OF APRAXIA: GOODGLASS/ KAPLAN AND DE RENZI

In 1963, Goodglass and Kaplan found some important behavioral associations and dissociations in patients with left hemisphere damage (LHD) that they believed supported Liepmann's movement representation model rather than a competing model that postulated that apraxia and aphasia share a central problem of symbols (asymbolia) (Goodglass & Kaplan, 1963). They tested patients with and without apraxia performing simple and complex gestures and found that the apraxic patients were impaired on tasks of motor skill relative to nonapraxic patients. The apraxic aphasic patients had more difficulty with gesture imitation compared to the nonapraxic aphasic patients. Both groups could use actual tools, and there was no relationship between severity of aphasia and apraxia. Others have found a close association between apraxia and aphasia (Dee, Benton, & Van Allen, 1970; Kertesz & Hooper, 1982); although there are instances of apraxia without aphasia. Perhaps the most compelling support for the idea that language and praxis representations are independent came from

Liepmann's original observation that only 14 of 20 patients with apraxia also had aphasia. Liepmann, however, believed that apraxic patients were clumsy with actual tools. The behavioral dissociation of apraxia and aphasia supports the current prevailing view that these two neural systems are anatomically and functionally distinct, although specific brain regions critical to these independent neural systems may be located in close proximity and, therefore, may be included in a common cortical lesion associated with acute vascular injury in post-stroke patients. This general view, however, is also subject to the idea that some common neurons may link specific features of behavior suggesting that indeed there may be areas of overlap in specific neural systems that share a common substrate.

De Renzi and colleagues (1980; 1985; 1988) provided additional empiric evidence to support the view that apraxia and aphasia are separable neural systems. De Renzi developed a 24-item test of apraxia to qualitatively examine gestures performed to imitation (De Renzi, Motti, & Nichelli, 1980). On the basis of scores from 100 healthy controls, De Renzi and colleagues found that 50 percent of LHD patients and 20 percent of the right hemisphere damaged (RHD) patients met the clinical criteria of apraxia. They found that the RHD patients had a less severe form compared to the LHD patients who often had severe apraxia and were nearly always aphasic. De Renzi and colleagues speculated that the two symptoms were likely co-occurring in individual patients because of the contiguity of the underlying neuroanatomical substrates rather than a common defect at the level of processing. They distinguished between two levels of gestural processing including: (1) *action semantics,* which refer to the long-term conceptual representations of gesture; and (2) *motor control,* which includes action execution (De Renzi, 1985; De Renzi & Lucchelli, 1988). Based on this approach, De Renzi proposed that a deficit in the conceptual representation would result in impaired classification of gestures and deficits to command but not to imitation. In contrast, he postulated that a deficit in motor control would induce errors on both command *and* imitation. In order to evaluate conceptual aspects of the praxis system, De Renzi and Lucchelli (1988) examined 20 LHD patients with a multiple object use test and a single object use test. Both of these subtests require the ability to demonstrate how the objects are used. These tests were designed to assess ideational apraxia defined as the inability to demonstrate the use of objects. Neither of these tests of conceptual knowledge correlated with the De Renzi test of gestures to imitation which evaluates ideomotor apraxia. There was also a reported relationship to lesion location with ideational apraxia frequently, but not exclusively, associated with a lesion to the left temporo-parietal junction. Therefore, they concluded that ideational apraxia is an autonomous syndrome that occurs independent of ideomotor apraxia. They postulated that the localization of the predominant lesion site is associated with semantic memory disorders more than defective motor control.

HEILMAN-ROTHI DUAL COMPONENT MODEL OF LIMB APRAXIA

Liepmann's theory of gesture production distinguished between the formulation of a motor program and the implementation of the spatial-temporal sequence. Heilman, Rothi, & Valenstein (1982) directly examined this idea in 20 patients with unilateral left hemisphere stroke using a gesture to command and a gesture discrimination task. Patients with lesions to the left parietal cortex were impaired in both gesture production and gesture discrimination, whereas patients with frontal lesions were impaired in gesture production but not gesture discrimination. Based on this relationship between task and lesion location (i.e., double dissociation), they posited that there are at least two mechanisms that can account for performance deficits in limb apraxia: (1) a *praxis production system* and (2) a *praxis reception system* (Heilman, Rothi, & Valenstein, 1982). Based on their model, variance in the expression of apraxia is related to destruction of the movement representations themselves, via damage to the inferior parietal lobule (SMG), or to disconnection of the inferior parietal lobule from other critical modules of the praxis system. Although the studies of Liepmann and others cited above were the critical initial steps toward the development of a model of praxis systems, Rothi, Ochipa, and Heilman developed a more comprehensive cognitive neuropsychological model of praxis based on a model of language production and comprehension, designed to account for dissociations within the praxis system (Rothi, Ochipa, & Heilman, 1991).

The Heilman-Rothi praxis model is a dual-component model for the organization of action including an *action production system* and a *conceptual system* (Heilman, 1979; Heilman & Gonzalez Rothi, 2003; Heilman, et al., 1982; Ochipa, Rothi, & Heilman, 1989; Rothi, et al., 1991). This model accounts for modality specific input differences with a further distinction between dysfunction caused by destruction of the parietal areas that store the spatial-temporal representations and the deficit resulting from the disruption of the frontal motor areas. Because learned skilled movements are also dependent on the conceptual knowledge of tools, objects and actions, there is some interaction between action semantics and the action lexicon.

Two other models warrant comment. These models include the models developed by Roy and colleagues (Roy, 1985; Roy, Clark, Aigbogun, & Square-Storer, 1992; Roy et al., 2000; Roy, Square-Storer, Hogg, & Adams, 1991; Stamenova, Roy, & Black, 2009) and the Cubelli-Della Sala model (Cubelli, Marchetti, Boscolo, & Della Sala, 2000). Roy and colleagues originally thought that apraxia could result from disruption of the conceptual system and/or the production system (Roy, 1985). Based on this model Roy and colleagues made specific predictions and examined patients performing a variety of tasks in order to test their hypotheses (Roy, 1985; Roy, et al., 2000; Roy, et al., 1991). Most recently, they presented a model-based approach to understand apraxia in corticobasal degeneration (Stamenova, et al., 2009). Cubelli et al developed a model that is an extension of the Heilman-Rothi dual-component model. This model proposes a separate visuo-motor conversion mechanism while maintaining modality-specific input systems and the secondary level of modality-specific analysis before action semantic processing (Cubelli, et al., 2000). A modified Heilman-Rothi-Roy-Cubelli model of the praxis system is shown in Figure 9.2. Based on this model, four different apraxia subtypes can be identified (refer to Table 9.1). These subtypes are theoretically based and can be classified in patients based on performance on apraxia subtests. There continues to be some lack of clarity between cognitive and anatomical categories within the model; thus, specific cognitive-motor apraxia types may not be completely dissociated by lesion location (Barrett & Foundas, 2004; Heilman & Gonzalez Rothi, 2003; Petreska, Adriani, Blanke, & Billard, 2007; Watson, Fleet, Gonzalez-Rothi, & Heilman, 1986).

KINEMATICS AND MOTOR CONTROL IN APRAXIA

Fisk and Goodale were the first to use kinematic methods to examine visually guided limb movements (Fisk & Goodale, 1988). They studied 17 LHD and 11 RHD patients performing a task with the ipsilesional limb compared to controls performing the tasks with each limb in order to contrast right- and left-hand performance in each brain damaged group. Participants were instructed to point to a target while sitting in front of a monitor with the head stabilized. At the beginning of each trial, participants were instructed to fixate on a central point and then point to a series of targets at various angles from the point of fixation. LHD patients did not show any gross disruption in the morphology of the velocity wave form as the expected bell-shaped acceleration and deceleration phases were seen. This result suggested that there was relative preservation of the global elements of the movement representation. However, there was a prolonged phase of low-velocity movement at the end of the pointing task. This final movement was attributed to one of two potential mechanisms. Either the LHD patients had difficulty monitoring and adjusting the motor program online or had difficulty utilizing sensory feedback to monitor the limb movement. Both explanations support the idea that the movement abnormality was associated with a closed-loop processing defect. However, the LHD group also attained a lower peak velocity at the end of the acceleration phase. This movement anomaly may be associated with a different type of "movement formula" or "innervatory pattern" reflecting a problem with open-loop processing.

In order to evaluate these competing hypotheses, Haaland and Harrington conducted a series of experiments to study the kinematics of movement trajectory during a simple aiming task (Harrington & Haaland, 1997). The task involved the use of a vertical stylus initially centered inside a start circle. One or two seconds

Table 9.1 **Cognitive-Motor Apraxia Types**

Type 1: Impaired gesture-to-command, gesture-imitation preserved: Impairments to command reflect a disruption in the motor representation and may be associated with an inability to access the representation from memory. Deficits can exist in the lexical and/or nonlexical route. Lesions may be small in size and disconnect posterior from anterior regions within left frontal-parietal circuits. Lexical and nonlexical routes may be impaired in lesions that extend to callosal fibers that disconnect the right hemisphere.
Type 2: Impaired gesture-to-command and gesture-imitation: Impairments on gesture-imitation may reflect an inability to implement, execute, or control learned skilled movements. Deficits on gesture-imitation may be associated with degraded nonrepresentational movements, and then the patient may have a more basic disorder of motor programming. Deficits can exist in the lexical and/or nonlexical route.
Type 3: Impaired gesture-to-command, impaired gesture recognition-discrimination: Lesions are more likely to be large middle cerebral artery (MCA) territory and posterior in location including the inferior parietal lobe (Brodmann's area—BA 39, 40) with extension to periventricular white matter (PVWM) and/or to ventral temporal regions. There may be dissociations with lexical and nonlexical deficits seen with lesions to both of these regions whereas lesions restricted to areas 39/40 may affect the lexical but spare the nonlexical route.
Type 4: Impaired gesture-to-command, intact gesture recognition-discrimination: Lesions will be more likely to involve anterior frontal sites within the MCA territory (peri-rolandic).

later, a target circle appeared at varying distances from the start circle. The participant was instructed to move the stylus as quickly and accurately as possible to the target. Participants sat in front of a monitor to perform the task while reaction time, velocity and the initial and secondary components of the movement were recorded. Eleven LHD and 14 RHD stroke patients participated in this study. The RHD subjects were able to perform this simple aiming task without any disturbance in the movement trajectory. In contrast, the LHD subjects were slower to initiate the movement, and showed deficits in the initial but not the secondary movement component. These results support the idea that the left hemisphere regulates some aspects of open-loop processing. Visual feedback was not manipulated in this study; therefore, it was unclear whether some of these effects could be influenced by specific visual feedback conditions. Unfortunately, because of the small sample size, participants were not divided into apraxic and nonapraxic groups. These results suggest that LHD patients with paresis have ipsilateral dynamic deficits in trajectory control based on impaired modulation of torque amplitude as response amplitude increases.

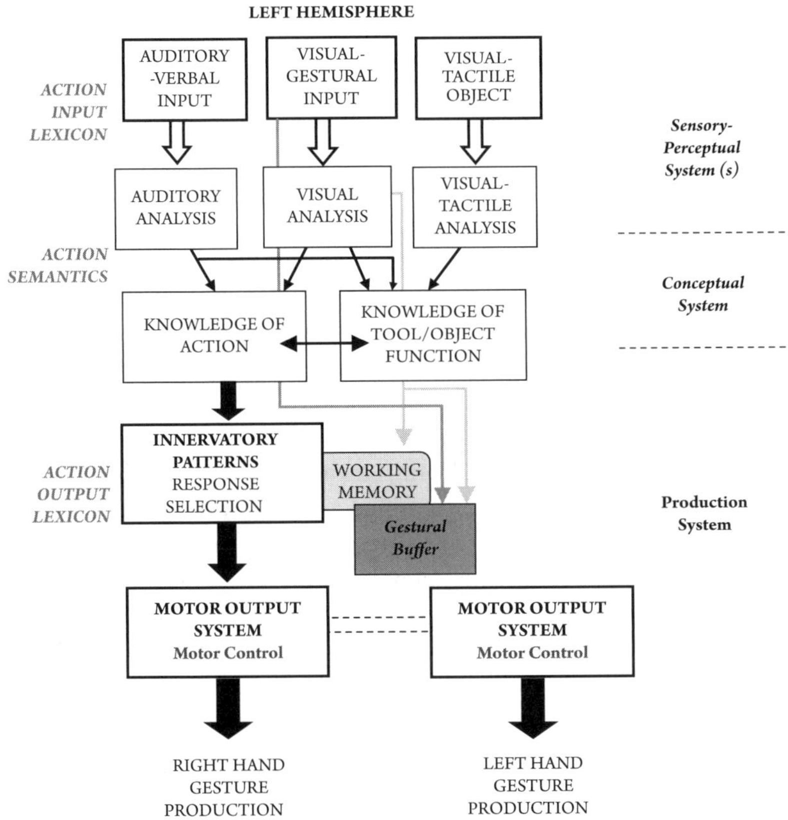

Figure 9.2 Praxis Cognitive-Process Model. This figure is presented to show a current "box diagram" that depicts the praxis system based on a modified Heilman-Rothi-Roy-Cubelli model.

The specific nature of these ipsilateral motor deficits was directly examined in a study that evaluated several aspects of motor control in LHD and RHD stroke patients (Schaefer, Haaland, & Sainburg, 2007). Healthy controls, LHD and RHD patients were observed producing targeted single-joint elbow movements of different amplitude in ipsilesional space. LHD, but not RHD, patients had reduced acceleration amplitude. RHD, but not LHD, patients made errors at the end of the movement with reduced amplitude. These results support the idea that the right and left hemisphere contribute different types of actions to the movement trajectory. Specifically, LHD patients had more difficulty with the initiation of movements, and RHD patients had more difficulty with the final movement position. In another study, Haaland and colleagues examined ipsilesional trajectory control in LHD patients with and without hemiparesis and in a group of controls in order to evaluate the lateralized contribution of the left hemisphere to this aspect of motor control (Schaefer, Haaland, & Sainburg, 2009). Only the paretic group showed dynamic deficits of movement characterized by reduced modulation of the peak torque. These results could not be attributed to lesion volume or to peak velocity as these variables did not differ between the groups. Lesion location differed with the paretic group having involvement of motor cortical areas. In summary, these studies have shown that limb apraxia may induce a deficit in the ability to parse serial movements within a hierarchical structure. Specific aspects of motor programming may be associated with disorders of learned skilled movements in individuals with LHD with and without apraxia. Ipsilesional motor deficits may differ by hemisphere and may explain the ipsilesional deficits in motor control post-stroke (Haaland, 2006). These hemispheric differences may also be manifested by the different types of errors seen during gesture production in LHD versus RHD stroke patients.

Kinematic studies also show some differences in motor control and motor programming during learned skilled movements. In order to evaluate movement trajectories, Clark and colleagues examined the kinematics of limb movements with the production of a "slicing" movement required to cut a loaf of bread into slices (Clark, et al., 1994). The spatiotemporal features of the movements were examined in a series of conditions in which contextual cues were introduced in a graded fashion. Three patients with limb apraxia associated with left parietal stroke and four healthy controls were studied. The apraxic patients, who performed the task with the ipsilesional limb, had a decoupling of the spatiotemporal relationships across cue conditions. These patients showed some improvement in movement amplitude and speed with the addition of the object being acted upon, but did not show as much benefit with the addition of the actual tool. These results are interesting and important to reconcile with the motor control studies of Haaland and colleagues that show different amplitude and movement trajectory impairments in movements performed with the ipsilesional limb. In another study, Poizner and colleagues analyzed joint-coordination deficits in these same apraxic patients (Poizner, et al., 1995). This study showed that these patients had deficits in the spatial plan of the movement and had difficulty translating these action plans into the angular motions at the joint even when physically manipulating the actual tool/object.

In a recent study, Jacobs and colleagues (2009) investigated object manipulation by examining the relationship between the ability to integrate an object into a coordinated movement, and then related this performance directly to tool use. LHD patients with and without apraxia were studied. Participants were asked to point to targets located at various distances using either their finger (body-part as tool) or using one of two sticks (i.e., tools) of different lengths (23 and 53 cm). Movement kinematics were analyzed with an emphasis on the position of the tool/finger in relation to the target, defined as the working point of the action. The LHD patients without apraxia produced similar kinematic movement characteristics across all conditions and they were slightly less accurate with the stick relative to the finger. In contrast, the performance of the LHD patients with apraxia was more variable. They concluded that this impairment may be related to disruption of dynamic body representation (Jacobs, Bussel, Combeaud, & Roby-Brami, 2009). It may be that this type of performance indicates a problem with extra-corporal space and the trajectory. Indeed, this movement type may be characteristic of a body-part-as tool problem with the internal configuration and movement of the limb in relation to the object being acted upon. An alternative explanation could be that action execution (motor control) and action observation (visual transcoding of the movement representation to the motor plan) may be partially mediated by mirror neurons that link action observation to action execution (Agnew, Brownsett, Woodhead, & de Boissezon, 2008; de Jong, van der Graaf, & Paans, 2001; Freund, 2001; Pazzaglia, Pizzamiglio, Pes, & Aglioti, 2008; Rothi, Heilman, & Watson, 1985).

The Heilman-Rothi praxis model attempts to reconcile conceptual and preparatory aspects of the motor program with perceptual and kinematic features, and is designed to account for abstract concepts such as praxis imagery and object imagery. A study of a patient with selective deficits in praxis imagery illustrates how visual object imagery may be independent of the ability to visualize the kinematics of a movement sequence required to produce a goal-directed movement (Ochipa, et al., 1997). Imagery for learned skilled movement (praxis imagery) was studied in a patient with severe limb apraxia. This patient, who made predominantly spatial and movement errors when performing transitive (tool) limb movements to command, was also impaired in her ability to answer imagery questions about joint movement or the spatial position of the hands during an action. Visual object imagery was spared. The finding of these parallel praxis production and praxis imagery deficits supports the idea that the same representations used for gesture production are activated during imagery of motor acts. Functional imaging studies have supported this view (de Jong, et al., 2001; Freund, 2001). These findings also suggest that certain aspects of motor imagery may be dissociable from general object imagery (Ochipa, et al., 1997).

Apraxia Assessment

One of the earliest observations about apraxia was that impairments can be seen under some performance conditions and not others (for review, Heilman, 1979). There are patients that can perform gestures-to-imitation but not to command. Other patients may not have deficits when performing gestures-to-command, but may have impaired gesture-recognition discrimination. Each of these types of deficits can be examined with tasks that probe specific cognitive and motor operations within a praxis model. Thus, different gesture types elicited under a variety of performance conditions should be administered when conducting a comprehensive assessment of a patient with limb apraxia. Table 9.2 includes a list of some common examples of gestures elicited to command and to imitation in patients with limb apraxia. In the research setting, these tasks are videotaped for later scoring by trained raters. The approach may vary in the clinical setting where limb apraxia is most commonly examined by having a patient pantomime-to-command a series of tool-gestures. For example, the clinician would ask the patient to "show me how you would use a hammer to hammer a nail into the wall." As the patient is performing the gesture, the clinician observes the performance of this gesture-to-command and scores the limb movement as apraxic or not apraxic. This type of gesture-to-command task is considered the most sensitive test of ideomotor apraxia, as many apraxic patients improve when gesturing to imitation, and improve further when performing gestures with the actual tool (Heilman, 1979).

LIMB APRAXIA SUBTESTS AND ERROR TYPES

There is considerable inconsistency in the literature with respect to the methods used to assess apraxia. In most studies, the predominant focus has been on the assessment of gesture production, elicited with tests of gesture-to-command and/or gesture imitation. While this method is essential to the evaluation, it does not challenge the full range of functional elements that comprise the cognitive praxis model. A more comprehensive approach will permit a more detailed analysis of discrete deficits that may be tied to specific components of the praxis neural system (refer to Table 9.1). For example, some praxis assessment methods evaluate a combination of representational and/or nonrepresentational movements. Representational gestures can be subdivided into *transitive* gestures that involve the manipulation of an object, often a tool (e.g., showing the examiner how to use a hammer, how to use a key to unlock a door), and *intransitive* gestures that do not require the use of an object, but are more abstract representational or emblematic movements (e.g., showing the examiner how to salute, how to wave good-bye). Nonrepresentational movements can include single static hand-limb postures and movement sequences. Examination of these aspects of functioning is important for an understanding of the subject's ability to produce specific motor movements independent of lexical processing, which may be disrupted following LHD (Rothi, Raymer, & Heilman, 1997). Another important consideration in praxis testing relates to the limb evaluated. In unilateral stroke patients, it is critical that the unaffected, ipsilesional limb is used when assessing praxis performance. This instruction is important, especially when examining unilateral stroke patients, in order to control for potential confounds of weakness, sensory loss, or movement disorder. The operational definition of apraxia requires the exclusion of these neurological deficits in the limb that is being examined for apraxia. The examiner may focus on an examination of the dominant hand-limb or may evaluate

Table 9.2 **Examples of Stimuli Used in Apraxia Assessment**

Transitive Limb Movements—Gestures that require a tool or implement
• Show me how you would use a hammer to pound a nail into the wall.
• Show me how you would use a saw to cut a piece of wood.
• Show me how you would use a glass to drink some water.
• Show me how you would use a spoon to stir a cup of coffee on the table.
• Show me how you would use a comb to fix your hair.
• Show me how you would use a toothbrush to clean your teeth.
Intransitive Limb Movements—Gestures that do not require a tool or implement
• Show me how you would wave good-bye.
• Show me come here.
• Show me stop.
• Show me be quiet.
Action Schema—Gesture Action Sequences for Complex Movements
• Write and post a letter (paper, pen, envelope, stamp)
1. Write the letter.
2. Sign the letter.
3. Fold the piece of paper.
4. Put the paper in the envelope.
5. Seal the envelope.
6. Write the address on the envelope.
7. Lick the stamp.
8. Put the stamp on the envelope.
• Make toast (bread, toaster, plate, butter, jelly, knife)
1. Get a slice of bread.
2. Put the piece of bread in the toaster.
3. Press the toaster on (push the lever).
4. Wait for the bread to toast.
5. Put the toast on to the plate.
6. Put butter on the bread.
7. Put jelly on the bread.

both limbs in patients without sensorimotor deficits (e.g., Alzheimer's disease). The patient must be able to comprehend the task. It is essential that patients with apraxia are evaluated clinically. including a neurological examination of cranial nerves, sensorimotor function, coordination and balance, gait, and reflexes. In some instances, a comprehensive neuropsychological evaluation is necessary in patients with limb apraxia and related disorders of movement action and planning. This examination should assess attention and memory, language, visuospatial and executive functions, and motor dexterity and skill.

An additional dimension of analysis concerns the evaluation of error types in apraxia. Several scoring systems have been developed. One of the most systematic of the available scoring systems is that developed by Rothi and colleagues (Rothi, Mack, Verfaellie, Brown, & Heilman, 1988). This scoring system is based on American Sign Language with gestures analyzed qualitatively within four general domains: *spatial, temporal, content,* and *other.* A list of the error types and operational definitions as described by Rothi and colleagues (1988) is depicted in Table 9.3. Some of these error types are more common than others. For example, Goodglass & Kaplan (1963) found that when pantomiming to command, many patients with LHD produced errors in which they used a body part as if it were the tool (body-part-as-tool, BPT). These authors suggested that this error type may be pathognomonic of limb apraxia. Raymer and colleagues examined BPT gestures in LHD and healthy control subjects (Raymer, Maher, Foundas, Heilman, & Rothi, 1997). Two performance conditions were examined. In one of the conditions the subject was "reinstructed" to modify the inappropriate BPT error and in the other condition no instructions were given when BPT errors were made. The results of this study showed that patients with more severe apraxia were less likely to improve with prompting in contrast to the less severely impaired patients and controls who did use this instruction to self-correct. These results support the hypothesis that BPT errors may be associated with a more severe form of limb apraxia (although not pathognomnic), and that many patients who self-correct with reinstruction may not have a clinical diagnosis of limb apraxia.

STANDARDIZED APRAXIA BATTERIES

There are only a few standardized apraxia scales commercially available. Two of these, the Test of Oral and Limb Apraxia (TOL A) (Helm-Estabrooks, 1998) and the Kertesz apraxia subtest provided with the Western Aphasia Battery (Kertesz, 2006) have been widely used by clinicians and researchers. However, these tests do not cover all domains and semantic features of gesture production. In addition, these tests include both limb and buccofacial movements when deriving an overall apraxia score. This practice of collapsing across gesture types can limit the utility of the test score. The De Renzi tests of ideomotor and ideational apraxia are also widely used to evaluate apraxia (De Renzi, et al., 1980; De Renzi, Pieczuro,

Table 9.3 **Limb Apraxia: Error Types and Operational Definitions**

I. Content	*P*	*perseverative*	*A response that includes all or part of a previously produced pantomime*
	RC	*related content*	*Accurately produced pantomime associated in content to the target. For example, the subject might pantomime playing a trombone for a target of a bugle.*
	NC	*non-related content*	*Accurately produced pantomime not associated in content to the target. For example, the subject might pantomime playing a trombone for a target of shaving.*
II. Temporal	*S*	*sequence*	*Some pantomimes require multiple positioning of joints performed in a characteristic sequence. Sequencing errors involve any perturbation of this sequence including addition, deletion, or transposition of movements with the overall movement structure recognizable.*
	T	*time*	*Alterations from the typical timing or speed of a pantomime and may include an abnormally increased, decreased, or irregular rate of production.*
	O	*occurrence*	*A response that includes single (i.e., unlocking a door with a key) or repetitive (i.e., screwing in a screw with a screwdriver) movement cycles. This error reflects any multiplication of single cycles or reduction of a repetitive cycle to a single event.*
III. Spatial	*A*	*amplitude*	*Any amplification, reduction, or irregularity of the characteristic amplitude of a target pantomime.*
	IC	*internal configuration*	*When pantomiming, the fingers/hand must be in a specific spatial relation to one another to accommodate the imagined tool. This error type reflects any abnormality of the required finger/hand posture and its relationship to the target tool. For example, when asked to pretend to brush teeth, the subject's hand may be fisted with no space for the imagined toothbrush handle.*
	BPT	*body-part-as tool*	*The subject uses his/her finger/hand/arm as the imagined tool. For example, when asked to smoke a cigarette, the subject might puff on his index finger.*

(continued)

Table 9.3 **(Continued)**

	ECO	*external configuration orientation*	*When pantomiming, the fingers/hand/arm and the imagined tool must be in a specific relationship to the "object" receiving the action. Errors include difficulties orienting to the "object" or in placing the "object" in space. For example, the subject might pantomime brushing teeth by holding his hand next to his mouth without reflecting the distance needed to accommodate a toothbrush.*
	M	*movement*	*When acting on an object with a tool, a movement characteristic of the action and necessary to achieve the goal is required. A movement error is any disturbance of the characteristic movement. When pantomiming a screwdriver, a subject may orient the imagined tool correctly relative to the imagined screw, but instead of stabilizing the shoulder-wrist and twisting at the elbow, the subject stabilizes the elbow and twists at the wrist or shoulder.*
IV. Other	*NR*	*no response*	*No response is elicited.*
	UR	*unrecognizable response*	*A response is not recognizable and shares no temporal or spatial features of the target.*

Source: Modified from Rothi et al. (1988).

& Vignolo, 1968). One potential limitation is that gesture scoring is not segregated into command and imitation subtests, but these instructions are included as sequential probes depending on task performance. This scoring system can mask potentially important differences across these types of gesture production and may overestimate praxis severity.

Two comprehensive limb apraxia scales have recently been described and validated. One is a revision of the Rothi-Heilman comprehensive Florida Apraxia Battery (Power, Code, Croot, Sheard, & Gonzalez Rothi, 2009), and the other is a short-version designed to examine upper limb apraxia (Vanbellingen, et al., 2009). This newly developed test of upper limb ideomotor apraxia (TULIA) was administered to a sample of 50 healthy adults, 84 LHD and 49 RHD patients. The test is comprehensive, but still short to administer. The TULIA consists of 48 items including imitation and pantomime domains of non-symbolic (meaningless), intransitive (communicative) and transitive (tool-related) gestures corresponding to 6 subtests. A 6-point scoring method (0–5) was used (score range 0–240) to score videotaped performances of these subjects. The raters were blinded and had mostly good-to-excellent internal consistency, inter- and intra-rater (test-retest) reliability, both at the level of the six subtests and at the individual item level. Construct validity was demonstrated by a high correlation with the De Renzi apraxia test. The second comprehensive battery was developed by Rothi and colleagues (Power, et al., 2009). This battery extends and is a revision of the experimental Florida Apraxia Battery (Rothi, et al., 1992). This theoretically motivated comprehensive clinical assessment of limb apraxia includes subtests designed to distinguish components of the praxis system based on the Rothi-Heilman cognitive model of apraxia. It includes subtests that examine gesture-to-command and to imitation. Gesture recognition and discrimination are evaluated. Transitive and intransitive limb movements are evaluated and scored separately and together to yield a total apraxia score. Conceptual aspects of apraxia are evaluated and gesture naming is also tested. Responses are scored as correct or incorrect (i.e., apraxic) and an error analysis is used to examine specific error types and error domains as listed earlier in Table 9.3.

Many clinicians and researchers have speculated about age, education, and sex-related differences in praxis performance. Because apraxia is left-lateralized in most individuals, it is also important and interesting to evaluate potential factors that may modify these systems and/or that may be associated with atypical praxis laterality (i.e., bilateral or rightward). Some studies have evaluated praxis performance in left-handers and in women. Women may have an advantage in the ability to rapidly and accurately learn gesture sequences compared to men (Chipman & Hampson, 2006), however, another study did not find any performance differences when healthy men and women were compared on a praxis test (Rodrigues Cavalcante & Caramelli, 2009). This study also evaluated the effects of age and education. Ninety-six individuals were divided into two age groups (60–74 and 75–88 years). Each group included equal numbers of men and women. Individuals were asked to carry out tasks on verbal command and to imitation. There were no differences between the performance of men and women. Older individuals, however, performed more poorly than their younger counterparts. As far as educational level, three major groups emerged with performance differences across the education groups defined as follows: illiterate, individuals with 1–7 years of education, and those with 8 or more years of education. These results suggest that age and education significantly influenced the performance of individuals in limb praxis tests. Differences in lateralization of motor and praxis representations may be more common in non-right-handers. Therefore, it is important to evaluate hand preference and hand skill in individuals with limb apraxia.

In summary, limb apraxia is classified by accuracy and the nature of the errors made by the patient and the means by which these errors are elicited, but there is no widely used *standardized* test for limb apraxia. In the ideal situation, the apraxia examination would challenge all modules of functioning proposed by the cognitive model: gesture reception, gesture conceptualization and gesture production: (1) gesture-to-command; (2) gesture-imitation; and (3) gesture recognition-discrimination. Further division of representational gestures into transitive and intransitive categories allows for more refined hypotheses regarding lesion localization (hemispheric, cortical-subcortical).

Localization of Apraxia

Although estimates vary across studies (i.e., 40–70 percent of unilateral LHD patients have limb apraxia), there is considerable evidence that praxis systems are lateralized to the left cerebral hemisphere in most right-handers (Haaland & Flaherty, 1984; Haaland & Harrington, 1996; Hanna-Pladdy, Daniels, et al., 2001; Poizner, Mack, Verfaellie, Rothi, & Heilman, 1990; Poizner, et al., 1998; Rapcsak, Ochipa, Beeson, & Rubens, 1993; Roy, et al., 2000). Differences in these estimates relate to criteria for establishing apraxia, mode of gesture elicitation, the duration post-stroke, and other factors (e.g., atypical cerebral laterality). In general, the left hemisphere appears to be dominant for transitive limb movements, and for the imitation of complex limb movements (Rapcsak, et al., 1993; Schnider, Hanlon, Alexander, & Benson, 1997). There is conflicting evidence regarding the contributions of the right hemisphere in mediating movement sequences, especially intransitive movements (Foundas, Henchey, Gilmore, Fennell, & Heilman, 1995; Hanna-Pladdy, Daniels, et al., 2001). Some have suggested that the left-hemisphere is dominant for preparing and programming of movements (Haaland, Harrington, & Knight, 2000), and for learning to select the limb movement associated with the action of a specific object (Rushworth, Nixon, Wade, Renowden, & Passingham, 1998).

PRAXIS NETWORKS AND HEMISPHERIC DIFFERENCES

The regions important in the praxis network are depicted in Figure 9.3 based on a left-lateralized praxis system. The critical regions include the inferior parietal lobe (SMG), inter-hemispheric white matter connections (including cortical-cortical and cortical-subcortical pathways), and premotor regions with a special role for the supplementary motor area (SMA). In order to examine lesion differences in unilateral LHD and RHD stroke patients, Haaland, Harrington, and Knight compared areas of lesion overlap in patients with and without limb apraxia (based on a gesture imitation task). Those with limb apraxia were found to have damage to a left hemispheric network involving the middle frontal gyrus (MFG) and the anterior bank of the intra-parietal sulcus region within the SMG. The SMA was not a common lesion site in their patients with apraxia. Because these patients were examined many months

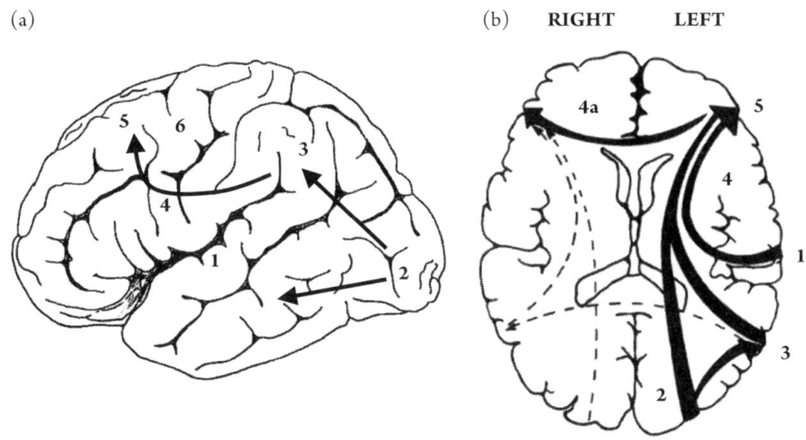

Neural systems implicated in right limb movements depicted in:

(a) lateral view of the left hemisphere
(b) axial view in the left hemisphere

Figure 9.3 Anatomy of Limb Apraxia. This figure shows the anatomy of limb apraxia localized to a left hemisphere network. The critical cortical and subcortical neuroanatomical areas and the white matter pathways involved in limb movements are listed by number. Brodmann's areas (BA) are also provided for each of these regions

1 = Auditory representations	(BA 41, 42, 22) – Temporal cortex
2 = Visual representations	(BA 17, 18, 19, 37) – Occipital cortex
3 = Cross-modal associations	(BA 39, 40) – Inferior Parietal Lobule
4 = White matter (WM) connections	Inter- & Intra-hemispheric WM, PVWM
5 = Motor-Frontal representation	(BA 6, SMA, 9, 46) – Premotor/Motor planning
6 = Primary motor cortex	(BA 4) – Motor homunculus/Hand-Arm area

When the praxis representations are lateralized to the left cerebral hemisphere, the information must pass from the left hemisphere via the corpus callosum (4a) to the right hemisphere motor regions (BA 6, 4, SMA), to produce the movements with the left hand. Frontal regions (BA 9, 46) are also implicated in this action schema.

post-stroke, it may be that other systems may take over the role of this region, or the SMA may be more important in mediating gestures-to-command (Watson, et al., 1986) than to imitation. Given the role of the MFG in working memory, the authors posited that this region may maintain the gesture representation while the motor program is being accessed. Functional neuroimaging and transcranial magnetic stimulation methods have provided converging evidence that these frontal-parietal circuits are critical for the mediation of learned skilled limb movements (Fadiga, Fogassi, Pavesi, & Rizzolatti, 1995; Gerloff, Uenishi, & Hallett, 1998; Rizzolatti, Fadiga, Gallese, & Fogassi, 1996) with the left-hemisphere dominant for the production of complex (Jancke, Kleinschmidt, Mirzazade, Shah, & Freund, 2001; Moll, et al., 2000) and simple (Kim, et al., 1993) movement sequences.

A number of studies have attempted to disentangle the role of the right hemisphere in learned skilled movement. Rapcsak and colleagues (1993) reported observations on a strongly right-handed man who had a massive left hemispheric stroke that resulted in almost complete destruction of that hemisphere. Therefore, his examination may reflect the abilities that were preserved in the right cerebral hemisphere and those functions destroyed in the left hemisphere or some compensation following the brain injury. This patient was severely impaired in his ability to perform transitive limb movements to command, although he could perform intransitive movements and he was able to manipulate and use real objects. Gesture recognition and discrimination were relatively preserved. Whole body types of axial commands were also preserved. Based on these observations, Rapcsak and colleagues postulated that the right hemisphere is critically dependent on the left hemisphere for the transcallosal transfer of stored representations of the motor program and for the abstract production of learned skilled movements. Context-dependent movements, however, were relatively preserved especially in over-learned movements like the manipulation of common tools suggesting that the right hemisphere may play a role in these specific conditions. This study also supported the idea that the right hemisphere may play an important role in gesture recognition/discrimination in some individuals.

In another study, error types were compared in a control group and in a sample of LHD and RHD stroke patients evaluated within 10 days post-stroke (Hanna-Pladdy, Daniels, et al., 2001). Overall, the LHD patients made significantly more apraxic errors compared to the RHD patients and controls on both transitive and intransitive limb movements. The LHD group made more body-part as object and spatial errors, including difficulty orienting the hand to the tool (internal configuration error), and in orienting the tool to the object being acted upon. RHD patients made more timing errors than controls. The finding that body-part as object and internal configuration errors were associated with LHD supports the contention that postural representations are stored in the left hemisphere. In contrast, alterations in the timing or speed of limb movements were the best predictors of RHD. These findings support the postulate that the left hemisphere stores the spatiotemporal and conceptual representations of learned skilled movements, although several components of action programs, such as limb orientation and timing, may have bilateral hemispheric representations.

To further examine the laterality of action programs, the production of learned skilled movement was documented in a study of nine patients performing gestures-to-command with the contralateral limb during selective right- and left-hemispheric anesthesia (Foundas, Henchey, et al., 1995). Results showed that praxis networks were lateralized to the left hemisphere in 7 of the 9 patients (78 percent), and were bilaterally represented in the other 2 (22 percent) participants. The full-range of spatial-temporal movement errors were elicited with left hemisphere injection. Amplitude and timing errors were uncommon overall but were found proportionally more often following right hemisphere injection. All participants were right-handed and had language lateralized to the left hemisphere. These results have been replicated (Meador, et al., 1999), and support the hypothesis that praxis networks are left-lateralized in most right-handed adults with some movement types specific to left-hemisphere networks while other components of action planning may require input from the right hemisphere (Heilman, 1997).

SUBCORTICAL BRAIN STRUCTURES IN LIMB APRAXIA

There is controversy regarding the importance of subcortical gray matter structures and cortical-subcortical white matter connections in the formulation of learned skilled movement. In a study of 699 LHD patients, Papagno and colleagues found that apraxia was mild to moderate in patients with subcortical lesions, and more severe in the cases with cortical lesions (Papagno, Della Sala, & Basso, 1993). Two other studies found that lesions to subcortical pathways were more common in patients without apraxia (Basso, Luzzatti, & Spinnler, 1980; Haaland et al, 2000). In a review of 82 cases of "subcortical" apraxia, Pramstaller and Marsden found that large left-hemisphere lesions with subcortical extension were more likely to induce apraxia than purely subcortical lesions of the putamen, thalamus. or lenticular nuclei (Pramstaller & Marsden, 1996).

In another study of patients with LHD cortical stroke, patients were evaluated on gesture-to-command, gesture-imitation, and gesture-discrimination tasks. Task performance was compared to a group of patients with purely subcortical left hemispheric lesions examined within 6 months post-stroke (Hanna-Pladdy, Heilman, & Foundas, 2001). The cortical stroke patients were impaired on all three tasks. In contrast, subcortical stroke patients had mild production-execution deficits with transitive limb movements, but normal performance of gestures to imitation and with gesture discrimination. Both groups made spatial and temporal errors, whereas only the subcortical group made postural and sequencing errors, and produced some unrecognizable gestures. In a study of 50 patients with CT scan-demonstrated LHD stroke, seven patients with lesions limited to the basal ganglia and/or thalamus were found to have ideomotor apraxia on gesture-to-command and to imitation, but performed normally with the actual object (Agostoni, Coletti, Orlando, & Tredici, 1983). Based on these results, it may be hypothesized that postural movements are mediated by frontal-subcortical networks, whereas visuo-motor transformations for reaching and the internal representation of the action plan are mediated by a left lateralized frontal-parietal network.

Lesion size and location was examined in unilateral LHD stroke patients with apraxia examined on oral and limb gestures-to-command (Kertesz &

Ferro, 1984). As predicted, lesion size and apraxia severity were positively correlated at 1 and 3 months post-stroke, although lesion size accounted for only 25 percent of the variance in apraxia. The authors found that some patients with small lesions had severe apraxia, and some patients with large lesions were not apraxic. Anterior portions of the periventricular white matter (PVWM) pathways were the most common lesion site in the apraxic patients with small lesions. Other investigators have also found that apraxia can occur in patients with small lesions of the PVWM without cortical involvement (Alexander, Baker, Naeser, Kaplan, & Palumbo, 1992; Kertesz & Ferro, 1984; Roy, Black, Blair, & Dimeck, 1998); (Freund, 2001; Freund & Hummelsheim, 1985; Kroliczak & Frey, 2009; Leiguarda, 2001). Taken together, results from these studies offer support for the postulate that lesions to white matter pathways, including small lesions at cortical and subcortical convergence points within the praxis network, can induce severe and persistent apraxia (Kertesz & Ferro, 1984). The lesions of the deep parietal, occipitofrontal and anterior callosal fibers seem to be particularly crucial in the manifestation of limb apraxia. The Geschwind and Kertesz "disconnection" models of apraxia support the postulate that some small lesions of white matter pathways are associated with apraxia. The proposed mechanism is that discrete lesions to these white matter pathways induce cortical hypoperfusion of critical sites, although this hypothesis has not been directly tested.

Our group has found differences in cortical (anterior, posterior) versus subcortical lesion location and apraxia severity (Foundas, et al., 2002). In this study, 23 LHD ischemic stroke patients and 23 healthy, matched controls were examined performing a series of gestures-to-command with no overlap between the LHD stroke patients and the controls on the gesture performance. The LHD stroke patients were then categorized as having mild (9 patients), moderate (8 patients) or severe (6 patients) apraxia. The severely apraxic patients were more likely to have lesions of the inferior parietal lobe (BA 39, 40) with extension to adjacent PVWM pathways compared to the moderate and mildly apraxic patients who did not have lesions that extended into these sites. In contrast, the moderately apraxic patients were more likely to have lesions to the somatosensory cortex compared to the other two groups, whereas the mildly apraxic patients were most likely to have purely subcortical lesions. We also found that the severely apraxic patients had lesions involving ventral temporal and visual pathways (areas 37, 18, 19) (Figure 9.4 a,b). These results support current anatomic models of apraxia, and provide evidence that there may be a *caudal-rostral* (posterior-anterior) and *cortical-subcortical* gradient of lesion site and praxis severity (Figure 9.5). Based on the finding that lesions to visual association and ventral temporal cortex resulted in severely degraded gesture production, we postulate that patients with this lesion profile may have lost the ability of the motor programs to access the visual representations of the movements. It is still unclear whether these lesion

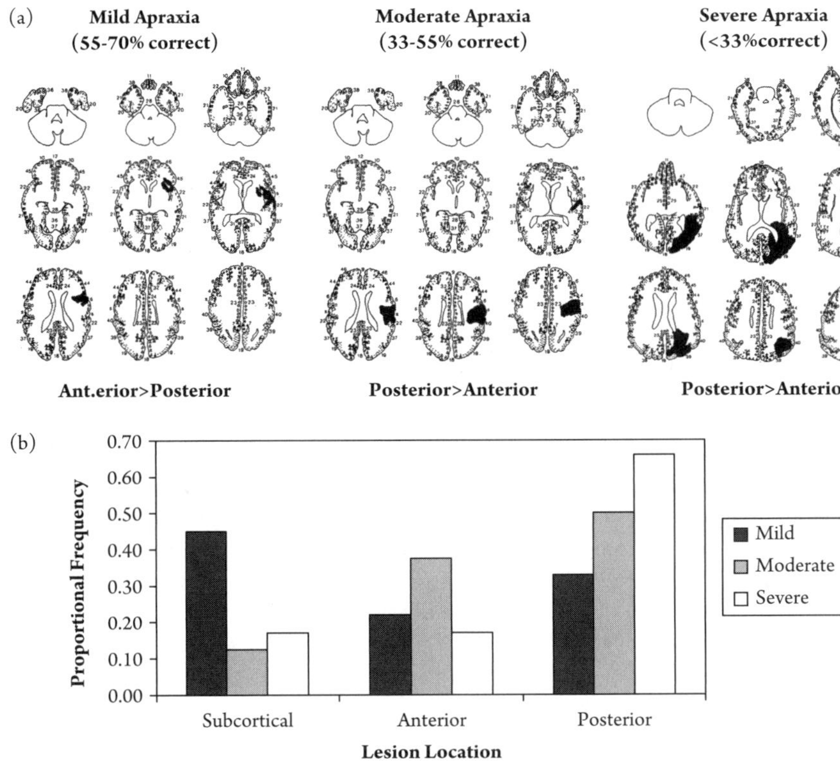

Figure 9.4 Lesion location varied in patients defined as having mild, moderate, and severe limb apraxia. Overlapping lesion sites are depicted in Figure 9.4(a) by severity subgroup (mild, moderate, severe apraxia) and the proportional frequency by lesion location is shown in Figure 9.4(b). (a) lesion mapping of lhd stroke patients with mild, moderate and severe (b) lesion localization in lhd stroke patients with apraxia.

sites are associated with persistent apraxia, as the patients were examined at 2 to 7 weeks post-stroke.

CONCEPTUAL APRAXIA AND TOOL KNOWLEDGE

Cognitive models and behavioral studies of apraxia have shown that the praxis production, reception, and conceptual systems are partially dissociable. One study examined conceptual apraxia in unilateral stroke patients (Heilman, Maher, Greenwald, & Rothi, 1997). Four groups were examined including: LHD patients with apraxia, LHD without apraxia, RHD stroke patients, and controls. Praxis conceptual systems were examined by assessing tool-action and tool-object relationships, and mechanical-tool knowledge. The

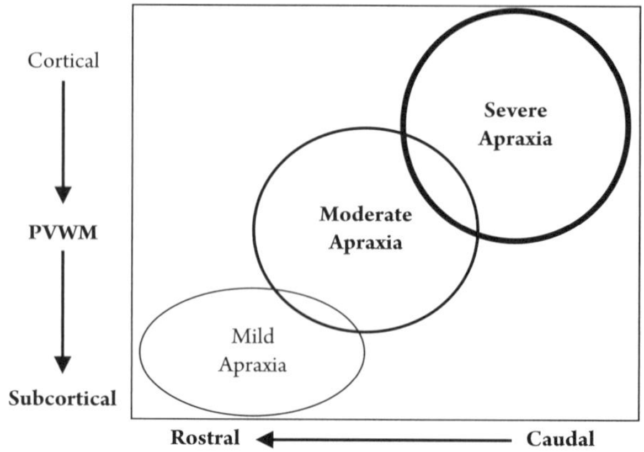

Figure 9.5 Rostral-Caudal and Vertical Gradient of Apraxia Severity. Differences in lesion location by apraxia severity suggest that there may be a severity gradient as depicted in Figure 9.5. Our data suggest that patients with large posterior lesions with subcortical extension would have a more severe type of limb apraxia compared to patients with small purely subcortical anterior lesions who would be expected to have a milder type of apraxia. It is important to note, however, that small lesions to convergence zones have been associated with moderate to severe limb apraxia.

LHD group with apraxia was more impaired on the tasks compared to all the other groups, but within the left hemisphere specific lesion sites were not associated with conceptual apraxia. The results also showed that tool knowledge (action semantics) was independent of the movement representations and verbal semantics. A functional MRI adaptation paradigm was used to test for brain regions that exhibit action-specific activity in order to evaluate brain regions that may be specific to action recognition (Kable & Chatterjee, 2006). Subjects watched a series of different types of action sequences. The results of this study showed that the representations stored in the superior temporal sulcus, human motion-sensitive cortex (middle to superior temporal), and extrastriate body area abstract actions from agents involved in the action. These brain regions also distinguished between different actions.

The ability to access tool-use-knowledge and to integrate this information into a movement plan is frequently disrupted in patients with limb apraxia. A recent study was designed to examine potential differences between these types of tasks (Randerath, Li, Goldenberg, & Hermsdorfer, 2009). Twenty controls, 17 LHD, and 10 RHD patients were evaluated performing gestures with the tool presented with the handle oriented away from the participant, and with the tool in the correct orientation. Participants were asked to grasp the tool and to demonstrate its typical "use" or to "transport" the tool into a container. Task content influenced the way the object was grasped. Nearly all participants, except for a few LHD subjects, produced a functional grasp during all of the "use"-task conditions. Non-functional grasping was always followed by apraxic tool use. These results suggest that grasping a tool is task specific. Selection of the grasp seemed to be influenced by several factors, including knowledge about the function of the object, structural tool characteristics, biomechanical cost of the movement, and prior experience. Perception and integration of tool structure plus specific tool-related functional knowledge are necessary for accurate or functional goal-directed movements and may need to be processed synchronously. These results support the idea that lesions to visual association and ventral temporal cortex may be associated with severely degraded gesture production because of the inability of the motor programs to access the visual representation of the movement.

Conceptual apraxia was studied in 32 patients with probable Alzheimer's disease (AD) and 32 matched controls by testing tool knowledge including: tool-action relationships, tool-object associations, and mechanical tool knowledge (Ochipa, Rothi, & Heilman, 1992). The AD patients were subdivided into four groups based on the presence or absence of ideomotor apraxia and the presence or absence of a lexical-semantic deficit. Results indicated that *each* of the four AD subgroups differed from controls on at least one measure of conceptual apraxia. Some AD patients had conceptual apraxia without ideomotor apraxia, but there were no patients with the opposite finding. Based on these results, the authors postulated that conceptual apraxia may be an early marker of AD, and may occur before the development of limb apraxia. These results suggest that lexical-semantic functions may be at least partially dissociable from the praxis conceptual system.

MODALITY-SPECIFIC AND SUPRA-MODAL MECHANISMS OF APRAXIA

The unity between perception and action continues to be an important concept that may be influenced by the capacity to transform sensory information concerning the object to be grasped into an accurate hand position, and the ability to generate independent finger movements. Thus, exploratory information is tightly coupled to tactile perception, independent finger movement, and the hand-object interaction. As discussed above, higher-order object knowledge produces patterns of manual exploratory movements that lead to haptically driven object representations. Klein (1931) introduced the term "tactile apraxia" to describe patients with disturbed transitive exploratory hand movements and preserved intransitive expressive and symbolic movements (Klein, 1931). Some patients with apraxia have difficulty recognizing their own hand movements (Sirigu, Daprati, Pradat-Diehl, Franck, & Jeannerod, 1999). Unimodal disorders of tactile object exploration have been reported in patients with parietal lobe lesions (Binkofski, Kunesch, Classen, Seitz, & Freund, 2001). In this study, effective grasping and object manipulation were evaluated in healthy controls and in a series of patients with focal lesions of the parietal, anterior frontal, and motor cortex. The patients with parietal lesions could produce rapid alternating finger movements even though they had sensory deficits including astereognosia. Anterior versus posterior parietal lesions showed somewhat different behaviors. Those with posterior parietal lesions had less spatial exploration behavior, whereas the anterior parietal lesion patients had a marked increase in the exploration of space. Both of these parietal lesion subgroups had difficulty with frequency and regularity of manipulative movements. In contrast, patients with frontal lesions were very impaired in the performance of contralesional manipulation and rapid alternating movements. The authors concluded that tactile apraxia represents a deficit in the programming of exploratory movements mediated by the parietal lobe. It is interesting that the posterior parietal group was also identified as having apraxia.

Other modality specific inputs may be essential to the performance of accurate, skilled, purposeful movements. Studies in nonhuman and human primates have shown that sound-producing actions are mapped on the same mirror circuits that are activated during the visual recognition and execution of actions (Galati, et al., 2008; Kohler, et al., 2002; Lahav, Saltzman, & Schlaug, 2007; Lewis, Brefczynski, Phinney, Janik, & DeYoe, 2005; Pizzamiglio, et al., 2005). However, no putative link between auditory recognition and execution of actions has been shown. A recent study examined the recognition of sounds specifically linked to human actions (Pazzaglia, et al., 2008). They evaluated twenty-eight LHD patients with or without limb and/or buccofacial apraxia and seven RHD patients with no apraxia. Participants were asked to match sounds evoking human-related actions or nonhuman action sounds with specific visual pictures. Hand and mouth action-related sound recognition were specifically impaired in limb and buccofacial apraxia patients, respectively. Lesion mapping showed that the left frontal-parietal cortex was crucial for recognizing the sound of limb movements. In contrast, the left inferior frontal gyrus and adjacent insular cortex were associated with the recognition of buccofacial-related action sounds. These behavioral and neuroanatomical double dissociations indicate that a left-lateralized multimodal mirror network may be actively involved in the body-part-specific motor mapping of limb and mouth action-related sounds, and in turn may influence the execution of the very same actions.

Patients with apraxia may have deficits at the level of motor planning or sensorimotor integration (Beauchamp & Martin, 2007). This aspect was examined in a functional MRI study with a repetition suppression task for hand gestures using a rapid event related design with pseudo-random stimulus order (Hamilton & Grafton, 2009). Brain areas associated with action retrieval were identified by comparing trials where an action was repeated to trials that involved a new action. Performance of a novel action, collapsed across individual actions, showed greater left hemisphere activation within a predominant frontal-parietal circuit involving inferior frontal gyrus and the inferior parietal cortex (SMG). Because of this study design and because the study participants were all normal adults, these effects cannot be ascribed to kinematic differences, simple action related activity, or differences of cognitive set. In summary, there is a general consensus that a necessary condition for persistent and severe apraxia is a cortical lesion to a critical frontal-parietal region with extension to adjacent white matter pathways. Isolated cortical lesions or purely subcortical lesions are less likely to be associated with severe and persistent apraxia. Modality-specific and supra-modal aspects of goal directed behaviors are important to consider when constructing a cognitive-behavioral-anatomical model of action/praxis.

Real World Effects of Limb Apraxia

Since many patients with apraxia use tools without difficulty, some investigators have postulated that apraxia is not problematic within natural contexts (De Renzi, 1985). Others have found that patients with apraxia are impaired in natural situations (Schwartz, 1995; Schwartz, et al., 1995). Action deficits in the natural environment have been observed in traumatic brain injury and in stroke patients with apraxia. Many patients with limb apraxia have difficulty eating a meal or making a cup of coffee (Foundas, Macauley, Raymer, Maher, Heilman, & Gonzalez Rothi, 1995; Schwartz, 1995). Even simple tasks of daily living such as shaving or brushing teeth can be poorly performed or may be dangerous if the incorrect tool is selected (Schwartz & Buxbaum, 1997). For example, stroke patients have been observed to incorrectly select a comb instead of a toothbrush when intending to brush teeth (Ochipa, et al., 1989).

Spatiotemporal characteristics of gestural movements of apraxic patients, like slicing bread or carving a turkey, have shown alterations in the plane of motion, decoupling of hand speed and the trajectory curvature, changes in the wrist trajectory, and loss of inter-joint coordination (Poizner, et al., 1990; Poizner, et al., 1998). These findings, as well as analysis of action errors observed while LHD stroke subjects with apraxia were eating, suggest that limb apraxia may adversely influence activities of daily living (Foundas, Macauley, Raymer, Maher, Heilman, & Gonzalez Rothi, 1995). This view is also supported by the findings of Sundet and colleagues (Sundet, Finset, & Reinvang, 1988), who investigated the relationship between neuropsychological deficits of brain-damaged patients and their need for supervision in everyday life. They found that among LHD patients, apraxia scores correlated significantly with the level of dependence defined as an increase in caregiver burden.

In a study of ten unilateral LHD stroke patients, eight of whom were apraxic, disturbances in tool use and disruption of the infrastructure of mealtime activities were noted when they were compared to healthy matched controls (Foundas,

Macauley, Raymer, Maher, Heilman, & Gonzalez Rothi, 1995). Furthermore, a relationship was found between mealtime action errors and the severity of the apraxia suggesting that limb apraxia may adversely influence activities of daily living. Although these results demonstrated that ideomotor apraxia can have real-world effects, the patients studied were successful in completing the overall action goal and caregivers did not report difficulty in the natural context. Furthermore, previous investigations have not eliminated alternative explanations for deficits in activities of daily living such as associated motor and cognitive impairment. Consequently, whether the spatiotemporal motor deficits associated with apraxia result in dependency in activities of daily living which require remediation, remains largely unanswered.

In another study, the relationship between limb apraxia and dependency, in terms of increased caregiver assistance in the performance of physical activities of daily living, was assessed while controlling for elementary motor deficits, extent of cognitive impairment, post-stroke depression, lesion size, and stroke-test interval (Hanna-Pladdy, Heilman, & Foundas, 2003). The relationship between apraxia severity, based on scores from a verbal gesture-to-command task and the dependency score as defined by increased caregiver assistance on the Physical Self-Maintenance Scale (PSMS), was evaluated in 10 unilateral LHD stroke patients and 10 matched controls. There was a significant relationship between apraxia severity and dependency in PSMS score. Impairment on the PSMS in the apraxic patients could not be accounted for on the basis of overall cognitive impairment, post-stroke depression, elementary motor impairment, lesion size, or stroke-test interval. Analysis of categories comprising the PSMS revealed that the patients with apraxia had increased dependency in grooming, bathing, and toileting relative to age matched controls. One of the secondary goals of this study was to eliminate alternative explanations such as depression, and motor dysfunction as an explanation for the real world deficits. Therefore, patients meeting diagnostic criteria for depression were excluded. Elementary motor function was measured by a test of speed requiring independent finger movements. These deficits did not account for the severity of deficits in learned skilled movements. It is also interesting that there was no relationship between apraxia and dependence in either ambulating or dressing, two major rehabilitation targets for stroke patients. It may be that the ability to dress independently is related to perceptual deficits instead of deficits in skilled movements, as suggested by others (Baum & Hall, 1981; Warren, 1981; Williams, 1967).

The relationship between apraxia severity and dependency across a number of physical activities of daily living emphasizes the ecological implications of apraxia. This relationship suggests that rehabilitation strategies are needed to improve the execution and efficiency of coordinated skilled movements in LHD stroke patients. There is some evidence that higher order motor deficits like apraxia increase caregiver burden more than hemiparesis (Bjorneby & Reinvang,

1985; Sundet, et al., 1988). Apraxia is also associated with impaired gestural communication (Barrett, Dore, Hansell, & Heilman, 2002; Borod, Fitzpatrick, Helm-Estabrooks, & Goodglass, 1989; Foundas, Macauley, Raymer, Maher, Heilman, & Rothi, 1995). Limb apraxia is common in stroke patients with estimates that 70 percent of LHD and 30 percent of RHD patients make errors when performing learned skilled movements (Donkervoort, Dekker, van den Ende, Stehmann-Saris, & Deelman, 2000). Apraxia is also common in neurodegenerative disorders like Alzheimer's disease, corticobasal degereration, and Parkinson's disease (Cummings, 2004; Gross & Grossman, 2008; Stamenova, et al., 2009; Zadikoff & Lang, 2005). Future investigations directly measuring the performance of learned skilled movements in the natural context are needed to more specifically determine targets for treatment planning (Buxbaum, et al., 2008).

References

Agnew, Z. K., Brownsett, S., Woodhead, Z., & de Boissezon, X. (2008). A step forward for mirror neurons? Investigating the functional link between action execution and action observation in limb apraxia. *Journal of Neuroscience, 28*(31), 7726–7727.

Agostoni, E., Coletti, A., Orlando, G., & Tredici, G. (1983). Apraxia in deep cerebral lesions. *Journal of Neurology, Neurosurgery, and Psychiatry, 46*(9), 804–808.

Alexander, M. P., Baker, E., Naeser, M. A., Kaplan, E., & Palumbo, C. (1992). Neuropsychological and neuroanatomical dimensions of ideomotor apraxia. *Brain, 115 Pt 1*, 87–107.

Barrett, A. M., Dore, L. S., Hansell, K. A., & Heilman, K. M. (2002). Speaking while gesturing: the relationship between speech and limb praxis. *Neurology, 58*(3), 499–500.

Barrett, A. M., & Foundas, A. L. (2004). Apraxia. In M. Rizzo & P. Eslinger (eds.), *Principles and Practice of Behavioral Neurology and Neuropsychology* (pp. 409–422). Philadelphia: W.B. Saunders Co.

Basso, A., Luzzatti, C., & Spinnler, H. (1980). Is ideomotor apraxia the outcome of damage to well-defined regions of the left hemisphere? Neuropsychological study of CAT correlation. *Journal of Neurology, Neurosurgery, and Psychiatry, 43*(2), 118–126.

Baum, B., & Hall, K. M. (1981). Relationship between constructional praxis and dressing in the head-injured adult. *American Journal of Occupational Therapy, 35*(7), 438–442.

Beauchamp, M. S., & Martin, A. (2007). Grounding object concepts in perception and action: evidence from fMRI studies of tools. *Cortex, 43*(3), 461–468.

Binkofski, F., Kunesch, E., Classen, J., Seitz, R. J., & Freund, H. J. (2001). Tactile apraxia: unimodal apractic disorder of tactile object exploration associated with parietal lobe lesions. *Brain, 124*(Pt 1), 132–144.

Bjorneby, E. R., & Reinvang, I. R. (1985). Acquiring and maintaining self-care skills after stroke. The predictive value of apraxia. *Scandinavian Journal of Rehabilitation Medicine, 17*(2), 75–80.

Borod, J. C., Fitzpatrick, P. M., Helm-Estabrooks, N., & Goodglass, H. (1989). The relationship between limb apraxia and the spontaneous use of communicative gesture in aphasia. *Brain and Cognition, 10*(1), 121–131.

Buxbaum, L. J., Haaland, K. Y., Hallett, M., Wheaton, L., Heilman, K. M., Rodriguez, A., et al. (2008). Treatment of limb apraxia: moving forward to improved action. *American Journal of Physical Medicine & Rehabilitation* 87(2), 149-161.

Chipman, K., & Hampson, E. (2006). A female advantage in the serial production of non-representational learned gestures. *Neuropsychologia, 44*(12), 2315–2329.

Clark, M. A., Merians, A. S., Kothari, A., Poizner, H., Macauley, B., Gonzalez Rothi, L. J., et al. (1994). Spatial planning deficits in limb apraxia. *Brain, 117 (Pt 5),* 1093–1106.

Cubelli, R., Marchetti, C., Boscolo, G., & Della Sala, S. (2000). Cognition in action: testing a model of limb apraxia. *Brain and Cognition, 44*(2), 144–165.

Cummings, J. L. (2004). Drug Therapy: Alzheimer's disease. *New England Journal of Medicine, 351*(1), 56–67.

de Jong, B. M., van der Graaf, F. H., & Paans, A. M. (2001). Brain activation related to the representations of external space and body scheme in visuomotor control. *Neuroimage, 14*(5), 1128–1135.

De Renzi, E. (1985). Methods of limb apraxia examination and their bearing on the interpretation of the disorder. In E. A. Roy (ed.), *Neuropsychological studies of apraxia and related disorders* (pp. 45–64). Amsterdam: Elsevier Science Publishers.

De Renzi, E., & Lucchelli, F. (1988). Ideational apraxia. *Brain, 111 (Pt 5),* 1173–1185.

De Renzi, E., Motti, F., & Nichelli, P. (1980). Imitating gestures. A quantitative approach to ideomotor apraxia. *Archives of Neurology, 37*(1), 6–10.

De Renzi, E., Pieczuro, O., & Vignolo, L. A. (1968). Ideational apraxia: A quantitative study. *Neuropsychologia, 6,* 41–52.

Dee, H. L., Benton, A. L., & Van Allen, M. W. (1970). Apraxia in relation to hemispheric locus of lesion and aphasia. *Transactions of the American Neurological Association, 95,* 147–150.

Donkervoort, M., Dekker, J., van den Ende, E., Stehmann-Saris, J. C., & Deelman, B. G. (2000). Prevalence of apraxia among patients with a first left hemisphere stroke in rehabilitation centres and nursing homes. *Clinical Rehabilitation, 14*(2), 130–136.

Fadiga, L., Fogassi, L., Pavesi, G., & Rizzolatti, G. (1995). Motor facilitation during action observation: a magnetic stimulation study. *Journal of Neurophysiology, 73*(6), 2608–2611.

Fisk, J. D., & Goodale, M. A. (1988). The effects of unilateral brain damage on visually guided reaching: hemispheric differences in the nature of the deficit. *Experimental Brain Research, 72*(2), 425–435.

Foundas, A. L., Daniels, S. K., Maher, L. M., Raymer, A. M., Rothi, L. J., & Heilman, K. M. (2002). Lesion localization in ideomotor limb apraxia: A relationship to praxis. *Neurology, 58.*

Foundas, A. L., Henchey, R., Gilmore, R. L., Fennell, E. B., & Heilman, K. M. (1995). Apraxia during Wada testing. *Neurology, 45*(7), 1379–1383.

Foundas, A. L., Macauley, B. L., Raymer, A. M., Maher, L. M., Heilman, K. M., & Gonzalez Rothi, L. J. (1995). Ecological implications of limb apraxia: evidence from mealtime behavior. *Journal of the International Neuropsychological Society, 1*(1), 62-66.

Foundas, A. L., Macauley, B. L., Raymer, A. M., Maher, L. M., Heilman, K. M., & Rothi, L. J. (1995). Gesture laterality in aphasic and apraxic stroke patients. *Brain and Cognition, 29*(2), 204–213.

Freund, H. J. (2001). The parietal lobe as a sensorimotor interface: a perspective from clinical and neuroimaging data. *Neuroimage, 14*(1 Pt 2), S142–146.

Freund, H. J., & Hummelsheim, H. (1985). Lesions of premotor cortex in man. *Brain, 108 (Pt 3),* 697–733.

Galati, G., Committeri, G., Spitoni, G., Aprile, T., Di Russo, F., Pitzalis, S., et al. (2008). A selective representation of the meaning of actions in the auditory mirror system. *Neuroimage, 40*(3), 1274–1286.

Gerloff, C., Uenishi, N., & Hallett, M. (1998). Cortical activation during fast repetitive finger movements in humans: dipole sources of steady-state movement-related cortical potentials. *Journal of Clinical Neurophysiology, 15*(6), 502–513.

Geschwind, N. (1965). Disconnexion syndromes in animals and man. *Brain, 88*(2), 237–294.

Geschwind, N., & Kaplan, E. (1962). A human cerebral deconnection syndrome. A preliminary report. *Neurology, 12,* 675–685.

Gogol, N. (1873). *Ein Beitrag zur lehre von der Aphasie.* Breslau, Inaugural Dissertation.

Goodglass, H., & Kaplan, E. (1963). Disturbance of Gesture and Pantomime in Aphasia. *Brain, 86,* 703–720.

Gross, R. G., & Grossman, M. (2008). Update on apraxia. *Current Neurology and Neuroscience Reports, 8*(6), 490–496.
Haaland, K. Y. (2006). Left hemisphere dominance for movement. *Clinical Neuropsychology, 20*(4), 609–622.
Haaland, K. Y., & Flaherty, D. (1984). The different types of limb apraxia errors made by patients with left vs. right hemisphere damage. *Brain and Cognition, 3*(4), 370–384.
Haaland, K. Y., & Harrington, D. L. (1996). Hemispheric asymmetry of movement. *Current Opinion in Neurobiology, 6*(6), 796–800.
Haaland, K. Y., Harrington, D. L., & Knight, R. T. (2000). Neural representations of skilled movement. *Brain, 123 (Pt 11)*, 2306–2313.
Hamilton, A. F., & Grafton, S. T. (2009). Repetition suppression for performed hand gestures revealed by fMRI. *Human Brain Mapping, 30*(9), 2898–2906.
Hanna-Pladdy, B., Daniels, S. K., Fieselman, M. A., Thompson, K., Vasterling, J. J., Heilman, K. M., et al. (2001). Praxis lateralization: errors in right and left hemisphere stroke. *Cortex, 37*(2), 219–230.
Hanna-Pladdy, B., Heilman, K. M., & Foundas, A. L. (2001). Cortical and subcortical contributions to ideomotor apraxia: analysis of task demands and error types. *Brain, 124*(Pt 12), 2513–2527.
Hanna-Pladdy, B., Heilman, K. M., & Foundas, A. L. (2003). Ecological implications of ideomotor apraxia: evidence from physical activities of daily living. *Neurology, 60*(3), 487–490.
Harrington, D. L., & Haaland, K. Y. (1997). Representations of actions in ideomotor limb apraxia: Clues from motor programming and control. In L. J. Rothi & K. M. Heilman (eds.), *Apraxia: The Neuropsychology of Action* (pp. 111–147). East Sussex UK: Psychology Press.
Heilman, K. M. (1979). Apraxia. In K. M. Heilman & E. Valenstein (eds.), *Clinical Neuropsychology* (pp. 159–185). New York: Oxford University Press.
Heilman, K. M. (1997). Handedness. In L. J. Rothi & K. M. Heilman (Eds.), *Apraxia: The neuropsychology of action* (pp. 19–28). East Sussex: Psychology Press.
Heilman, K. M., & Gonzalez Rothi, L. J. (2003). Apraxia. In K. M. Heilman & E. Valenstein (eds.), *Clinical Neuropsychology* (4th ed., pp. 215–235). Oxford: Oxford University Press.
Heilman, K. M., Maher, L. M., Greenwald, M. L., & Rothi, L. J. (1997). Conceptual apraxia from lateralized lesions. *Neurology, 49*(2), 457–464.
Heilman, K. M., Rothi, L. J., & Valenstein, E. (1982). Two forms of ideomotor apraxia. *Neurology, 32*(4), 342–346.
Helm-Estabrooks, N. (1998). Test of Oral and Limb Apraxia (TOLA). Austin: PRO-ED.
Jacobs, S., Bussel, B., Combeaud, M., & Roby-Brami, A. (2009). The use of a tool requires its incorporation into the movement: evidence from stick-pointing in apraxia. *Cortex, 45*(4), 444–455.
Jancke, L., Kleinschmidt, A., Mirzazade, S., Shah, N. J., & Freund, H. J. (2001). The role of the inferior parietal cortex in linking the tactile perception and manual construction of object shapes. *Cereb Cortex, 11*(2), 114–121.
Kable, J. W., & Chatterjee, A. (2006). Specificity of action representations in the lateral occipitotemporal cortex. *Journal of Cognitive Neuroscience, 18*(9), 1498–1517.
Kertesz, A. (2006). Western Aphasia Battery—Revised (WAB-R). San Antonio: Psychological Corporation.
Kertesz, A., & Ferro, J. M. (1984). Lesion size and location in ideomotor apraxia. *Brain, 107 (Pt 3)*, 921–933.
Kertesz, A., & Hooper, P. (1982). Praxis and language: the extent and variety of apraxia in aphasia. *Neuropsychologia, 20*(3), 275–286.
Kim, S. G., Ashe, J., Hendrich, K., Ellermann, J. M., Merkle, H., Ugurbil, K., et al. (1993). Functional magnetic resonance imaging of motor cortex: hemispheric asymmetry and handedness. *Science, 261*(5121), 615–617.

Klein, R. (1931). Zur symptomatologie des parietallappens. *Zeitschrift fur gesamte neurologie und psychiatrie, 135*, 589–608.

Kohler, E., Keysers, C., Umilta, M. A., Fogassi, L., Gallese, V., & Rizzolatti, G. (2002). Hearing sounds, understanding actions: action representation in mirror neurons. *Science, 297*(5582), 846–848.

Kroliczak, G., & Frey, S. H. (2009). A common network in the left cerebral hemisphere represents planning of tool use pantomimes and familiar intransitive gestures at the hand-independent level. *Cerebral Cortex, 19*(10), 2396–2410.

Lahav, A., Saltzman, E., & Schlaug, G. (2007). Action representation of sound: audiomotor recognition network while listening to newly acquired actions. *Journal of Neuroscience, 27*(2), 308–314.

Leiguarda, R. (2001). Limb apraxia: cortical or subcortical. *Neuroimage, 14*(1 Pt 2), S137–141.

Lewis, J. W., Brefczynski, J. A., Phinney, R. E., Janik, J. J., & DeYoe, E. A. (2005). Distinct cortical pathways for processing tool versus animal sounds. *Journal of Neuroscience, 25*(21), 5148–5158.

Liepmann, H. (1920). Apraxie. *Ergebnisse der Gesamten Medzin, 1*, 516–543.

Liepmann, H., & Mass, O. (1907). Fall von linksseitiger Agraphie und Apraxie bei rechsseitiger Lahmung. *Zeitschrift fur Psychologie und Neurologie, 10*, 214–227.

Meador, K. J., Loring, D. W., Lee, K., Hughes, M., Lee, G., Nichols, M., et al. (1999). Cerebral lateralization: relationship of language and ideomotor praxis. *Neurology, 53*(9), 2028–2031.

Moll, J., de Oliveira-Souza, R., Passman, L. J., Cunha, F. C., Souza-Lima, F., & Andreiuolo, P. A. (2000). Functional MRI correlates of real and imagined tool-use pantomimes. *Neurology, 54*(6), 1331–1336.

Ochipa, C., Rapcsak, S. Z., Maher, L. M., Rothi, L. J., Bowers, D., & Heilman, K. M. (1997). Selective deficit of praxis imagery in ideomotor apraxia. *Neurology, 49*(2), 474–480.

Ochipa, C., Rothi, L. J., & Heilman, K. M. (1989). Ideational apraxia: a deficit in tool selection and use. *Annals of Neurology, 25*(2), 190–193.

Ochipa, C., Rothi, L. J., & Heilman, K. M. (1992). Conceptual apraxia in Alzheimer's disease. *Brain, 115 (Pt 4)*, 1061–1071.

Papagno, C., Della Sala, S., & Basso, A. (1993). Ideomotor apraxia without aphasia and aphasia without apraxia: the anatomical support for a double dissociation. *Journal of Neurology, Neurosurgery & Psychiatry, 56*(3), 286–289.

Pazzaglia, M., Pizzamiglio, L., Pes, E., & Aglioti, S. M. (2008). The sound of actions in apraxia. *Current Biology, 18*(22), 1766–1772.

Petreska, B., Adriani, M., Blanke, O., & Billard, A. G. (2007). Apraxia: a review. *Progress in Brain Research, 164*, 61–83.

Pizzamiglio, L., Aprile, T., Spitoni, G., Pitzalis, S., Bates, E., D'Amico, S., et al. (2005). Separate neural systems for processing action- or non-action-related sounds. *Neuroimage, 24*(3), 852–861.

Poizner, H., Clark, M. A., Merians, A. S., Macauley, B., Gonzalez Rothi, L. J., & Heilman, K. M. (1995). Joint coordination deficits in limb apraxia. *Brain, 118 (Pt 1)*, 227–242.

Poizner, H., Mack, L., Verfaellie, M., Rothi, L. J., & Heilman, K. M. (1990). Three-dimensional computergraphic analysis of apraxia. Neural representations of learned movement. *Brain, 113 (Pt 1)*, 85–101.

Poizner, H., Merians, A. S., Clark, M. A., Macauley, B., Rothi, L. J., & Heilman, K. M. (1998). Left hemispheric specialization for learned, skilled, and purposeful action. *Neuropsychology, 12*(2), 163–182.

Power, E., Code, C., Croot, K., Sheard, C., & Gonzalez Rothi, L. J. (2010). Florida Apraxia Battery-Extended and Revised Sydney (FABERS): Design, description, and a healthy control sample. *Journal of Clinical and Experimental Neuropsychology, 32(1)*, 1–18.

Pramstaller, P. P., & Marsden, C. D. (1996). The basal ganglia and apraxia. *Brain, 119 (Pt 1)*, 319–340.

Randerath, J., Li, Y., Goldenberg, G., & Hermsdorfer, J. (2009). Grasping tools: effects of task and apraxia. *Neuropsychologia, 47*(2), 497–505.

Rapcsak, S. Z., Ochipa, C., Beeson, P. M., & Rubens, A. B. (1993). Praxis and the right hemisphere. *Brain and Cognition, 23*(2), 181–202.

Raymer, A. M., Maher, L. M., Foundas, A. L., Heilman, K. M., & Rothi, L. J. (1997). The significance of body part as tool errors in limb apraxia. *Brain and Cognition, 34*(2), 287–292.

Rizzolatti, G., Fadiga, L., Gallese, V., & Fogassi, L. (1996). Premotor cortex and the recognition of motor actions. *Brain Research Cognitive Brain Research, 3*(2), 131–141.

Rodrigues Cavalcante, K., & Caramelli, P. (2009). Evaluation of the performance of normal elderly in a limb praxis protocol: influence of age, gender, and education. *Journal of the International Neuropsychological Society, 15*(4), 618–622.

Rothi, L. J., Heilman, K. M., & Watson, R. T. (1985). Pantomime comprehension and ideomotor apraxia. *Journal of Neurology, Neurosurgery, & Psychiatry, 48*(3), 207–210.

Rothi, L. J., Mack, L., Verfaellie, M., Brown, P., & Heilman, K. M. (1988). Ideomotor apraxia: error pattern analysis. *Aphasiology, 2*, 381–388.

Rothi, L. J., Ochipa, C., & Heilman, K. M. (1991). A cognitive neuropsychological model of limb praxis. *Cognitive Neuropsychology, 8*, 443–458.

Rothi, L. J., Raymer, A. M., & Heilman, K. M. (1997). Limb praxis assessment. In L. J. Rothi & K. M. Heilman (eds.), *Apraxia: The Neuropsychology of Action* (pp. 61–73). East Sussex UK: Psychology Press.

Rothi, L. J., Raymer, A. M., Ochipa, C., Maher, L. M., Greenwald, M. L., & Heilman, K. M. (1992). *Florida Apraxia Battery, Experimental Edition.*

Roy, E. A. (1985). *Neuropsychological studies of apraxia and related disorders.* New York: Elsevier Science.

Roy, E. A., Black, S. E., Blair, N., & Dimeck, P. T. (1998). Analyses of deficits in gestural pantomime. *Journal of Clinical and Experimental Neuropsychology, 20*(5), 628–643.

Roy, E. A., Clark, P., Aigbogun, S., & Square-Storer, P. A. (1992). Ipsilesional disruptions to reciprocal finger tapping. *Archives of Clinical Neuropsychology, 7*(3), 213–219.

Roy, E. A., Heath, M., Westwood, D., Schweizer, T. A., Dixon, M. J., Black, S. E., et al. (2000). Task demands and limb apraxia in stroke. *Brain and Cognition, 44*(2), 253–279.

Roy, E. A., Square-Storer, P., Hogg, S., & Adams, S. (1991). Analysis of task demands in apraxia. *International Journal of Neuroscience, 56*(1–4), 177–186.

Rushworth, M. F., Nixon, P. D., Wade, D. T., Renowden, S., & Passingham, R. E. (1998). The left hemisphere and the selection of learned actions. *Neuropsychologia, 36*(1), 11–24.

Schaefer, S. Y., Haaland, K. Y., & Sainburg, R. L. (2007). Ipsilesional motor deficits following stroke reflect hemispheric specializations for movement control. *Brain, 130*(Pt 8), 2146–2158.

Schaefer, S. Y., Haaland, K. Y., & Sainburg, R. L. (2009). Hemispheric specialization and functional impact of ipsilesional deficits in movement coordination and accuracy. *Neuropsychologia, 47*(13), 2953–2966.

Schnider, A., Hanlon, R. E., Alexander, D. N., & Benson, D. F. (1997). Ideomotor apraxia: behavioral dimensions and neuroanatomical basis. *Brain and Language, 58*(1), 125–136.

Schwartz, M. F. (1995). Re-examining the role of executive functions in routine action production. *Annals of the New York Academy of Science, 769*, 321–335.

Schwartz, M. F., & Buxbaum, L. J. (1997). Naturalistic Action. In L. J. Rothi & K. M. Heilman (eds.), *Apraxia: The Neuropsychology of Action* (pp. 269–289). East Sussex UK: Psychology Press.

Schwartz, M. F., Montgomery, M. W., Fitzpatrick-DeSalme, E. J., Ochipa, C., Coslett, H. B., & Mayer, N. H. (1995). Analysis of a disorder of everyday action. *Cognitive Neuropsychology, 12*, 863–892.

Sirigu, A., Daprati, E., Pradat-Diehl, P., Franck, N., & Jeannerod, M. (1999). Perception of self-generated movement following left parietal lesion. *Brain, 122 (Pt 10)*, 1867–1874.

Stamenova, V., Roy, E. A., & Black, S. E. (2009). A model-based approach to understanding apraxia in Corticobasal Syndrome. *Neuropsychologyl Review, 19*(1), 47–63.
Sundet, K., Finset, A., & Reinvang, I. (1988). Neuropsychological predictors in stroke rehabilitation. *Journal of Clinical and Experimental Neuropsychology, 10*(4), 363–379.
Vanbellingen, T., Kersten, B., Van Hemelrijk, B., Van de Winckel, A., Bertschi, M., Muri, R., et al. (2009). Comprehensive assessment of gesture production: a new test of upper limb apraxia (TULIA). *European Journal of Neurology, 17*(1), 59–66.
Warren, M. (1981). Relationship of constructional apraxia and body scheme disorders in dressing performance in adult CVA. *American Journal of Occupational Therapy, 35*(7), 431–437.
Watson, R. T., Fleet, W. S., Gonzalez-Rothi, L., & Heilman, K. M. (1986). Apraxia and the supplementary motor area. *Archives of Neurology, 43*(8), 787–792.
Williams, N. (1967). Correlation between copying ability and dressing activities in hemiplegia. *American Journal of Physical Medicine, 46*(4), 1332–1340.
Zadikoff, C., & Lang, A. E. (2005). Apraxia in movement disorders. *Brain, 128*(Pt 7), 1480–1497.

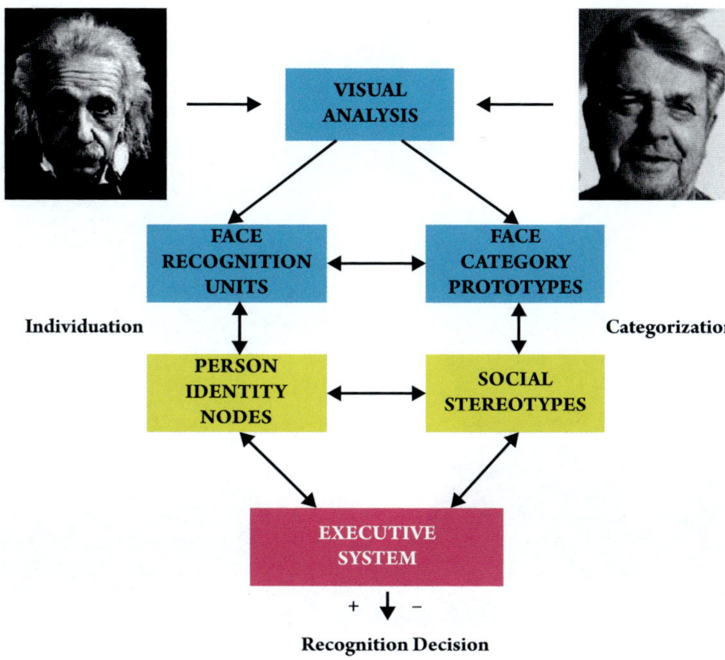

Figure 6.1 Cognitive model of face recognition memory. Recognition performance is the integrated product of individuation and categorization and involves distinct visual, (blue), semantic (yellow), and executive (magenta) operations.

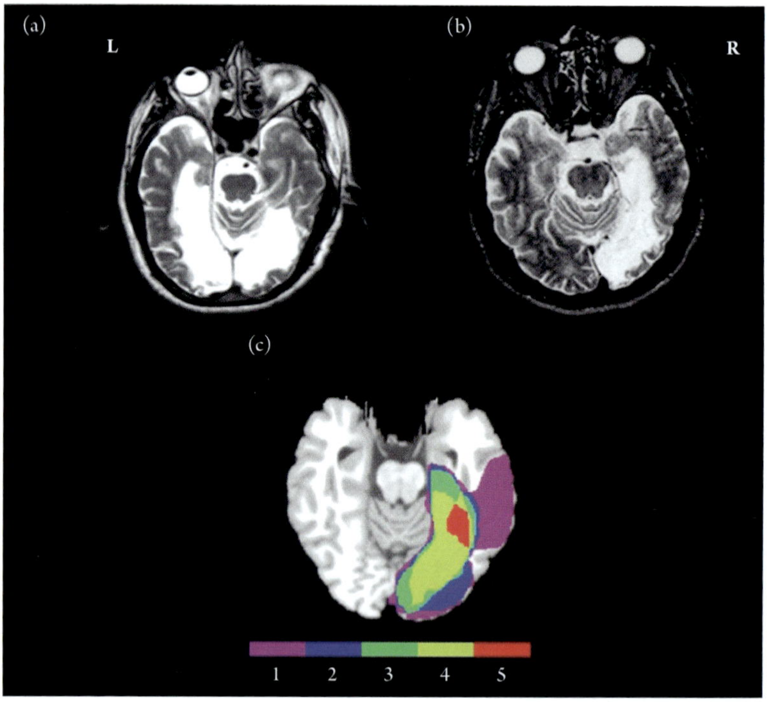

Figure 6.2 Bilateral (a) and unilateral right-sided (b) occipito-temporal lesions in patients with prosopagnosia following PCA strokes. Lesion overlap map of five patients with prosopagnosia due to unilateral right occipito-temporal damage (c). The area of maximum damage (red) includes right mid-fusiform cortex corresponding to the location of the fusiform face area (FFA) in functional neuroimaging studies.

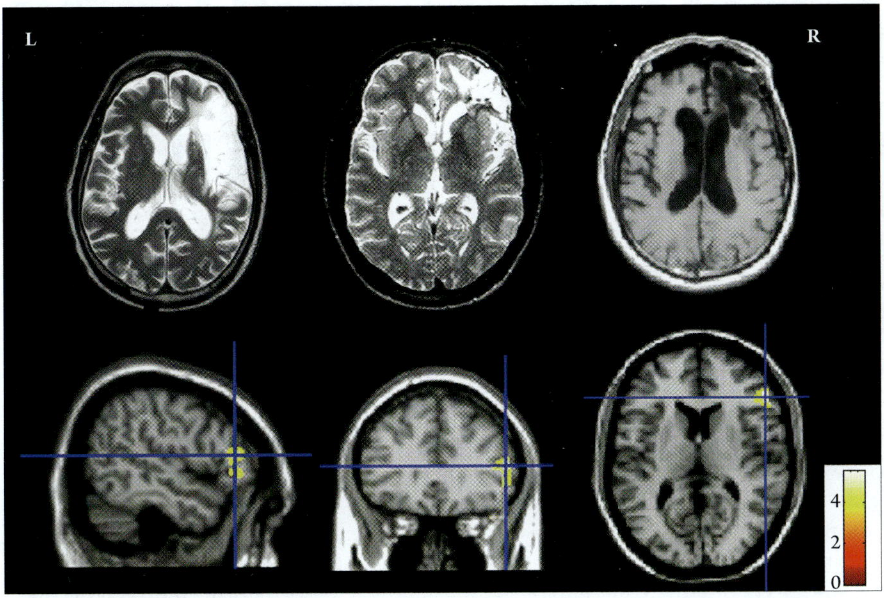

Figure 6.4 Right prefrontal cortex (PFC) lesions in patients with false facial recognition (top). Damage involves a ventrolateral frontal lobe region that shows activation during face recognition performance in normal subjects (bottom).

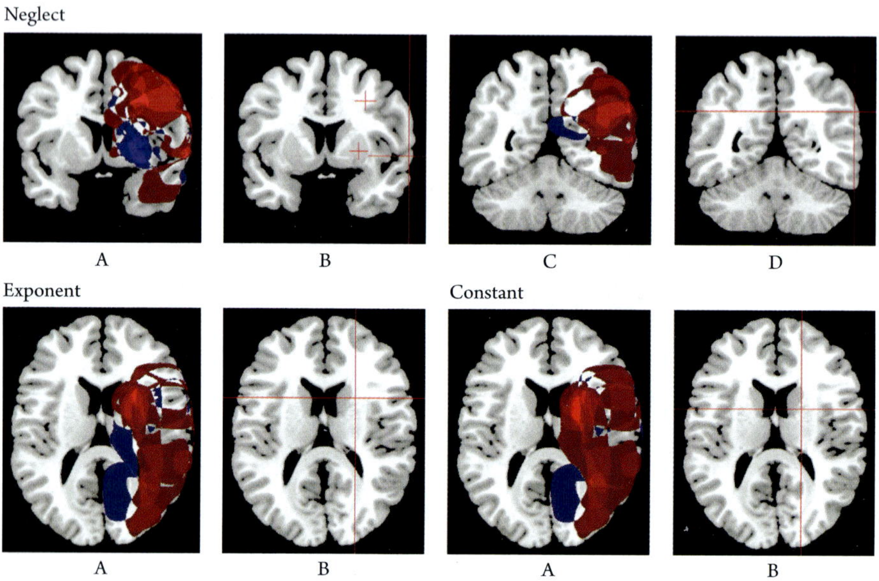

Figure 7.7 Results of a lesion subtraction analysis for 17 patients with right hemisphere lesions. The top row of pictures (Neglect) shows subtraction of RHL- from RHL+ scans. Brighter red areas indicate lesions common to RHL+ but not RHL-. Brighter blue indicates the opposite. Figure A shows brighter red areas—one involving white matter beneath BAs 6, 4 and 3 and another involving BA 38/21 in the anterior temporal lobe – and one area of brighter blue centered on the putamen. Crosshairs in figure B show the center of these areas, respectively. Figure C shows area of red overlap involving BA 39 with corresponding crosshair in Figure D. The bottom row of pictures (Exponents) show scans of RHL patients with normal or high power function exponents subtracted from those with decreased exponents and (Constants) of patients with normal or low constants subtracted from those with high constants. Figure A under exponent shows a brighter red area centered on the anterior limb of the internal capsule. [Similar involvement of the thalamic radiations was observed in higher slices (not shown).] Figure A under constant shows a brighter red area centered on the anterior limb and genu of the internal capsule.

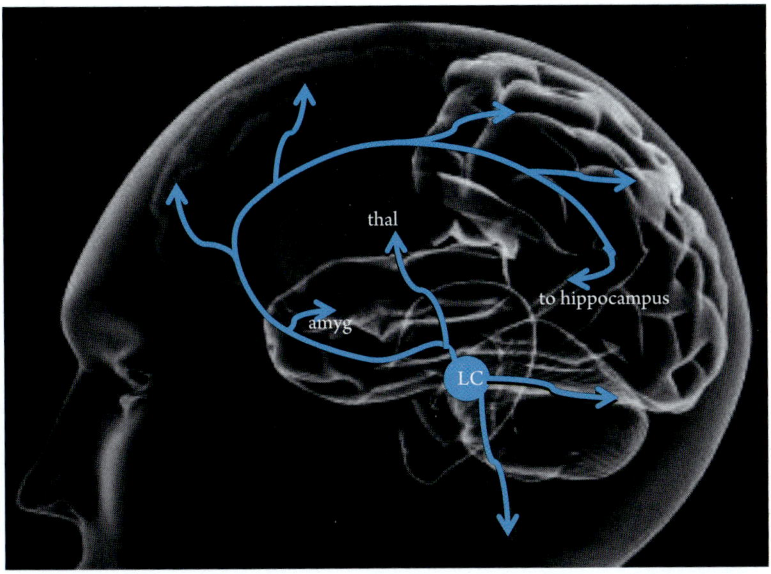

Figure 14.1 Noradrenergic pathways. The locus coeruleus (LC) projects posteriorly to the cerebellum and up to the thalamus (thal) and amygdala (amyg), as well as throughout the neocortex along a pericingular tract, also terminating posteriorly at the hippocampus (Heimer, 1995). The descending fibers to the spinal cord are also shown. Not shown is the lateral tegmental noradrenergic system which also projects to the amygdala and down to the spinal cord.

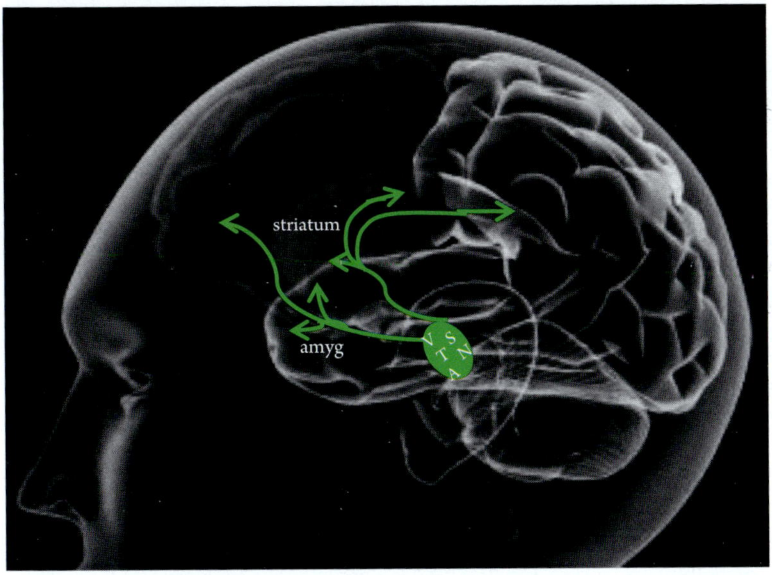

Figure 14.2 Dopaminergic pathways. Projections from the substantia nigra (SN) to the striatum are demonstrated, as are projections from the ventral tegmental area (VTA) to the amygdala (amyg), ventral striatum, and frontal cortex (Heimer, 1995). Not shown are the tuberoinfundibular and posterior hypothalamic dopaminergic systems.

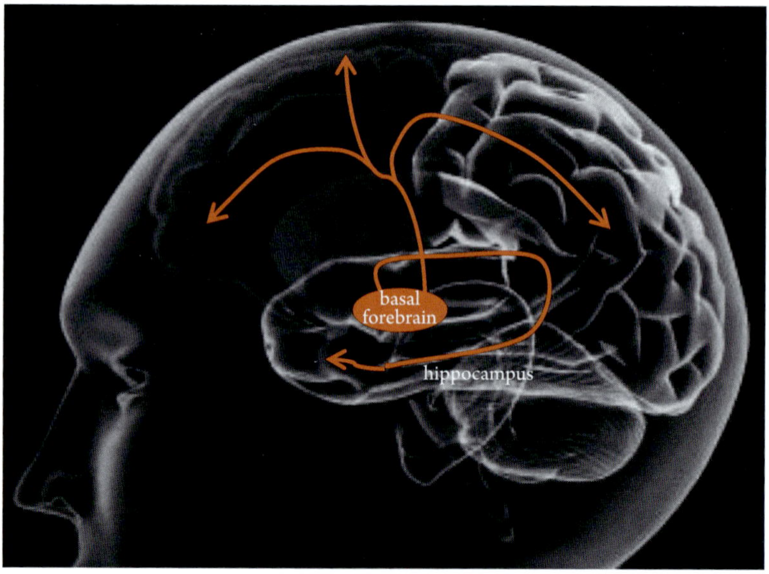

Figure 14.3 Cholinergic pathways. Cortical projections from the basal forebrain are demonstrated to the cingulate, and pericingulate cortex, as well as the mesial frontal cortex along a mesial pericingular tract, and laterally through the external capsule and claustrum to the capsular region and lateral neocortex (Selden et al., 1998).

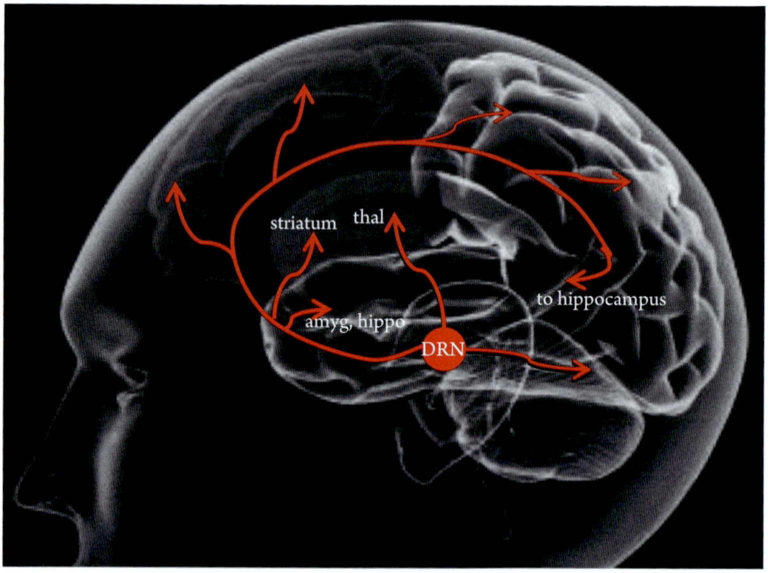

Figure 14.4 Serotonergic pathways. The dorsal raphe nuclei (DRN) project posteriorly to the cerebellum and intracerebellar nuclei, and up to the thalamus (thal), with projections also to the amygdala (amyg), hippocampus (hippo), hypothalamus, olfactory and entorhinal cortices, then to the ventral striatum as well as throughout the neocortex along a pericingular tract, also terminating posteriorly at the hippocampus (Heimer, 1995). Not shown is the caudal raphe nuclei, which also project to the cerebellum and intracerebellar nuclei, and down to the spinal cord.

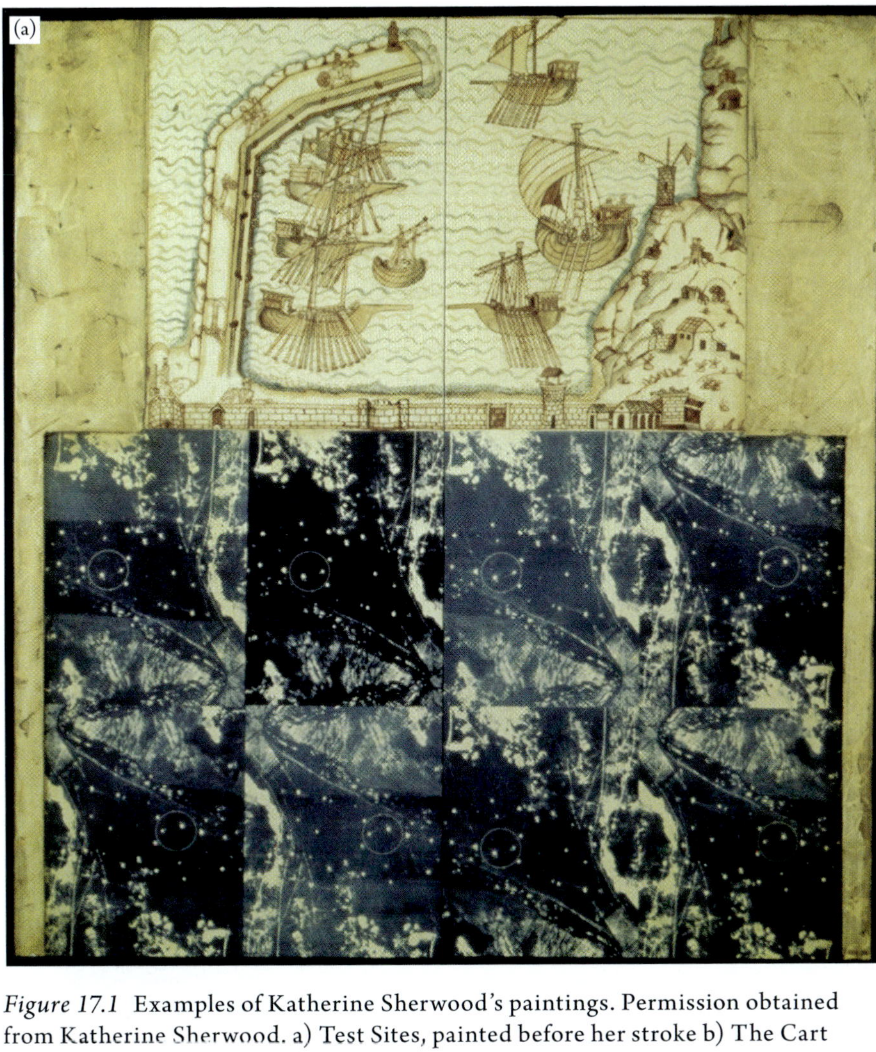

Figure 17.1 Examples of Katherine Sherwood's paintings. Permission obtained from Katherine Sherwood. a) Test Sites, painted before her stroke b) The Cart Before the Horse, painted after her stroke.

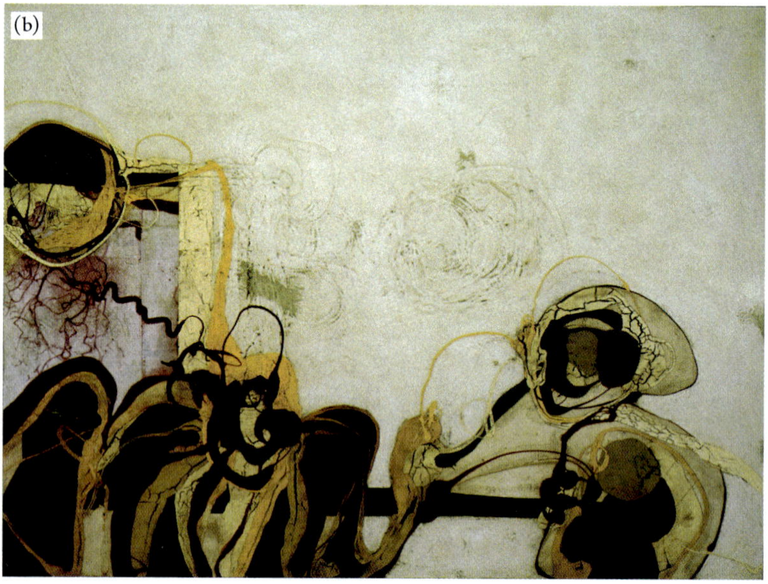

Figure 17.1 (Continued)

CHAPTER 10

Body Representations: Updating a Classic Concept

H. Branch Coslett

Introduction

An internal representation of the human body is crucial for a wide range of activities such as planning action, registering the location of sensory input, and making judgments about whether one could fit into a particularly appealing item of clothing. Given the central role of body representations in these and many other behaviors, it is not surprising that the issue was addressed by a number of investigators in the early part of the 20th century (e.g., Pick, 1922; Head & Holmes, 1911–1912). In this chapter, I first review evidence supporting the existence of multiple discrete, but interacting, representations of the human body. In the second section of the chapter, I will elaborate on the "body schema," a representation of particular relevance for sensory-motor processing as it mediates between perception and action. As will become clear, the accounts developed are heavily influenced by the work of neurologists and psychiatrists from the 19th and early part of the 20th centuries—the original cognitive neuroscientists.

Evidence for Multiple, Dissociable Body Representations

Following in the tradition of Head and Holmes (1911–12) and Pick (1922) and drawing on the contributions of Sirigu et al. (1991), we have argued for at least three distinct types of body representations: the *body schema, body structural description,* and *body image.* (See Table 10.1) We first introduce these constructs and provide evidence from investigations of patients with brain lesions for the distinctions between these putative representations. We then review data from

Table 10.1 **Putative Body Representations**

A.	Body Structural Description: topological map of the human body
B.	Body Image: semantic and lexical information about the body
C.	Body Schema: on-line representation of the body in space
1.	Primary somatosensory representation
2.	Body form representation
3.	Body postural representation

a group study that supports the tripartite distinction. Finally, we review recent work suggesting that the body schema or on-line sensory-motor representation may be further fractionated.

It should be noted that this domain of research has and continues to be plagued by confusing and inconsistent terminology. For example, the terms "body schema" and "body image," which we use to refer to quite different representations, have been taken to be interchangeable by some investigators; rather than create a different nosology, we employ traditional terminology, but attempt to introduce a principled distinction between the "body schema," "body image," and "body structural description."

BODY SCHEMA: ON-LINE SENSORIMOTOR REPRESENTATIONS

Following Head and Holmes (1911–1912) among others, we take the *body schema* to be a dynamic, on-line representation of the relative positions of body parts derived from multiple sensory and motor inputs (e.g., proprioceptive, vestibular, tactile, visual, efference copy) that interacts with motor systems in the genesis of action (e.g., Schwoebel, Boronat, & Coslett, 2002). A compelling demonstration of the "body schema" is provided by the "Pinocchio Illusion" reported by Lackner (1988). Vibrating a static muscle produces the illusion that the muscle is being stretched; the application of 80 Hz vibration to the triceps of a blindfolded person, for example, is associated with a feeling that one's arm is being extended at the elbow. The Pinocchio illusion arises when a subject is touching their nose and a vibrator is placed in touch with their triceps. The resulting sensation of extension of the arm is associated with the feeling that one's nose is elongating in concert with arm extension. As forcefully argued by Lackner (1988), the demonstration that manipulating the apparent position of the arm influences the perceived dimensions of the nose requires a representation of the body that is malleable and updated in real-time.

We suggest that a number of clinical disorders such as phantom limb, somatoparaphrenia, and supernumerary limbs are characterized by a disruption of the body schema. We have demonstrated that the body schema may be disrupted in patients with neglect (Coslett, 1998). In this study, subjects with neglect were asked to judge the laterality of a visually presented picture of a hand shown with the wrist toward the subject—that is, in an anatomically plausible position. Parsons and others have argued that the body schema underlies simulated movements of the body as well (Schwoebel, Boronat, et al., 2002; Schwoebel, Coslett, Bradt, Freidman, & Dileo, 2002; Schwoebel, Friedman, Duda, & Coslett, 2001; Coslett, 1998; Parsons, 1987, 1994). Data from a series of experiments examining the time required for subjects to determine the laterality of pictured hands suggest that participants confirm laterality judgments by imagining their hand moving from its current position into the orientation of a stimulus hand. Thus, response times depend on whether a participant's own hand is palm-up or palm-down and its degree of angular disparity from the stimulus hand. Furthermore, the response times for such imagined movements reflect the human body's biomechanical constraints on movement and are highly correlated with actual movement times. These findings suggest that the simulated hand movements rely on a dynamic internal representation of hand position, which may be derived from proprioceptive input as well as efference copy information (i.e., body schema). We found that subjects with neglect, but not subjects with right hemisphere lesions without neglect or subjects with left hemisphere lesions, exhibited a selective deficit in identifying the left hand. We (Coslett, 1998) interpreted these data as evidence that the body schema was disrupted in neglect in that the representation of the left hand was either absent or inaccessible.

We suggest that the body schema also provides an on-line representation of sensory input that articulates with spatial systems that permits one to localize stimuli both with respect to the body surface and peripersonal space. Support for this assertion comes from a number of sources. For example, we (Schwoebel et al., 2001; Coslett et al., 2008) reported a 77-year-old woman with a left temporal-parietal-occipital junction infarct who was not able to compute a representation of the body surface. Although she reliably detected tactile stimuli delivered to any location on her body, she was unable to localize the stimuli on her body surface. For example, when touched twice in succession and asked to determine if she had been touched in the same or different places, her performance was influenced not by distinctions between body parts (e.g., thigh versus forearm) but strictly by the distance between the touched locations; that is, unlike normal controls who show sensitivity to distinctions between body parts, she was as likely to report that successive touches were in the same location if one was on her thigh and the other on her forearm as compared to trials on which both touches were on her thigh. Strikingly, her performance in pointing to locations on her body surface that were touched by the examiner with her eyes closed was dramatically affected by the size and familiarity of the room in which she was tested: she performed significantly better in her small, familiar bedroom than in a large, less familiar room. These and other data are consistent with the claim that she compensated for a disrupted body surface representation by employing a relatively preserved spatial representation.

One final issue regarding this patient (Shoebill, Coslett, & Boxhaul, 2001) bears comment. Visual and proprioceptive information are often assumed to be crucial for reaching. The patient, however, exhibited profound tactile and proprioception deficits, yet reached to targets accurately without vision of her hand. One possible explanation for this finding is that a "forward model" derived from efference copy predicts the consequences of action, thereby providing information about the anticipated location of the arm during and after movement. To test the hypothesis that the "forward model" provides information that updates a representation of arm position, the patient performed a double-start task. In one condition she reached from a starting position to the tip of her nose and then to a remembered target; in a second condition, her hand was passively moved from the same initial starting position to the tip of her nose and she then reached to the remembered target. She was dramatically impaired in the second condition, often groping blindly for the target (see Coslett et al., 2008 for detail). These data suggest that the forward model can provide at least relatively accurate information about the on-line position of the hand.

We have recently reported evidence suggesting a relationship between the representations underlying performance on the hand laterality task and the ability to produce spatially and temporally accurate movements (Schwoebel, Boxhaul, & Coslett, 2004). In a group of 55 unilateral left hemisphere stroke patients, multiple regression analyses demonstrated that performance on the hand laterality task was a significant predictor of performance on tasks requiring the production of meaningful gestures to command and imitation, as well as tasks requiring the imitation of meaningless movements. This suggests that components of the body schema (i.e., representations derived from efference copy) may, in part, underlie performance on tasks requiring both imagined and real actions. Functional neuroimaging findings further suggest that the performance of hand laterality judgments as well as explicit motor imagery are associated with activation in inferior and superior parietal areas as well as motor and premotor areas (e.g., Parsons et al., 1995) and that these brain regions overlap substantially with the areas activated during actual movements (e.g., Grazes & Decay, 2001; Jeanne rod, 2001; Parsons & Fox, 1998; Gerard in et al., 1996). Consistent with these findings, Sirigu et al. (1995, 1996) have noted that although strong correlations between the times required to imagine and execute sequential finger movements are observed in normal subjects and patients with motor cortex damage, patients with parietal damage exhibit poor correlations, suggesting an impaired ability to accurately simulate action. Taken together, these findings suggest that both actual and mentally simulated movements may depend on the body schema and that the posterior parietal cortex may serve as an integral component of the neural substrate underlying body schema representations.

BODY IMAGE: SEMANTIC AND LEXICAL REPRESENTATIONS OF THE BODY

We postulate that a second distinct representation, the "body image," encodes conceptual, propositional knowledge about the human body as well as the emotional attitude towards and beliefs about one body. The latter is one aspect of what is commonly called one's "self-image". We believe that the body image is linked to the verbal system and is accessible to consciousness. It includes information about the role and function of body parts. The body image may be interrogated by language tasks such as naming body parts and comprehending names of body parts.

Evidence for a distinct propositional, conscious representation of the body that is accessible to consciousness comes from studies of patients with brain lesions. Several disorders are consistent with the hypothesis that the body image may be selectively impaired. The Eastman syndrome, for example, is characterized by an inability to point to or name fingers (and, typically, other body parts) sometimes in the absence of a significant impairment in sensation and action. Dennis et al., (1976) reported a patient who could reach to touched body parts, but could not name or point to named body parts.

There is also evidence that knowledge of the body is a distinct semantic domain. Suzuki et al. (1997) reported a patient with Boca's aphasia and left-hemisphere infarctions, which included the frontal operculum, who exhibited impaired body part name comprehension despite preserved comprehension of words from other semantic categories and a preserved ability to point to visually identified body parts on himself (i.e., he was not autotopagnosic). For example, when asked to point to a named picture among distracters from the same category, he correctly identified 2 of 10 body parts, but identified at least 8 of 10 stimuli in all ten additional semantic categories tested. In contrast, Shelton et al. (1998) and Coslett et al. (2002) reported patients with selective preservation of body knowledge. The patient reported by Coslett et al. (2002), who exhibited semantic dementia (Hodges et al., 1992) was significantly better in comprehending, reading and writing names for body parts as compared to stimuli matched for frequency and imageability. For example, when asked to point to named pictures of body parts and non-body part stimuli that were matched for frequency and familiarity, the patient correctly identified 12 of 12 body parts and 4 of 8 stimuli from other categories. A similar pattern of performance was also observed on comprehension and oral reading tasks (see also Shelton, Fouch, & Caramazza, 1998).

BODY STRUCTURAL DESCRIPTION: A TOPOLOGICAL MAP OF THE BODY

The third putative representation, the *body structural description,* is a topological map of the human body derived primarily from visual input that defines body part boundaries and proximity relationships (e.g., Boxhaul & Coslett, 2001; Sirigu et al., 1991). Support for the existence of the body structural description comes from clinical syndromes such as autotopagnosia, a disorder in which patients may be unable to point to named human body parts (Pick, 1922; Ogden, 1985; Boxhaul & Coslett, 2001). Consistent with Pick's (1922) original account of the syndrome, recent findings suggest that autotopagnosia may be attributable to a selectively impaired representation of the structure of the human body. In contrast to the body schema, which appears to be derived from multiple sensory and motor inputs, the body structural description is postulated to be derived primarily from visual input (Boxhaul & Coslett, 2001; Sirigu et al., 1991). We (Boxhaul & Coslett, 2001) reported an autotopagnosic patient (G.L.) with a left parietal hemorrhagic contusion who was impaired relative to controls when asked to point to named or visually identified body parts on himself or others; he was also impaired in matching pictures of body parts across view shifts but exhibited no difficulty with objects; for example, when shown a the sole of a foot, he could not match this to a picture of a foot, yet when shown the bottom of a coffee cup, he recognized the relationship of the stimulus to a cup presented in a canonical orientation. The impairment in pointing to body parts was specific to the human body; although unable to point an ear on a mannequin or the examiner, he correctly pointed to the ear of horse (cf. Ogden, 1985). These findings suggest that G.L.'s ability to access structural descriptions of human body parts may be selectively disrupted. G.L. also performed flawlessly when asked to point to the part of the body associated with objects; that is, when touched on his wrist and asked to point to the corresponding body part on the examiner he was significantly impaired; he was perfect, however, in pointing to the examiner's wrist when asked to demonstrate where a watch would be worn.

GROUP STUDY OF BODY REPRESENTATIONS

In the preceding discussion, we argued that classical accounts of neurologic syndromes as well as detailed investigations of single subjects with brain dysfunction support the view that three distinct types of knowledge of the human body may be identified. In this section, we describe results from a group study that support this conclusion. We examined the performance of 70 patients with single hemisphere stroke and 18 age-matched normal controls on a battery of tasks developed to assess the body schema, body structural description, and body image.

The battery included 7 tasks, none of which required a verbal response, designed to assess the putative distinct body representations. The *body schema* was assessed by two tasks. On the "Matching Body Parts by Function" test subjects were shown a target body part and three additional body parts and asked to indicate which one of 3 depicted body parts was most similar with respect to function or "things that they do." For example, on one trial, the target was an elbow; response options included a knee (the correct choice), a forearm, and a nose.

The second task required subjects to match body parts to clothing and objects. On each of 20 trials, an item of clothing was displayed along with 4 body parts. Subjects were asked to point to the picture of the body part with which the item of clothing or accessory was most closely associated. Foils included conceptually related, unrelated, and contiguous body parts. For example, for watch, the associated stimuli would include pictures of a wrist, elbow, ankle, and ear.

The *body structural description* was assessed with three tasks. On one task, pictures of 24 individual body parts were presented and subjects were asked to point to the same part of their own body. On a second task, a suprathreshold tactile stimulus was presented to the subject's body, and the subject was asked to point on a mannequin to the location that had been touched on their own body. Finally, in the third task, a target body part was visually presented and subjects were asked to point to one of three pictured body parts that was closest on the body surface to the target body part. Stimuli for this task were the same as those used in the matching body part by function task described above.

The *body schema* was assessed with two mental motor imagery tasks. The hand lateralization task of Parson (1987) described above was employed. Subjects were shown a picture of a hand and asked to indicate if the stimulus is the right or left hand. Pictures of hands were presented in the palm-up or palm-down condition, and in one of four orientations: fingers pointing away, fingers pointing toward the subject, fingers pointing to the left, and fingers pointing to the right. There were 64 trials; subjects responded by moving the appropriate hand or, if hemiplegic, by pointing to the contralesional hand when appropriate. The second task was adapted from Sirigu et al. (1996). In this task, four movements ranging in difficulty from repetitive touching of the index and thumb to the independent extension of the index and little fingers were included. Subjects were tested with both hands independently in each of two conditions; hemiplegic subjects were tested with the ipsilesional hand only. In one condition, subjects were asked to imagine making a specified movement 5 times, as quickly and as accurately as possible; in the second condition, subjects were asked to execute the same movement 5 times. The examiner gave a verbal signal to initiate each trial and movement times were recorded with a stopwatch; for imagined movements, subjects indicated when they had completed the movement. Each imagined and executed movement was tested twice. For those subjects unable to produce the more difficult movements, easier movements were substituted so that all subjects were tested 8 times in both conditions with each hand. For both the ipsilesional and contralesional hands, the ratio of imagined to executed movement was calculated.

Several different analyses were performed. First, a principal components analysis was performed. We reasoned that tasks designed to assess a particular body representation would be strongly correlated with one another rather than with tasks designed to assess a different representation (i.e., the tasks would form a factor). The factor analysis strongly supported the claim that discrete and dissociable body representations may be identified. For example, support for the claim that the body structural description represents a distinct representation comes from the fact that the three tasks assessing the body structural description exhibited substantial internal consistency; the first factor (sum of squared loadings, or SSLs = 2.49) was primarily defined by the three body structural description tasks. Additionally, the two tasks assessing the body image comprised factor 4 (SSL = 1.73). Contrary to our expectations, the tasks designed to assess the body schema (hand laterality and hand imagery/action tasks with both the right and left hands) did not load onto the same factor. The hand laterality judgment with the contralesional and ipsilesional hands constituted the second component (SSL = 1.75), whereas the hand imagery/action task with the contralesional and ipsilesional hands constituted the third component (SSL = 1.75). Indeed, a striking double dissociation between the two body schema tasks was observed. Twenty-six subjects performed abnormally (i.e., below the range of scores for normal controls) on either the hand laterality or hand imagery/action task; nine could not perform the hand imagery/action task with the contralesional hand because of hemiplegia. Of the 17 subjects for whom data on both tasks is available, only one performed abnormally on both tasks. Eight of 16 patients performed abnormally on the hand laterality task, but normally on the hand imagery/action task, (t (7) = 3.03, p <.02) and 8 of 16 performed abnormally on the hand imagery/action task, but normally on the hand laterality task, (t (7) = 8.62, p < .001).

A second analysis was performed in which we examined whether there were selective deficits on the tasks assessing the three putative body representations. To this end, the performance of each of the 70 patients was compared to control means. First, mean scores were calculated for the body structural description (3 tasks) and body image (2 tasks) measures; these measures, along with performance on the hand laterality (ipsi- and contralesional hands) and hand imagery/action tasks (ipsi- and contralesional hand) were then compared with control performance. Patient scores that fell below the range of scores for the normal controls were considered impaired. Several interesting observations emerged from this comparison. First, the analysis of the performance of individual subjects suggests that the body schema, body structural description, and body image are dissociable representations. Seven subjects exhibited impairment on the hand imagery/action task but performed normally on all other body representation measures. Similarly, 6 subjects performed abnormally on only the hand laterality task and two subjects abnormally only on the body structural description measure. Finally, three subjects were impaired only on the body image measure. Consistent with the hypothesis that the body schema, body image, and body structural description are distinct representations, subjects with selective impairment of all three putative representations were identified.

Neuroimaging was available for 54 subjects with stroke. We used these data to explore the anatomic bases of body representations. There were several interesting findings. First, disorders of the body structural description and body image were strongly associated with left hemisphere lesions; for example, 16/18 subjects with abnormal performance on body structural description and 15/16 subjects with disorders of the body schema had left hemisphere lesions. Although not significant, we found that deficits on the hand action/imagery task were likely to be associated with left hemisphere lesions (7/9 subjects); there was no tendency for deficits on the hand lateralization task to be associated with lesions of the left hemisphere. Although quantitative analyses using new techniques such as Voxel-based lesion-symptom mapping could not be performed because of the lack of high-resolution imaging, there was a clear tendency for impairment of the body structural description and body image to be associated with lesions of the temporal lobe; in contrast, impairment in the measures of body schema were associated with lesions in sensory-motor cortices. In summary, both the principal components analysis as well as the comparison of individual subjects to the control group provided support for the claim that at least three distinct body representations could be identified.

CURRENT ACCOUNT OF BODY REPRESENTATIONS

The data described above provide support for the distinction between information regarding knowledge of the body, the form of the human body, and an on-line, often unconscious representation of the body that mediates between perception and action. Of these representations, the body schema is of greatest relevance with respect to understanding and potentially remediating clinical disorders. In the following section, we describe recent work that has attempted to unpack the body schema. More specifically, we provide a brief account of the multiple representations that we take to comprise the "body schema." Our account of the body schema (see Medina & Coslett, 2010) incorporates three distinct but highly interactive components: primary somatosensory, body form, and body postural representations.

PRIMARY SOMATOSENSORY REPRESENTATIONS

Tactile and proprioceptive stimuli are first processed at the cortical level in the post-central gyrus (BA 3b, 3a, 2, 1). As in BA4, there is clear evidence of somatotopic organization with areas that have a greater sensory acuity (e.g., fingertips and face) having disproportionately large cortical representations. A substantial amount of work during the last decades has demonstrated that the architecture of somatosensory cortices is experience-dependent. From relatively early work with monkeys (Merzenich et al., 1983, 1984; see Calford, 2002 for a review) to more recent work with humans, multiple studies have demonstrated that the somatosensory cortex remaps in response to both peripheral (Gandevia &

Phegan, 1999) and central lesions (Ramachandran et al., 1992; Medina & Rapp, 2008). Furthermore, changes in somatosensory cortical organization in humans may be induced by motor (e.g., Braun et al., 2001) and sensory (Schaefer et al., 2008) activity. Finally, although the primary somatosensory cortex had long been regarded as unimodal, neurons responding to multiple sensory inputs have been described in this region (see Ghazanfar & Schroeder, 2006).

BODY FORM REPRESENTATION

Despite the striking differences in cortical representations between "sensitive" regions such as the fingertip or face and less "sensitive" regions such as the back, subjects are at least relatively good at judging the size of stimuli or the distance between two points for stimuli presented at both locations. Taylor-Clarke et al. (2004) presented two tactile stimuli to points on the skin surface with high (fingertips) and low (forearm and back) cortical representations. Although normal subjects consistently judged the distance to be greater on the regions with high cortical representation, the differences were substantially less than would have been predicted by the differences in cortical magnification. On the basis of these findings, the investigators argued that, just as the visual system scales inputs from the fovea and periphery to achieve size constancy, information from primary somatosensory representations must be rescaled to a second, higher-order body representation; we term this the *body form representation*. This representation is assumed to be multisensory in nature (see also Medina & Coslett, 2010; Longo, Azanon, & Haggard, 2010).

A striking demonstration of the body form representation is provided by the Pinocchio illusion (Lackner, 1988) briefly described above. Vibrating a muscle tendon stimulates muscle spindles, causing the sensation that the body has moved to a different position. When the biceps tendon is vibrated in blindfolded subjects who are touching their nose, the subjects not only report the arm extending, but also feel their nose extending. This illusion demonstrates a fundamental point. First, the effect demonstrates the necessity of a representation of the body form; the illusory extension of the nose cannot be attributed to alterations in primary somatosensory cortex as tactile input did not change.

Alterations in the perception of the body that may represent a distortion of the body form are observed in clinical populations (e.g., microsomatagnosia; phantom limb) as well as after nerve block or anesthesia (e.g., Gandevia & Phegan, 1999).

The neural correlate of the body form representation is unclear, perhaps because studies of persistent distortions of the body form are relatively uncommon. Ehrsson et al. (2005) performed an fMRI study in which subjects experienced a vibration-induced illusion that caused them to perceive their arm moving and, in some conditions, their waist shrinking. They found that the sensation of waist shrinking was associated with activity at the junction of the post-central gyrus and the intraparietal sulcus. Different regions were active for illusory arm movements without illusory shrinking of the waist, suggesting separable functional subcomponents for body form versus body posture representation. We have recently completed a study involving Transcranial Magnetic Stimulation in normal subjects that suggests that the anterior intraparietal sulcus is important for this representation (see below).

BODY POSTURAL REPRESENTATION

As described above, the body form representation makes explicit the shape, size, texture, and location of stimuli on the surface of the body. Whereas such a representation is crucial, it is not sufficient. As noted by Pick (1922) and Head and Holmes (1911–12), an on-line representation of the position of the body in real time is essential to account for the performance of routine motor acts such as reaching to a coffee cup while reading the newspaper; the fact that such movements may be performed quickly, accurately, and effortlessly without attending to the initial position of the torso, arm, or hand suggests that a representation of the body in space is computed and maintained on-line and is incorporated into motor control systems directly (that is, without conscious planning of the motor act). We term this the body postural representation.

This representation is generated from several different types of inputs. Proprioceptive feedback is crucial as witnessed, for example, by the devastating consequences of its loss. Cole and Paillard (1995), for example, reported two patients who were deprived of sensory input (including proprioception) from the extremities as a consequence of a severe sensory neuropathy; although not weak, these patients experienced profound impairments on routine motor tasks including walking and reaching to objects in the environment. Such acts could be performed only with considerable effort and the use of visual monitoring of the movements. Indeed, sitting in a chair without falling required constant vigilance (see also Medina, Jax, & Coslett, 2009). Even in normal subjects, proprioception is not sufficient as, over time and with inactivity, body position defined by proprioception may "drift" (Wann & Ibrahim, 1992).

At least three other types of input inform the body postural representation. First, in most real world situations visual information is crucial to the representation of the body in space. Although the relative contributions of vision and proprioception may vary depending on the task at hand (van Beers, Wolpert, & Haggard, 2002; Shenton, Schwoebel, & Coslett, 2004), in many contexts, visual information overrides proprioceptive information (Graziano et al., 2000). Indeed, visual "dominance" over proprioception is evident in a number of phenomena to be considered below, such as the "rubber hand" (Botvinick & Cohen, 1998; Tsakiris & Haggard, 2005) and "mirror box" illusions (Ramachandran & Altschuler, 2009).

We suggest that BA 5 is a crucial element in the neural instantiation of the body postural representation. This region receives direct, robust input from primary as well as secondary sensory cortices. Furthermore, electrophysiologic work in monkeys has demonstrated neurons that would appear to be well-suited to this task. For example, neurons in BA5 respond to both vision as well as somatosensory input, respond to touch only when in a certain position in space (Macaluso & Maravita, 2010) and fire when a visualized and realistically (but not implausibly) positioned fake limb is stimulated (Rizzolatti, Fogassi, & Gallese, 2002). Wolpert, Goodbody & Husain (1998) reported a subject with a large left superior parietal cyst who was unable to maintain a stable representation of limb location, suggesting its involvement in maintaining a representation of body posture.

We have recently completed a study involving Transcranial Magnetic Stimuluation (TMS) that also speaks to the anatomic underpinnings of the body structural description and the body form representation. Yamamoto and Kitazawa (2001a; see also 2001b) performed a temporal order judgment task in which suprathreshold tactile stimuli were presented to each hand at varying temporal intervals and subjects were asked to judge the order of the stimuli (right versus left hand). With the arms uncrossed, the just noticeable difference (JND) between stimuli was as low as 70 msec. However, when the arms were crossed, the JND was much longer (up to 1 sec); additionally, some subjects consistently inverted the correct temporal order on trials with small temporal discrepancies between the stimuli. The authors concluded that initial processing of hand location does not take into account limb position (and relies strictly on the initial, somatotopic representation), and then subsequently takes into account limb position in external space (i.e., the body postural representation, see also Ehrsson et al., 2005; Makin et al., 2007).

We recently repeated this experiment in 12 normal subjects before and after 20 minutes of 1 Hz TMS at 90 percent motor threshold delivered to either the BA 5 (anterior superior parietal lobule), the putative substrate for the body postural description, or the anterior intraparietal sulcus, the putative substrate for the body form representation. Consistent with the claim that the body postural representation integrates proprioceptive and tactile information to generate a representation of the body in space, TMS to BA 5 significantly impaired performance on the hands crossed, but not hands uncrossed condition. Additionally, TMS to the anterior intraparietal sulcus impaired performance in both conditions as would be expected if it interfered with the registration of tactile information. These data support the claim that the body form and body postural representations serve different roles in the genesis of the integrated body schema; furthermore, the lesion approach, here instantiated in a TMS paradigm, provides novel information regarding the anatomic bases of these putative body representations that has not been available from imaging studies.

RELATIONSHIP TO OTHER ACCOUNTS OF BODY REPRESENTATIONS

We have argued for the principled distinction between three putative body representations. As one would expect (and hope), however, a number of alternative accounts of body knowledge have been developed. Perhaps the most influential account of body representations proposes a fundamental distinction between representations computed in the service of action as opposed to perception (Paillard, 1999; Dijkerman & DeHaan, 2007). Modeled on the influential account of visual processing that postulates a fundamental distinction between the ventral "what" and dorsal "where" (Ungerleider & Mishkin, 1982) or "how to" (Milner & Goodale, 1995) systems, the Dijkerman and DeHaan account distinguishes between a conscious "body image" that provides information regarding object identity and a typically unconscious "body schema" that represents body location.

Although there are clear similarities in our account and that of Dijkerman and DeHaan (2007), important differences may be identified. In contrast to the perception/action account, we propose that primary somatosensory information maps onto representations of the body form that encodes location relative to the body (not external space) and, in parallel, onto the body postural representation that encodes body position in external space. On our view, both the body form and postural representations may be accessible to both perception and action systems; similarly, both may operate without awareness or, depending on task demands, be accessible to consciousness. Additional investigations will be needed to adjudicate between these accounts.

In conclusion, we have argued that multiple distinct representations of one's body are computed, each of which provides information relevant to different goals and behaviors. Under normal circumstances these representations appear to interact seamlessly. We suggest that, as in many other cognitive and behavioral domains, brain dysfunction has unearthed the fault lines in the system, thereby permitting the modularity of the representations to be recognized. Future investigations, including theoretically motivated explorations of patients with brain lesions, will be required to fully characterize these representations and explore their implications for accounts of brain function and rehabilitation.

References

Botvinick, M., & Cohen, J. (1998). Rubber hands "feel" touch that eyes see. *Nature, 391*, 756.

Braun, C., Heinz, U., Schweizer, R., Wiech, K., Birbaumer, N., & Topka, H. (2001). Dynamic organization of the somatosensory cortex induced by motor activity. *Brain, 124*, 2259–2267.

Buxbaum, L., & Coslett, H. (2001). Specialized structural descriptions for human body parts: evidence from Autotopagnosia. *Cognitive Neuropsychology, 18*, 289–306.

Calford, M. B. (2002). Dynamic Representational Plasticity in Sensory Cortex. *Neuroscience, 4*, 709–738.

Cole, J., & Paillard, J. (1995). Living without touch and peripheral information about body position and movement: Studies with deafferented subjects. In J. L. Bermudez, A. Marcel & N. Eilan (eds.), *The Body and the Self* (pp. 245–266). Cambridge, MA: MIT Press.

Coslett, H. (1998). Evidence for a disturbance of the body schema in neglect. *Brain and Cognition, 37*(3), 527–544.

Coslett, H., Buxbaum, L., & Shoebill, J. (2008). Accurate Reaching after Active but not Passive Movements of the Hand: Evidence for Forward Modeling. *Behavioral Neurology, 19*(3), 117–125.

Coslett, H. B., Saffran, E. M., & Shoebill, J. (2002). Knowledge of the human body: a distinct semantic domain. *Neurology, 59*(3), 357–363.

Dennis, M. (1976). Dissociated naming and locating of body parts after left anterior temporal lobe resection: an experimental case study. *Brain and Language, 3*(2), 147–163.

Dijkerman, H., & de Haan, E. (2007). Somatosensory processes subserving perception and action. *Behavioral and Brain Sciences, 30*(2), 189–201.

Ehrsson, H. H., Kito, T., Sadato, N., Passingham, R. E., & Naito, E. (2005). Neural substrate of body size: Illusory feeling of shrinking of the waist. *PLOS Biology, 3*(12), 2200–2207.

Gandevia, S. C., & Phegan, C. M. L. (1999). Perceptual distortions of the human body image produced by local anaesthesia, pain and cutaneous stimulation. *Journal of Physiology—London, 514*(2), 609–616.

Ghazanfar, A. A., & Schroeder, C. E. (2006). Is neocortex essentially multisensory? *Trends in Cognitive Sciences, 10*(6), 278–285.

Graziano, M. S. A., Cooke, D. F., & Taylor, C. S. R. (2000). Coding the location of the arm by sight. *Science, 290*(5497), 1782–1786.

Head, H., & Holmes, G. (1911). *Sensory Disturbances from Cerebral Lesions. Brain, 34*, 103–254.

Gerardin, E., Sirigu, A., Lehéricy, S., Poline, J. B., Gaymard, B., Marsault, C., Agid, Y., et al. (1996). Partially overlapping neural networks for real and imagined hand movements. *Cerebral Cortex (New York, N.Y.: 1991), 10*(11), 1093–1104.

Grèzes, J., & Decety, J. (2001). Functional anatomy of execution, mental simulation, observation, and verb generation of actions: a meta-analysis. *Human Brain Mapping, 12*(1), 1–19.

Hodges, J. R., Patterson, K., Oxbury, S., & Funnell, E. (1992). Semantic dementia. Progressive fluent aphasia with temporal lobe atrophy. *Brain: a journal of neurology, 115 (Pt 6)*, 1783–1806.

Jeannerod, M. (2001). Neural simulation of action: a unifying mechanism for motor cognition. *NeuroImage, 14*(1 Pt 2), S103–109.

Lackner, J. R. (1988). Some Proprioceptive Influences on the Perceptual Representation of Body Shape and Orientation. *Brain*, 111, 281–297.

Longo, M. R., Azanon, E., & Haggard, P. (2010). More than skin deep: Body representation beyond primary somatosensory cortex. *Neuropsychologia, 48*(3), 655–668.

Macaluso, E., & Maravita, A. (2010). The representation of space near the body through touch and vision. *Neuropsychologia, 48*(3), 782–795.

Makin, T., Holmes, N., & Zohary, E. (2007). Is that near my hand? Multisensory representation of peripersonal space in human intraparietal sulcus. *Journal of Neuroscience, 27*(4), 731–740.

Medina, J., Jax, S. A., & Coslett, H. B. (2009). Two-component models of reaching: Evidence from deafferentation in a Fitts' law task. *Neuroscience Letters, 451*, 222–226.

Medina, J., & Rapp, B. (2008). Phantom Tactile Sensations Modulated by Body Position. *Current Biology,18*(24): 1937–1942.

Merzenich, M. M., Kaas, J. H., Wall, J. T., Sur, M., Nelson, R. J., & Felleman, D. J. (1983). Progression of change following median nerve section in the cortical representation of the hand in areas 3b and 1 in adult owl and squirrel monkeys. *Neuroscience, 10*(3), 639–665.

Merzenich, M. M., Nelson, R. J., Stryker, M. P., Cynader, M. S., Schoppmann, A., & Zook, J. M. (1984). Somatosensory Cortical Map Changes Following Digit Amputation in Adult Monkeys. *Journal of Comparative Neurology, 224*(4), 591–605.

Milner, A. D., & Goodale, M. A. (1995). *The Visual Brain in Action*. New York: Oxford University Press.
Mishkin, M., & Ungerleider, L. G. (1982). Contribution of striate inputs to the visuospatial functions of parieto-preoccipital cortex in monkeys. *Behavioural Brain Research, 6*(1), 57–77.
Ogden, J. A. (1985). Autotopagnosia. Occurrence in a patient without nominal aphasia and with an intact ability to point to parts of animals and objects. *Brain: a journal of neurology, 108 (Pt 4)*, 1009–1022.
Paillard, J. (1999). Body schema and body image—A double dissociation in deafferented patients. In G. N. Gantchev, S. Mori, and J. Massion, (eds.), *Motor Control, Today and Tomorrow* (pp. 197–214). Akademicno Izdatelstvo: Sofia.
Parsons, L. M. (1987). Imagined spatial transformation of one's body. *Journal of Experimental Psychology. General, 116*(2), 172–191.
Parsons, L. M. (1994). Temporal and kinematic properties of motor behavior reflected in mentally simulated action. *Journal of Experimental Psychology. Human perception and performance, 20*(4), 709–730.
Parsons, L. M., & Fox, P. T. (1998). The neural basis of implicit movements used in recognizing hand shape. *Cognitive Neuropsychology*, 15, 583–615.
Parsons, L. M., Fox, P. T., Downs, J. H., Glass, T., Hirsch, T. B., Martin, C. C., Jerabek, P. A., et al. (1995). Use of implicit motor imagery for visual shape discrimination as revealed by PET. *Nature, 375*(6526), 54–58.
Pick, A. (1922). Storung der Orientierung am Eigenen Korper. Psychologische Forschung, 2, 303–318.
Ramachandran, V., & Altschuler, E. (2009). The use of visual feedback, in particular mirror visual feedback, in restoring brain function. *Brain, 132*, 1693–1710.
Ramachandran, V., Stewart, M., & Rogers-Ramachandran, D. (1992). Perceptual correlates of massive cortical reorganization. *Neuroreport, 3*(7), 583–586.
Rizzolatti, G., Fogassi, L., & Gallese, V. (2002). Motor and cognitive functions of the ventral premotor cortex. *Current Opinion in Neurobiology, 12*(2), 149–154.
Schaefer, M., Heinze, H. J., & Rotte, M. (2008). Observing the touched body magnified alters somatosensory homunculus. *Neuroreport, 19*(9), 901–905.
Schwoebel, J., Boronat, C., & Coslett, H. (2002). The man who executed "imagined" movements: Evidence for dissociable components of the body schema. *Brain and Cognition, 50*(1), 1–16.
Schwoebel, J., Buxbaum, L. J., & Coslett, H. B. (2004). Representations of the human body in the production and imitation of complex movements. *Cognitive Neuropsychology, 21*, 285–298.
Schwoebel, J., Coslett, H. B., Bradt, J., Friedman, R., & Dileo, C. (2002). Pain and the body schema: Effects of pain severity on mental representations of movement. *Neurology, 59*(5), 775–777.
Schwoebel, J., Coslett, H., & Buxbaum, L. (2001). Compensatory coding of body part location in autotopagnosia: Evidence for extrinsic egocentric coding. *Cognitive Neuropsychology, 18*(4), 363–381.
Schwoebel, J., Friedman, R., Duda, N., & Coslett, H. B. (2001). Pain and the body schema—Evidence for peripheral effects on mental representations of movement. *Brain, 124*, 2098–2104.
Shelton, J. R., Fouch, E., & Caramazza, A. (1998). The Selective Sparing of Body Part Knowledge: A Case Study. *Neurocase, 4*(4–5), 339–351.
Shenton, J. T., Schwoebel, J., & Coslett, H. B. (2004). Mental motor imagery and the body schema: evidence for proprioceptive dominance. *Neuroscience Letters, 370*(1), 19–24.
Sirigu, A., Duhamel, J. R., Cohen, L., Pillon, B., Dubois, B., & Agid, Y. (1996). The mental representation of hand movements after parietal cortex damage. *Science (New York, N.Y.), 273*(5281), 1564–1568.

Sirigum A., Grafman, J., Bressler, K., &Sunderland, T. (1991). Multiple Representations Contribute to Body Knowledge Processing: Evidence from a case of Autopagnosia. *Brain 114*: 629–642.

Suzuki, K., Okuda, J., Nakasato, N., Kanno, A., Hatanaka, K., Yamadori, A., Fujii, T., et al. (1997). Auditory evoked magnetic fields in patients with right hemisphere language dominance. *Neuroreport, 8*(15), 3363–3366.

Taylor-Clarke,M., Jacobsen, P., & Haggard, P. (2004). Keeping the world a constant size: object constancy in human touch. *Nature Neuroscience, 7*(3), 219–220.

Tsakiris, M., & Haggard, P. (2005). The rubber hand illusion revisited: Visuotactile integration and self-attribution. *Journal of Experimental Psychology: Human Perception & Performance, 31*, 80–91.

van Beers, R. J., Wolpert, D. M., & Haggard, P. (2002). When feeling is more important than seeing in sensorimotor adaptation. *Current Biology: CB, 12*(10), 834–837.

Wann, J. P., & Ibrahim, S. F. (1992). Does limb proprioception drift? *Experimental Brain Research. Experimentelle Hirnforschung. Expérimentation cérébrale, 91*(1), 162–166.

Wolpert, D. M., Goodbody, S. J., & Husain, M. (1998). Maintaining internal representations the role of the human superior parietal lobe. *Nature Neuroscience, 1*(6), 529–533.

Yamamoto, S., & Kitazawa, S. (2001a). Reversal of subjective temporal order due to arm crossing. *Nature, 4*(7), 759–765.

Yamamoto, S., & Kitazawa, S. (2001b). Sensation at the tips of invisible tools. *Nature Neuroscience, 4*(10), 979–980.

CHAPTER 11

The Neuropathologies of the Self

Todd E. Feinberg

The *neuropathologies of the self* (NPS; Table 11.1; Feinberg, 2001; 2009a; 2010; 2011) include disorders of the *bodily self* in which there is a transformation in the person's sense of their physical being; disorders of the *relational self* where the individual has a disturbance in the personal and autobiographical significance of the self in relation to the world; and pathologies of the *narrative self* that impact how the individual thinks about and describes personal past and present circumstances. I describe here several of the more common NPS and present a synopsis of a theory of their causation and mechanism. For additional clinical description of individual cases, see Feinberg, 2009a; 2010 For the relationship of these clinical disorders to a general model of the neurobiology of the self, see Feinberg, 2009a; 2011.

Disorders of the Bodily Self: Anosognosia for Hemiplegia (AHP), Asomatognosia and Somatoparaphrenia

Anosognosia, literally "lack of knowledge of the existence of disease," occurs in a wide variety of neuropsychiatric conditions (Feinberg & Roane, 2003) but anosognosia for hemiplegia (AHP) is the most common and best known form (for some recent reviews and studies of AHP, see Fotopoulou, Tsakiris, Haggard, Vagopoulou, Rudd, & Kopelman, 2008; Marcel, Tegnér, & Nimmo-Smith, 2004; Orfei, Robinson, Bria, Caltagirone, & Spalletta, 2008; Orfei, Robinson, Prigatano, Starkstein, Rüsch, Bria, Caltagirone, & Spalletta, 2007; Vallar & Ronchi, 2009; Vuilleumier, 2004). In the typical AHP patient, there is an acute lesion, most commonly a stroke in the non-dominant hemisphere that leads to left hemiplegia and hemispatial neglect. The diagnosis of AHP requires only a simple *unawareness of hemiplegia* (Levine, 1990; Levine, Calvanio, & Rinn, 1991), but

Table 11.1 **Some of the most widely reported neuropathologies of the self (NPS). The most delusional forms of these disorders are clinical end points on a multifactorial continuum that includes both negative and positive factors (see Figure 11.1). A subset of these conditions, most specifically related to *delusional misidentification syndromes* (DMS), have also been referred to or overlap with *reduplicative paramnesia or delusions* (Pick, 1903; Alexander et al., 1979; Weinstein & Burnham, 1991) *delusional paramnesic misidentification* (e.g., Burgess et al., 1996), *content-specific delusions* (e.g., Malloy & Richardson, 1994), or *monothematic delusions* (e.g., Davies et al., 2001). The confabulations associated with NPS are most commonly of the *fantastic* (Bonhoeffer, 1901; Schnider, 2008) or *personal* (Feinberg, 1997; Feinberg & Roane, 1997; Feinberg, 2009b) subtypes (modified from Feinberg, 2011).**

Syndrome	*Clinical features*
Delusional anosognosia	Delusional denial of paralysis, often accompanied by confabulation
Somatoparaphrenia	Delusional misidentification of the arm, often accompanied by confabulation
Delusional Misidentification Syndrome (DMS)	Persistent delusional under or over-related misidentification of a person, place, or thing
Capgras syndrome	Under-related DMS
syndrome	Over-related DMS
DMS for the mirror image	Under-related DMS for the mirror image
Phantom Boarder Syndrome	The delusional belief that a person (s) is living in the residence or close by to the patient
Nurturing Syndrome	The delusional belief that a deceased loved one (typically a spouse) is alive and the patient interacts with him or her
Delusional companion syndrome	The patient adopts a soft toy such as a teddy bear and treats it like a close companion or child

AHP may include a wide range of behaviors. Some patients when pressed may agree that the limb is immobile, or attribute this failure to trivial causes such as lack of effort, while others may claim that the limb indeed has moved (illusory or confabulatory limb movements) while they can see that it is in reality lying motionless at their side (Feinberg, Roane, & Ali, 2000). Even when the paralysis is repeatedly demonstrated, the patient may adamantly deny weakness, and here it is appropriate to characterize the belief as a delusion (see below, and Coltheart, 2007; Critchley, 1953; Davies, Aimola Davies, & Coltheart, 2005; Feinberg &

Roane, 1997; Feinberg & Roane, 2003; Gerstmann, 1942; McKay, Langdon, & Coltheart, 2005). A number of perceptual and neurocognitive deficits may facilitate AHP, including proprioceptive loss, hemispatial neglect, generalized confusion, and a host of others factors (Figure 11.1; for some of these see Critchley, 1953; Feinberg & Roane, 2003; Gerstmann, 1942; Heilman, 1991; Heilman, Barrett, & Adair, 1998; Levine et al., 1991; Marcel, Tegner, & Nimmo-Smith, 2004; Orfei et al., 2007; Orfei et al., 2008; Vallar & Ronchi, 2009; Vuilleumier, 2004). There remain, however, some unanswered questions regarding AHP. For instance, while the presence of hemispatial neglect is a common contributing factor, one can temporarily reverse the neglect in some anosognosic patients, yet the anosognosia itself improves only in some cases (Cappa, Sterzi, Vallar, & Bisiach, 1987; Bisiach, Rusconi, & Vallar, 1991), and patients with and without AHP may have similar lesions and degrees of hemispatial neglect (see Bisiach & Geminiani, 1991 and Feinberg & Roane, 2003 for reviews). Finally, there is a wide continuum of degrees and types of AHP. For these and other reasons, it is becoming increasingly evident that no single factor or mechanism can account for AHP (Feinberg & Roane, 1997; Marcel, Tegnér, & Nimmo-Smith, 2004; McKay, Langdon, & Coltheart, 2005; Orfei et al., 2007).

T *Asomatognosia* and somatoparaphrenia most commonly occur in the setting of right hemisphere damage, left hemiplegia, hemisensory deficits, and hemi-spatial neglect (Baier & Karnath, 2008; Critchley, 1953; 1955; Feinberg, 2009a; Feinberg, Haber, & Leeds, 1990; Feinberg, Venneri, Simone, Fan, & Northoff, 2010; Gerstmann, 1942; Halligan, Marshall, & Wade, 1995; Meador, Loring, Feinberg, Lee, & Nichols, 2000; Vallar, & Ronchi, 2009). As in anosognosia, there is considerable heterogeneity in the asomatognosic response (Feinberg et al., 2010). Critchley (1953) introduced the term *asomatognosia* to describe the more general feature of a "loss of awareness of one body-half" without other delusional features, and Gerstmann (1942) referred to *somatoparaphrenia* that was notable for the presence of prominent delusional and confabulatory features.

Disorders of the Relational Self: Delusional Misidentification Syndromes and Delusions and Fantasies about Imaginary Persons

The NPS overlap with several other syndromes, especially the *delusional misidentification syndromes* (DMS; Alexander, Stuss, & Benson, 1979; Capgras & Reboul-Lachaux, 1923; Christodoulou, 1976; 1977, 1986; Feinberg & Roane, 2003; 2005; Fleminger & Burns, 1993; Vie´, 1930; 1944) and *monothematic* (delusions on a single theme; Coltheart, 2007; Critchley, 1953; Davies, Aimola Davies, & Coltheart, 2005; McKay, Langdon, & Coltheart, 2005) or *content specific* (Malloy & Richardson, 1994) *delusions*. One commonly reported form of DMS in neurological patients is the Capgras syndrome (Capgras & Reboul-Lachaux, 1923), in which the individual claims that persons, places, or objects have been replaced by nearly identical "doubles." In the Frégoli syndrome, (Courbon & Fail, 1927) the patient claims that a known person is taking on the appearance of a stranger. Capgras syndrome represents an *under-personalized* and Frégoli syndrome an *over-personalized* misidentification (Feinberg & Roane, 1997; 2003; 2005). Somatoparaphrenia has been interpreted as a variant of Capgras syndrome for their arm in which patients misidentifies in a delusional and confabulatory fashion a part of their body (Vie′, 1930; 1944; Feinberg & Roane, 1997; 2003; 2005).

We described patient S.P. ("Susan") with *delusional misidentification of the self in the mirror* (mirror-image DMS; Gluckman, 1968; Feinberg & Shapiro, 1989; Spangenberg, Wagner, & Bachman, 1998). She was a woman in her 60s who was hearing impaired since the age of five and communicated by speaking, lip reading, and sign language (Feinberg &Shapiro, 1989; 2009a) who used sign language in the mirror with another "S.P." who was nearly identical to her in appearance, age, and background. MRI of the brain revealed right temporoparietal atrophy and neuropsychological testing revealed evidence of right hemisphere dysfunction. S.P.'s misidentification could not be solely due to a perceptual problem, as she readily acknowledged that she was looking in a mirror; she had no spatial confusion with mirrors (i.e., she did not display "mirror agnosia"; Ramachandran, Altschuler, & Hillyer; 1997) and she had no difficulty identifying any other persons in the mirror at the same time that she claimed her reflection belonged to "the other S.P." Therefore, the misidentification of her reflection could not be due to problem with mirrors per se, or a deficit in emotional relatedness per se but represented a selective disorder of relatedness restricted to her own mirror image. I will argue that S.P.'s mirror image is in nearly every respect akin to an *imaginary companion* as occurs in childhood.

In some NPS, also grouped within the DMS (Rubin, 1988; Hwang, Yang, & Tsai, 2003), individuals claim the existence of an imaginary person, often an imaginary child (Weinstein, Kahn, & Morris, 1956). A self-referential aspect of these delusions is that these patients often attributed to the "phantom child" the same illness or disability that the patient had. In another NPS, Shanks and Venneri (2002) described patients with *delusional companions* who claimed that an inanimate object was alive and they interacted with the object in a fashion commensurate with these beliefs. They described three patients, all women, with predominantly right hemisphere dysfunction who treated teddy bears, cloth toys, or dolls as persons. In light of the theory I will present later on, I point out the wishful nature of the beliefs, and that the delusional companions were a source of emotional comfort and companionship. Finally, Venneri and co-workers have also described a similar disorder they call *nurturing syndrome* (Venneri, Shanks, Staff, & Della Sala, 2000). They described two cases—also both women—who were in the early stages of dementia. SPECT scans in both patients demonstrated frontal dysfunction, right greater than left. After the deaths of their husbands, these women claimed that they were still alive. Both women tried to feed photographs of their husbands.

Disorders of the Narrative Self: Symbolic Representations of Personal Experiences

In some patients with *personal confabulation* (Feinberg & Roane, 1997; Feinberg, 2009b), while the narrative is obstensively about veridical personal events, it may also be an expression of the individual's feelings about the self. Feinberg, DeLuca, Giacino, Roane, & Solms (2005) described patient L.A., who had a ruptured arteriovenous malformation resulting in a right frontal intracranial hemorrhage ho adamantly denied his neurological deficits.

LA: *A couple of days ago people been telling me the things that happened to me and its possible that something happened to me.... People been telling me that they think there was a big explosion in one place I was at and that destroyed my mind. And that is one of the reasons I'm having now.... What do you call a person that is sleeping and starts to walk?*

TEF: *Sleep walking.*

LA: *Yeah I started to do that.... and that is causing all the disturbances in my mind.....People are saying, somebody said I was in a room like next door, a big explosion in there and I was in there, and that was going to destroy my mind, my personality. That might be what it is.....They said also that I was going to be sleeping and I was going to awake. But I didn't wake up and I started to walk* [starts to cry] *I never had it before.... The doctor said I was going to be sleeping and start walking in my sleep, and I don't understand because I never had it.*

TEF: *Are you sleep walking now?*

LA: *Not according to my parents and not according to me.*

TEF: *How is your actual walking?*

LA: *My actual walking is good.*

TEF: *Fine? So you can run and dance and jump?*

LA: *No problem....*

Although L.A. claims he is in good health and denies his gait impairment, he refers to his problems with "sleepwalking," and although he appears unaware of any of his cognitive problems or personality issues, he describes how the therapists have told him that an explosion had "destroyed his mind." In this way, the narrative appears to function on both an explicit and an implicit level with reference to the patient's self-awareness.

Explaining the Neuropathologies of the Self: The Ego Disequilibrium Theory

The NPS are distinguished from purely cognitive conditions in that these latter disorders are *neutral* with reference to the patient's self and personal relatedness, in contrast to the NPS which are specifically related to and often confined to something of *personal significance* to the individual (Feinberg & Roane, 1997). The confabulations in NPS also differ from the confabulations in purely amnestic confabulations in that in NPS the confabulations tend to be *less ad hoc, more personally idiosyncratic and motivated, less tied to a specific domain of neurological impairment (multimodal), and more enduring, resistant to correction, repeatable, and delusional;* Feinberg, 2010). The confabulations in NPS are related to or share particular features with *fantastic* (Bonhoeffer, 1901) or *motivated* (Conway & Tacchi, 1996) *confabulation*. The confabulations and delusions that I have posited are typical of the NPS could also be considered *fantastic, personal or motivated confabulations, delusional misidentifications, reduplicative paramnesia or delusions, monothematic delusions, content-specific delusions,* or simply *delusions* (Table 11.1). Regardless of how they are classified, the four essential features that distinguish the confabulations in NPS from errors based solely upon neurological and cognitive impairments are that they are simultaneously *multimodal, selective, personally significant,* and *delusional* (Feinberg, 2010; 2011).

The *negative features* (Jackson, 1884) that accompany many of the NPS cannot fully explain these syndromes (see for example Goldstein, 1939). For example, why are *the misbeliefs and misidentifications in DMS and NPS generally multimodal and selective*? Some patients with Capgras syndrome may have preserved overt facial recognition that permits accurate facial recognition, but an impairment in covert (emotional) responses to faces—a negative factor—leads them to deny that the individual is the one that they are normally related to (Ellis & Young, 1990; Ellis, et al., 1997; Ellis, 1998). While this finding could account for some aspects of the syndrome, it does not explain certain critical issues (Feinberg, 2010): 1) Capgras syndrome is a multimodal disorder and cannot be accounted for by dysfunction in a single sense modality (vision) or perceptual class (faces); 2) patients with the Capgras syndrome do not utilize readily available extra-facial visual and other non-visual information such as hair, clothing, voice, etc.—that also carry emotional value—to correct the error; 3) why is the misidentification typically confined to a single person or a few persons among the many emotionally significant persons in the patient's life? (Feinberg et al., 2005; although this may not be the case among some patients with primary psychiatric diagnoses; see for example Ellis, Young, Quayle, & DePauw, 1997); 4) this account may only be applied to under-personalized misidentification, as occurs in Capgras syndrome, but leaves unexplained over-personalized misidentification as occurs in the Frégoli syndrome or in some cases of NPS or DMS in which there is no misidentification at all; and 5) it is frequently noted that the confabulations and delusional misidentifications in these cases may be *wish-fulfilling* (Conway & Tacchi, 1996; Feinberg & Roane, 1997, 2003; Feinberg, DeLuca, Giacino, Roane, & Solms, 2005; Fotopoulou, Solms, & Turnbull, 2004; Fotopoulou, Conway, & Solms, 2007). A unified theory must also account for the role played by positive and motivational factors as well.

I have proposed a hypothesis called the *ego dysequilibrium theory* (Feinberg et. al., 2005; Feinberg, 2009 a & b) that attempts to satisfy these multiple constraints and unify the negative and positive factors in the origin of these conditions. According to this theory, the unique features of the adult neuropathologies of the self result from 1) a *neurologically derived* alteration in the self-boundaries 2) a *regression* to a developmentally earlier, hierarchically lower, or more primitive stage of psychological functioning and 3) a *recrudescence* of the patterns of thought and psychological defense typical of these earlier periods. The primitive defensive patterns in question include but are not limited to *denial, projection, splitting, fantasy,* and *paranoia,* functions that were dormant in the normal adult brain, but are now activated by the neurological lesion (Feinberg, 2009a; 2010).

The theory accepts the hypothesis that there is a hierarchy of defensive functions (see for example Vaillant, 1977, 1992, 1993), with denial, delusional projection (including delusional paranoia), and distortion the most primitive and hierarchically lowest defenses, followed by *projection* and *fantasy* that make their appearance somewhat later in child development (Cramer (1991; 2006). Cramer (1991; 2006) further points out that *denial through fantasy* is a coping strategy for the child, and (Taylor, 1999) describes how the fantasy of an *imaginary companions* serves important adaptive functions for the child, including alleviating loneliness, coping with trauma, and conquering fears, all motivational factors that are relevant to the adult NPS cases. Finally, it has been proposed that the psychological defense of *splitting* is another primitive defense relevant to the creation of imaginary companions in children (Taylor, 1999) and is also associated with the adult neuropathology cases (Berson, 1983).

A Four-tiered Hierarchical Model of the Neuropathologies of the Self

In Figure 11.1 I present a roughly hierarchical four-tiered model that can serve as a flowchart or template for the analysis of these syndromes (for a more detailed analysis, see Feinberg, 2010; 2011).

Level 1: Cognitive deficits are negative cognitive factors, the presence of which will vary depending upon the syndrome and case. In asomatognosia and somatoparaphrenia, sensory loss and neglect have been posited to play an essential role

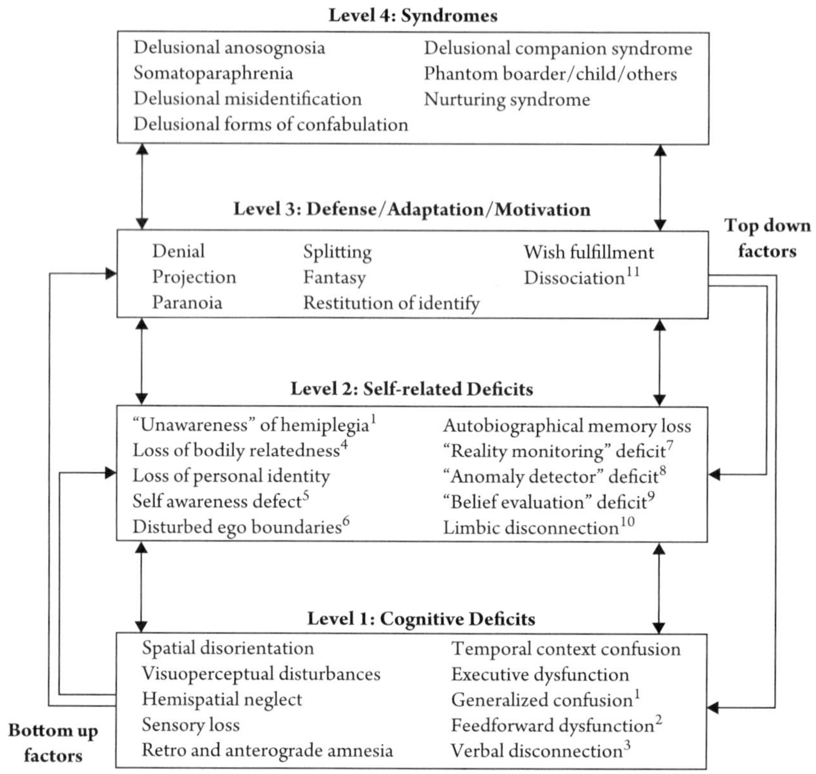

Figure 11.1 A hierarchical four-tiered model of representative factors contributing to the neuropathologies of the self. Specific cognitive deficits may only be relevant to certain conditions, while self-related deficits and positive features may be applied to all syndromes. Top-down and bottom-up factors contribute to the neuropathologies of the self. A temporal dimension emerges as syndromes evolve from the interaction of multiple lower-level negative and higher-level positive factors.

[1]Levine, 1990; Levine et al., 1991; [2]Heilman, 1991; Heilman et al., 1998. [3]With reference to anosognosia and asomatognosia see Geschwind, 1965; Gazzaniga, 2000; [4]For the neural representation of body ownership see Feinberg et al., 1990; Vallar & Ronchi, 2009; Tsakiris, 2009; [5]Stuss, 1991; [6]Feinberg et al., 2005; Feinberg, 2009a; 2009b; Feinberg et al., 2010; [7]Johnson, 1991; [8]Ramachandran, 1995; [9]Coltheart, 2007; Davies et al., 2005; McKay et al., 2005; [10]With reference to Capgras syndrome see Alexander et al., 1979; Ellis & Young, 1990; [11]With reference to DMS see Christodoulou, 1976;1977;1986.

(Vallar & Ronchi, 2009), while in confabulation and misidentification, memory disorders, executive dysfunction, and anatomical disconnection are noted to be contributing factors (see for example Alexander, Stuss, & Benson, 1979). ***Level 2: Self-related deficits*** are also negative factors, but are specifically *self-related*. Since these are negative factors, with reference to anosognosia for hemiplegia and asomatognosia, for example, I characterize this level of impairment as *unawareness of hemiplegia* and *loss of bodily relatedness* (i.e., negative factors, including personal neglect) as opposed to *delusional denial of hemiplegia* and *delusional denial of ownership* (delusional AHP and somatoparaphrenia at the top of the hierarchy, Figure 11.1). While right temporoparietal regions are central to the establishment of normal self-relatedness to the body (for a review see Tsakiris, 2009), and damage to this region is an essential negative factor in the creation of asomatognosia and somatoparaphrenia (Feinberg et al., 1990; Feinberg et al., 2010; Vallar & Ronchi, 2009), additional factors must be operative when this negative unawareness evolves into delusional misidentification of the body as occurs in somatoparaphrenia. Negative factors cited in case of DMS and confabulation include the dysexecutive syndrome after frontal damage (Stuss & Benson, 1985; Stuss, 1991; Stuss, Picton, & Alexander, 2001; Stuss, Rosenbaum, Malcolm, Christianna, & Keenan, 2005) a "reality monitoring defect" in confabulation (Johnson, 1991), an "anomaly detector" defect in anosognosia for hemiplegia (Ramachandran, 1995), or a deficit in a hypothetical "belief evaluation system" (Davies et al., 2005), Coltheart, 2005; 2007) and McKay et al., 2005) in anosognosia and DMS. An additional negative factor in the development of these disorders is that bilateral or right, especially frontal, pathology causes a *permeability of the ego boundaries* that results in an *ego dysequilibrium* that produces a *two-way disturbance* between the self and the environment, specifically with regard to personal relatedness. This could potentially lead to disorders of *both* under (e.g., Capgras syndrome) and over (e.g., Frégoli syndrome, Feinberg, Eaton, Roane, & Giacino, 1999) relatedness between the self and the world (Feinberg et al., 2005; Feinberg & Keenan, 2005, Feinberg, 2009a, 2010).

Level 3: Defense, adaptation, and motivation represent the way the damaged brain adapts—in a positive fashion—to the various cognitive and psychological deficits, but it does so in a regressed fashion. These primitive mechanisms according to Cramer (1991) are largely unconscious and automatic when compared to the mature defenses, which are held to be more conscious and voluntary. The developmental progression from primitive and immature to mature defenses may result from brain maturation and increasing cognitive skills (Cramer, 1991, 2006; Elkind, 1976; Laughlin, 1970). Another variable is the relationship between primitive and immature defenses and ego boundaries (Feinberg, 2009a; 2010; 2011). Immature or hierarchically lower order defenses are more likely to violate the boundary between self and non-self (Cramer, 1991), and the manifestations of both denial and projection involve treating that which actually pertains to the self as if it were only relevant to the external world (Breznitz, 1983).

Level 4: The syndromes are the result of numerous positive and negative factors and the lines of development for any given disorder of the self can be traced from lower to higher levels. For example, moving from bottom to top, asomatognosia may result from a large number of "cognitive deficits," such as sensory loss, neglect, and anatomical disconnection, and specific "self-related deficits," such as disturbed ego boundaries, self-monitoring defects, and loss of relatedness to a part of the body. To these negative defects are positive contributing factors such as the mobilization of immature defenses and adaptations (denial, projection, fantasy, splitting, etc.) If a sufficient number of these interacting factors are operative, the entire picture results in the full clinical syndrome of somatoparaphrenia, in which the patient not only misidentifies the arm, but it may be reduplicated or the subject of fantastic fantasy and confabulation (Feinberg et al., 2010). With regard to DMS, Staton, Brumback, & Wilson (1982) and Bouvier-Peyrou, Landis & Annoni (2000) reported single cases of young men with traumatic brain injuries and bifrontal damage and delusional misidentification of the self. In line with Figure 11.1, both Staton et al. and Bouvier-Peyrou et al. proposed that combined executive and memory impairments (level 1) resulted in a failure to integrate current experience with their past sense of who they were, a mechanism similar to the explanation of Alexander et al. (1979), who posited a temporo-limbic-frontal disconnection in their case of Capgras syndrome. This disconnect between "past" and "present" selves created a loss of personal identity (level 2), and the response and adaptation to this in the presence of the neurologically derived permeability in ego boundaries is the emergence of the primitive defenses of *dissociation* ("This must be a dream") *denial* ("this can't be really happening") *projection* ("it's the world that isn't real"; "it's my parents who are fake, not me") and *fantasy* ("another version of me will wake up from this nightmare and I'll be well" (level 3). The ultimate syndromes we call delusional misidentification, including Capgras syndrome, delusional reduplication, and delusional confabulation.

Ego Boundaries and Neuroanatomy

The NPS are associated with frontal, especially right hemisphere pathology (Alexander et al., 1979; Burgess, Baxter, Martyn, & Alderman, 1996; Feinberg & Shapiro, 1989; Fleminger & Burns, 1993; Förstl, Burns, Jacoby, & Levy, 1991; Malloy Cimino, & Westlake, 1992; Spangenberg, Wagner, & Bachman, 1998). Burgess et al. (1996) reviewed 41 cases of confabulation, paramnesias, and various DMS and found the highest percentage of cases had right frontal hemisphere (44 percent) or bilateral frontal (39 percent) lesions while only 9.7 percent had left frontal lesions. Feinberg et al., (2005), in a series of published cases of DMS or reduplication, found 15 (51.72 percent) had left hemisphere damage, but right frontal damage was present in 28 out of 29 cases (96.6 percent). Feinberg et al. (2010) analyzed cases of simple asomatognosia (errors regarding the ownership of the limb) and somatoparaphrenia (denial of arm ownership, delusions, and confabulations) in patients with right hemisphere strokes and left hemiplegia. When compared with right hemisphere control patients without asomatognosia or somatoparaphrenia, patients with asomatognosia and somatoparaphrenia had more medial frontal damage, indicating a role for medial frontal damage in the development of all forms of asomatognosia, but the somatoparaphrenia cases also had greater orbitofrontal damage, suggesting an additional role for an orbitofrontal lesion that could be due to the role that orbitofrontal damage plays in the development of confabulation (Deluca & Diamond, 1995; Ptak & Schnider, 1999). These results taken collectively support the role that the frontal lobes, especially medial zones (Feinberg, 2009a; Feinberg et al, 2010; Northoff & Bermpohl, 2004; Northoff, Heinzel, de Greck, Bermpohl, Dobrowolny, & Panksepp, 2006; Northoff et al., 2009) play more generally in a host of self-related functions (Stuss, 1991; Stuss, Picton, & Alexander, 2001; Stuss, Rosenbaum, Malcolm, Christianna, & Keenan, 2005).

Conclusions: The Right Hemisphere and Ego Disequilibrium

The *neuropathologies of the self* are a group of syndromes in which brain dysfunction causes a significant alteration in the individual's sense of self. The neuropathology particularly involves the frontal lobes, especially within the right hemisphere, and damage to these sectors results in a disorder of ego boundaries and ego functions (*ego disequilibrium*) that facilitates the emergence of developmentally immature styles of thought and ego functioning. This accounts for the striking resemblance between some of the patterns of behavior we see in the adult NPS cases to behaviors that are common in the normal child. Given that the primitive defenses are largely verbally expressed—*what people say to themselves and others about themselves and the world*—in the NPS cases it is possible that the preservation and activation of the primitive defenses (including denial, projection, splitting, and fantasy) could be due to the relatively intact left verbal hemisphere, and that the neural basis of the mature defenses may be lateralized to the non-dominant hemisphere.

References

Alexander, M. P., Stuss, D. T., & Benson, D. F. (1979). Capgras syndrome: A reduplicative phenomenon. *Neurology, 29*, 334–339.

Baier, B., & Karnath, H-0. (2008). Tight link between our sense of limb ownership and self-awareness of actions. *Stroke, 39*, 486–488.

Berson, R. J. (1983). Capgras' syndrome. *American Journal of Psychiatry, 140*, 969–978.

Bisiach, E., & Geminiani, G (1991). Anosognosia related to hemiplegia and hemianopia. In G. P. Prigatano & D. L. Schacter (Eds.), *Awareness of deficit after brain injury* (pp. 17–39). New York: Oxford University Press.

Bisiach, E., Rusconi, M. L., & Vallar, G. (1991). Remission of somatoparaphrenic delusion through vestibular stimulation. *Neuropsychologia, 29*, 1029–1031.

Bonhoeffer, K. (1901). *Die akuten Geisteskrankheiten der Gewohnheitstrinker*. Gustav Fischer, Jena.

Bouvier-Peyrou, M, Landis, T., & Annoni, J-M. (2000). Self-duplication shifted in time: A particular form of delusional misidentification syndrome. *Neurocase, 6*, 57–63.

Breznitz, S. (1983). *The Denial of Stress*. New York: International Universities Press.

Burgess, P. W., Baxter, D., Martyn, R., & Alderman, N. (1996). Delusional paramnesic misidentification. In P. W. Halligan & J. C. Marshall (Eds.), *Method in Madness: Case Studies in Cognitive Neuropsychiatry* (pp.51–78). East Sussex, UK: Psychology Press.

Capgras, J., & Reboul-Lachaux, J. (1923). L'illusion des "sosies"dans un delire systematize *Bulletin de Société Clinique de Médicine Mentale, 11*, 6–16.

Cappa, S., Sterzi, R., Vallar, G., & Bisiach, E. (1987). Remission of hemineglect and anosognosia during vestibular stimulation. *Neuropsychologia, 25*, 775–782.

Christodoulou, G. N. (1976). Delusional hyper-identifications of the Fregoli type *Acta Psychiatrica Scandinavica, 54*, 305–314.

Christodoulou, G. N. (1977). The syndrome of Capgras. *British Journal of Psychiatry, 130*, 556–564.

Christodoulou, G. N. (1986). Role of depersonalization-derealization phenomena in the delusional misidentification syndromes. *Bibliotheca Psychiatrica, 164*, 99–104.

Coltheart, M. (2005). Delusional belief. *Australian Journal of Psychology, 57*, 72–76.

Coltheart, M. (2007). The 33rd Bartlett Lecture: Cognitive neuropsychiatry and delusional belief. Quarterly Journal of Experimental Psychology, *60*, 1041–1062.

Conway, M. A., & Tacchi, P. C. (1996). Motivated confabulation. *Neurocase, 2*, 325–339.

Courbon, P., & Fail, G. (1927). Syndrome d'illusion de Frégoli et schizophrénie. *Bulletin de Société Clinique de Médicine Mentale, 15*, 121–124.

Cramer, P. (1991). *The Development of Defense Mechanisms: Theory, Research, and Assessment*. New York: Springer-Verlag.

Cramer, P. (2006). *Protecting the Self: Defense Mechanisms in Action*. New York: The Guilford Press.

Critchley, M. (1953). *The Parietal Lobes*. New York: Hafner Press.

Critchley, M. (1955). Personification of paralyzed limbs in hemiplegics. *British Medical Journal, 30*, 284–287.

Davies, M., Coltheart, M., Langdon, R., & Breen, N. (2001). Monothematic delusions: Towards a two-factor account. *Philosophy, Psychiatry & Psychology, 8*, 133–158.

Davies, M., Aimola Davies, A., & Coltheart, M. (2005). Anosognosia and the two-factor theory of delusion. *Mind and Language, 20*, 209–236.

Deluca, J., & Diamond, B. J. (1995). Aneurysm of the anterior communicating artery: A review of the neuroanatomical and neuropsychological sequelae. *Clinical and Experimental Neuropsychology, 17*, 100–121.

Elkind, D. (1976). Cognitive development and psychopathology: observations on egocentrism and ego defense. In E. Schopler & R. J. Reichler (Eds.), *Psychopathology and Child Development. Research and Treatment* (pp. 167–183). New York: Plenum.

Ellis, H. D. (1998). Cognitive neuropsychiatry and delusional misidentification syndromes: An exemplary vindication of the new discipline *Cognitive Neuropsychiatry, 3*, 81–90.

Ellis, H. D., & Young, A. W. (1990). Accounting for delusional misidentifications. *British Journal of Psychiatry, 157*, 239–248.

Ellis, H. D., Young, A. W., Quayle, A. H., & de Pauw, K. W. (1997). Reduced autonomic responses to faces in Capgras delusion. *Proceedings of the Royal Society of London: Biological Sciences, B264*, 1085–1092.

Feinberg, T. E. (1997). Anosognosia and confabulation. In T. E. Feinberg and M. J. Farah (Eds.), *Behavioral Neurology and Neuropsychology*, (1st ed., pp. 369–390). New York: McGraw Hill.

Feinberg, T. E. (2001). *Altered Egos: How the Brain Creates the Self*. New York: Oxford University Press.

Feinberg, T. E. (2009a). *From Axons to Identity: Neurological Explorations of the Nature of the Self.* New York: W.W. Norton.

Feinberg, T. E. (2009b). Confabulation, the self, and ego functions: The "Ego Dysequilibrium Theory." In W. Hirstein (Ed.), *Confabulation: Views from Neuroscience, Psychiatry, Psychology and Philosophy* (pp. 91–107). New York: Oxford.

Feinberg, T. E. (2011). Neuropathologies of the self: Clinical and anatomical features. *Consciousness and Cognition, 20,* 75–81.

Feinberg, T. E. (2010). Neuropathologies of the self: a general theory. *Neuropsychoanalysis,* 2, 133–158.

Feinberg, T. E., DeLuca, J., Giacino, J. T., Roane, D. M., & Solms, M. (2005). Right hemisphere pathology and the self: Delusional Misidentification and Reduplication. In T. E. Feinberg & J. P. Keenan (Eds.), *The lost self: Pathologies of the brain and identity* (pp. 100–130). New York: Oxford.

Feinberg, T. E., Eaton, L. A., Roane, D. M., & Giacino, J. T. (1999). Multiple Fregoli delusions after traumatic brain injury. *Cortex, 35,* 373–387.

Feinberg, T. E., Haber, L. D., & Leeds, N. E. (1990). Verbal asomatognosia. *Neurology, 40,* 1391–1394.

Feinberg, T. E., & Keenan, J. P. (2005). Where in the brain is the self? *Consciousness and Cognition, 14,* 661–678.

Feinberg, T. E., & Roane, D. M. (1997). Anosognosia, completion and confabulation: The neutral-personal dichotomy. *Neurocase, 3,* 73–85.

Feinberg, T. E., & Roane, D. M. (2003). Anosognosia. In T. E. Feinberg & M. J. Farah (Eds.), *Behavioral Neurology and Neuropsychology* (2nd ed., pp. 345–362). New York: McGraw-Hill.

Feinberg, T. E., & Roane, D. M. (2005). Delusional misidentification syndromes. *Psychiatric Clinics of North America, 28,* 665–683.

Feinberg, T. E., Roane, D. M., & Ali, J. (2000). Illusory limb movements in anosognosia for hemiplegia. *Journal of Neurology, Neurosurgery, and Psychiatry, 68,* 511–513.

Feinberg, T. E., & Shapiro, R. M. (1989). Misidentification reduplication and the right hemisphere. *Neuropsychiatry, Neuropsychology, and Behavioral Neurology, 2,* 39–48.

Feinberg, T. E., Venneri, A., Simone, A. M., Fan, Y., & Northoff, G. (2010). The neuroanatomy of asomatognosia and somatoparaphrenia. *Journal of Neurology, Neurosurgery and Psychiatry, 81,* 276–81.

Fleminger, S., & Burns, A. (1993). The delusional misidentification syndromes in patients with and without evidence of organic cerebral disorder: A structured review of case reports. *Biological Psychiatry* 33, 22–32.

Förstl, H, Burns, A, Jacoby, R, & Levy, R. (1991). Neuroanatomical correlates of clinical misidentification and misperception in senile dementia of the Alzheimer's type. *Journal of Clinical Psychiatry, 52,* 268–271.

Fotopoulou, A, Conway, M. A., & Solms, M. (2007). Confabulation: Motivated Reality Monitoring. Neuropsychologia, 45, 2180–2190.

Fotopoulou, A. Tsakiris, M., Haggard, P., Vagopoulou, A., Rudd, A., & Kopelman, M. (2008). The role of motor intention in motor awareness: An experimental study on anosognosia for hemiplegia, *Brain, 131,* 3432–3442.

Gazzaniga, M. S. (2000). Cerebral specialization and interhemispheric communication: Does the corpus callosum enable the human condition? *Brain, 123,* 1293–1326.

Gerstmann, J. (1942). Problem of imperception of disease and of impaired body territories with organic lesions. *Archives of Neurology and Psychiatry, 48,* 890–913.

Geschwind, N. (1965). Disconnexion syndromes in animals and man. *Brain, 88,* 585–644.

Gluckman, L. K. (1968). A case of Capgras syndrome. *Australian and New Zealand Journal of Psychiatry, 2,* 39–43.

Goldstein, K. (1939). *The Organism: A Holistic Approach to Biology Derived from Pathological Data in Man.* New York: American Book Company.

Halligan, P. W., Marshall, J. C., & Wade, D. T. (1995). Unilateral somatoparaphrenia after right hemisphere stroke: a case description. *Cortex, 31*, 173–182.
Heilman, K. M. (1991). Anosognosia: Possible neuropsychological mechanisms. In G. P. Prigatano & G. L. Schacter (Eds.), *Awareness of Deficit after Brain Injury: Clinical and Theoretical Issues* (pp.53–62). New York: Oxford University Press.
Heilman, K. M., Barrett, A. M., Adair, J. C. (1998). Possible mechanisms of anosognosia: a defect in self-awareness. *Philosophical Transactions Royal Society of London B, Biological Science, 353*, 1903–1909.
Hwang, J-P., Yang, C-H., and Tsai, S-J. (2003). Phantom boarder symptom in dementia. *International Journal of Geriatric Psychiatry, 18*, 417–420.
Jackson, J. H. Evolution and dissolution of the nervous system. Croonian Lectures delivered at the Royal College of Physicians, March 1884. Reprinted in J. Taylor (ed.), *Selected Writings of John Hughlings Jackson*, 1958, vol. 2, (pp. 45–75). New York: Basic Books.
Johnson, M. K. (1991). Reality monitoring: Evidence from confabulation in organic brain disease patients. In G. P. Prigatano & G. L. Schacter (Eds.), *Awareness of Deficit after Brain Injury: Clinical and Theoretical Issues* (pp.176–197). New York: Oxford University Press.
Laughlin, H. P. (1970). *The Ego and Its Defenses*. New York: Appleton-Century-Crofts.
Levine, D. N. (1990). Unawareness of visual and sensorimotor defects: A hypothesis. *Brain and Cognition, 13*, 233–281.
Levine, D. N., Calvanio, R., & Rinn, W. E. (1991). The pathogenesis of anosognosia for hemiplegia. *Neurology, 41*, 1770–1781.
Malloy, P., Cimino, C., and Westlake, R. (1992). Differential Diagnosis of primary and secondary delusions. *Neuropsychiatry, Neuropsychology, and Behavioral Neurology, 5*, 83–96.
Malloy, P. F., & Richardson, E. D. (1994). The frontal lobes and content-specific delusions. *The Journal of Neuropsychiatry and Clinical Neurosciences, 6*, 455–466.
Marcel, A. J, Tegnér, R, & Nimmo-Smith, I. (2004). Anosognosia for plegia: Specificity, extension, partiality and disunity of bodily unawareness. *Cortex, 40*, 19–40.
McKay, R., Langdon, R., & Coltheart, M. (2005). "Sleights of mind": Delusions, defences and self-deception. *Cognitive Neuropsychiatry, 10*, 305–326.
Meador, K. J., Loring, D. W., Feinberg, T. E., Lee, G. P., & Nichols, M. E. (2000). Anosognosia and asomatognosia during intracarotid amobarbital inactivation. *Neurology, 55*, 816–820.
Northoff, G., & Bermpohl, F. (2004). Cortical midline structures and the self. *Trends in Cognitive Sciences, 8*, 102–107.
Northoff, G., Heinzel, A., de Greck, M., Bermpohl, F., Dobrowolny, H., & Panksepp, J. (2006). Self-referential processing in our brain—a meta-analysis of imaging studies on the self. *Neuroimage, 31*, 440–457.
Northoff, G., Schneider, F., Rotte, M., Matthiae, C., Tempelmann, C., Wiebking, C., Bermpohl, F., . . . , Panksepp, J. (2009). Differential parametric modulation of self-relatedness and emotions in different brain regions *Human Brain Mapping, 30*, 369–382.
Orfei, M. D., Robinson, R. G., Bria, P., Caltagirone, C., & Spalletta, G. (2008). Unawareness of illness in neuropsychiatric disorders: Phenomenological certainty versus etiopathogenic vagueness. *The Neuroscientist, 14*, 203–222.
Orfei, M. D., Robinson, R. G., Prigatano, G. P., Starkstein, S., Rüsch, N., Bria, P. C., Caltagirone, C., & Spalletta, G. (2007). Anosognosia for hemiplegia after stroke is a multifaceted phenomenon: a systematic review of the literature. *Brain, 130*, 3075–3090.
Pick, A. (1903). On reduplicative paramnesia. *Brain, 26*, 260–267.
Ptak, R., & Schnider, A. (1999). Spontaneous confabulations after orbitofrontal damage: The role of temporal context confusions and self-monitoring. *Neurocase, 5*, 243–250.
Ramachandran, V. S. (1995). Anosognosia in parietal lobe syndrome. *Consciousness and Cognition, 4*, 22–51.
Ramachandran, V. S., Altschuler, E. L., & Hillyer, S. (1997). Mirror agnosia. *Proceedings of the Royal Society of London, B. 264*, 645–647.

Rubin, E. H., Drevets, W. C., & Burke, W. J. (1988). The nature of psychotic symptoms in senile dementia of the Alzheimer type. *Journal of Geriatric Psychiatry and Neurology, 1*, 16–20.

Schnider, A. (2008). *The confabulating mind: How the brain creates reality*. New York: Oxford.

Shanks, M. F., & Venneri, A. (2002). The emergence of delusional companions in Alzheimer's disease: An unusual misidentification syndrome. *Cognitive Neuropsychiatry, 7*, 317–328.

Spangenberg, K. B., M. T. Wagner, and D. L. Bachman (1998). Neuropsychological analysis of a case of abrupt onset mirror sign following a hypotensive crisis in a patient with vascular dementia. *Neurocase, 4*, 149–154.

Staton, R. D., Brumback, R. A., Wilson, H. (1982). Reduplicative paramnesia: A disconnection syndrome of memory. *Cortex, 18*, 23–36.

Stuss, D. T. (1991). Disturbances of self-awareness after frontal system damage. In G. P. Prigatano & G. L. Schacter (Eds.), *Awareness of Deficit after Brain Injury: Clinical and Theoretical Issues injury* (pp. 63–83). New York: Oxford University Press.

Stuss, D., & Benson, D. F. (1985). *The Frontal Lobes*. New York: Raven Press.

Stuss, D. T., Picton, T. W., & Alexander, M. P. (2001). Consciousness, self-awareness, and the frontal lobes. In S. P. Salloway, P. F. Malloy & J. D. Duffy, (Eds.), *The frontal lobes and neuropsychiatric illness* (pp. 101–109). Washington, DC: American Psychiatric Publishing.

Stuss, D. T., Rosenbaum, R. S., Malcolm, S. Christianna, W., & Keenan, J. P. (2005). The frontal lobes and self-awareness. In T. E. Feinberg & J. P. Keenan (Eds.), *The lost self: Pathologies of the brain and identity* (pp. 50–64). New York: Oxford University Press.

Taylor, M. (1999). *Imaginary companions and the children who create them*. New York: Oxford University Press.

Tsakiris, M. (2009). My body in the brain: A neurocognitive model of body-ownership. *Neuropsychologia, 48*, 703–712.

Turnbull, O. H., Berry, H., & Evans, C. E. Y. (2004). A positive emotional bias in confabulatory false beliefs about place. *Brain and Cognition, 55*, 490–494.

Vaillant, G. E. (1977). *Adaptation to Life*. Boston: Little, Brown.

Vaillant, G. E. (1992). *Ego Mechanisms of Defense: A Guide for Clinicians and Researchers*. Washington, DC: American Psychiatric Press.

Vaillant, G. E. (1993). *The Wisdom of the Ego*. Cambridge, MA: Harvard University Press.

Vallar, G., & Ronchi, R. (2009). Somatoparaphrenia: a body delusion. A review of the neuropsychological literature. *Experimental Brain Research, 192*, 533–551.

Venneri, A., Shanks, M. F., Staff, R. T., & Della Sala, S. (2000). Nurturing syndrome: a form of pathological bereavement with delusions in Alzheimer's disease. *Neuropsychologia, 38*, 213–224.

Vie ́ J. (1930). Un trouble de l'identification des personnes: L'illusion des sosies. *Annales Médico-Psychologiques, 88*, 214–237.

Vie ́ J. (1944). Les meconnaissances systematiques. *Annales Médico- Psychologiques* (Paris), *102*, 410–455.

Vuilleumier, P. (2004). Anosognosia: The neurology of beliefs and uncertainties. *Cortex, 40*, 9–17.

Weinstein, E. A., & Burnham, D. L. (1991). Reduplication and the syndrome of Capgras. *Psychiatry, 54*, 78–88.

Weinstein, E. A., Kahn, R. L., & Morris, G. O. (1956). Delusions about children following brain injury. *Journal of the Hillside Hospital, 5*, 290–298.

CHAPTER 12

The Neurology of Emotional Expression

Lee X. Blonder

Introduction

Patient-oriented research into impairments of emotional expression has both theoretical and clinical significance. The study of these disorders in individuals with neurologic disease has shed light on the neuroanatomic, neuropharmacologic, and neurobehavioral mechanisms that underlie emotional expression. Furthermore, an understanding of how these disorders manifest themselves in different patient populations has generated increased translational work including efforts to develop appropriate treatments. Some requirements in Positron Emission Tomography (PET) or functional Magnetic Resonance Imaging (fMRI), such as the positioning of the individual in a scanning device and restriction of head motion, limit the ability to design and conduct experiments on emotional expression. Hence, current knowledge regarding both the neural substrates of and the effects of neurologic disease on emotional expression derives almost exclusively from patient-oriented research conducted either at the bedside, in the clinic or laboratory, or in the home.

Channels of Emotional Expression

Humans express emotion via verbal and non-verbal channels. Verbal communication of emotion occurs through spoken and written language and appears to be uniquely human— i.e,. there is little evidence suggesting that the capacity to use semantic, phonologic, and syntactic processes to express emotion is present in non-human primates. In contrast, non-verbal expression of emotion appears more primitive, given its use by non-human primates and mammals to communicate internal states and to establish position in the social hierarchy. Non-verbal communication of emotion includes facial expression, prosodic expression (intonation, stress, pause, and rhythm in speech), and gesture (hand gestures and body posture). While verbal and non-verbal channels of emotional expression work in concert in the neurologically intact individual, research in behavioral neurology and neuropsychology suggests that they are often fractionated in the brain-damaged patient. Thus, a person might be capable of articulating an emotionally expressive sentence such as "That makes me happy" but with a monotone voice, a "masked" facial expression, or both. Furthermore, in the neurologically intact individual, verbal and non-verbal expressions of emotion communicate internal state, affirm socio-cultural expectations including social status, and/or deceive and manipulate others. In contrast, the expression of emotion by brain-damaged patients is made more complex in that reduced signal or channel inconsistent behavior may reflect neural dysfunction rather than the patient's feelings or communicative agenda. The remainder of this chapter will consist of a review of past and current research on the neurology of emotional expression including discussion of theoretical and clinical implications.

Prosody

Neurobehavioral research in stroke patients has shown that deficits in prosody often accompany damage to the right hemisphere. In 1947, Norwegian neurologist Monrad-Krohn used the term "aprosody" to describe loss of prosody following neurologic disease. In 1977, Tucker, Watson, and Heilman published the first experimental study describing emotional aprosody in patients with right temporo-parietal lesions and unilateral neglect. These patients were also impaired in the comprehension of emotional prosody. Following this, Ross & Mesulam (1979) reported two cases of patients with right hemisphere pathology in the supra-sylvian distribution who developed "motor aprosody"—loss of ability to express emotion through prosody. These patients retained the ability to comprehend the emotion conveyed via prosody, suggesting that expressive and receptive functions are mediated in different brain regions. In 1981, Ross described ten cases of emotional aprosody following right hemisphere disease that he found to be homologous to aphasic syndromes that typically accompany left hemisphere pathology. He suggested that the functional/anatomic organization of affective language in the right hemisphere mirrors that of the left. Subsequent research by Brådvik et al. (1991) failed to replicate this finding. However, additional studies have shown that anterior lesions tend to result in expressive prosodic deficits, while posterior lesions often result in receptive deficits (Borod et al., 1986; Heller et al., 1998; Ross, 1981; Ross & Mesulam, 1979). In a study of patients with cerebral infarcts located in different brain regions, Cancelliere & Kertesz (1990) found that disorders of emotional prosodic expression most often include damage to the basal ganglia. More recently, Heilman et al. (2004) reported aman who sustained a right medial frontal cerebral infarction that resulted in expressive aprosody.

Several studies have used acoustic quantification of speech to examine further the nature of aprosodic disorders in RHD patients and to corroborate clinicians' impressions of "flat affect." Kent & Rosenbek (1982) found that the speech of RHD patients strongly resembles that of Parkinson patients in that both had a normal or increased rate of speech and decreased fundamental frequency (*fo*) variation. Cooper et al. (1984) showed that RHD patients' intonation contours were flatter and the duration of their utterances and sentence final words slightly shorter than that of Wernicke's aphasics and normal controls. Ryalls, Joanette, & Feldman (1987) found a trend for RHD patients tested prior to 100 days post-onset, to have narrower *fo* ranges than those tested at 100 days or more post-onset. These results suggest that in some patients the disorder may resolve spontaneously. Ross et al. (1988) found significant differences in several measures of *fo* on an emotional prosodic repetition task administered pre- and post-Wada testing. Shapiro & Danly (1985) asked LHD patients and RHD patients with anterior, central, or posterior lesions, and a group of normal controls to read sentences using linguistic (interrogative, declarative) or emotional (happy, sad) prosody. They found that RHD patients with anterior and central lesions demonstrated more restricted *fo* range in both linguistic and emotional prosody, while patients with posterior RHD had exaggerated *fo* range during linguistic and emotional speech. The prosody of LHD patients was similar to that of normal controls.

Blonder et al. (1995) had the unique opportunity to evaluate spontaneous prosody in audiotapes of interviews with a 77-year-old right-handed woman recorded six months before and six weeks after she suffered a stroke affecting the right fronto-temporo-parietal regions and the right basal ganglia. Post-stroke, the patient had a normal Mini-mental Status Examination Score of 29, hemispatial neglect, and impairments in the comprehension of facial expression and prosody. Self-rated mood was within normal limits. We compared beginning, peak, and ending fundamental frequencies (fo) in breath groups, the timing of these fo changes, rate of speech, pause duration, and breath-group duration. Results indicated that post-stroke, the patient had a more restricted fo contour, no changes in the timing of peak fo, an increased rate of speech, less variability in pause duration, and no changes in breath-group duration.

Ross & Monnot (2008) conducted a lesion mapping study of affective aprosody using the aprosodia battery developed by Ross et al. (1997). They found that spontaneous expressive aprosody is associated with lesions in the right frontal operculum usually including the right anterior insula. Furthermore, their findings largely support those of Ross (1981) in that, with the exception of prosodic repetition, affective aprosody appears to be functionally homologous in organization to that of propositional language in the left hemisphere. Moreover, in contrast to the findings of Cancelliere & Kertesz (1990) described above, Ross & Monnot (2008) suggest that expressive aprosody evolved as a cortically-based function in the human brain— in concert with language.

There have been very few attempts to develop treatment protocols for disorders of affective communication such as the aprosodias. Recently however, Rosenbek et al. (2004) and Leon et al. (2005) published studies of mechanism-based treatments for expressive aprosodia. Leon et al. (2005) used a single subject design in which three patients with cerebral infarction in the right hemisphere that resulted in expressive aprosodia received two different treatments. One treatment was based on the hypothesis that aprosodia is due to motor programming deficits related to vocal selection and planning. Participants were required to imitate emotional prosody in audiotapes. The alternative treatment was based on a cognitive-linguistic approach and used cards with cue words that included emotion labels, descriptions of the vocal components of affective prosody, and depictions of emotional facial expressions. Results indicated that both treatments produced improvement in prosodic production as demonstrated by moderate to large effect sizes. In a subsequent study involving additional participants, Rosenbek et al. (2006) found that one or the other of these two treatments for expressive aprosodia showed evidence of significant improvement in twelve of fourteen patients with right hemisphere damage. A subset of participants who were available at three-month follow-up continued to retain training effects. These studies are among the first attempts by clinical investigators to translate the findings of decades of lesion research into effective interventions for neurologic patients who suffer from impairments of emotional expression in speech.

Disorders of prosody such as monopitch and loss of volume in the voice are also characteristic of Parkinson's disease (PD). These findings have been observed both clinically and experimentally. For example, Darley et al. (1969) performed a judgment study of speech characteristics in PD and found that monopitch, monoloudness, and increased rate were among the most pronounced prosodic abnormalities. Acoustic analyses of Parkinsonian speech have also found evidence of monotone production (Canter, 1963, Kent & Rosenbek, 1982).

Many consider speech disorders in PD a motor phenomenon. However, there is evidence that prosodic disturbances in PD may have an emotional dimension. Scott et al. (1984) found that PD patients had difficulty producing anger through prosody. Blonder et al. (1989) showed that PD patients' ability to convey different emotions through prosody was judged to be impaired, and the intensity of their emotional prosody was also rated as less expressive than that of normal controls. Möbes et al. (2008) compared phonation, repetition, and emotional prosodic expression in PD patients to probe the motor versus emotional nature of aprosodia. They found that patients performed comparably to normal controls in phonation and prosodic repetition, but had restrictions in fundamental frequency and intensity ranges when producing spontaneous emotional prosody. Taken together, these studies support the notion that the neuropathological changes associated with PD hinder patients' ability to express emotion through prosody. It is likely that dysfunction in mesocorticolimbic dopamine systems that regulate emotion play a role in Parkinsonian aprosodia.

Whether or not aprosodia in Parkinson's disease is emotional in nature or caused by rigidity and bradykinesia affecting the vocal apparatus, the impact is the same: the ability of these patients to express emotion nonverbally is compromised and this may result in mis-communication. Pentland et al. (1987) reported that Parkinson patients were perceived by observers as more anxious, hostile, suspicious, unhappy, bored, introverted, and tense than were normal controls. They were also perceived as less intelligent and less likeable than normal controls. More recently, Pell & Leonard (2005) found that naïve listeners had difficulty identifying the intended emotion in Parkinsonian prosody, and some utterances were characterized by naïve listeners as sad or devoid of emotion. These studies suggest that non-verbal communicative deficits in Parkinson's disease may convey mood-incongruent or ambiguous signals, and thus have a negative impact on interpersonal relations.

Facial Expression

In addition to emotional aprosody, RHD stroke patients often suffer from loss of ability to produce emotional facial expressions–both spontaneously and volitionally. In an early study, Buck & Duffy (1980) videotaped patients' reactions to emotionally-evocative films and found that those with right hemisphere stroke or Parkinson's disease were significantly less expressive than left hemisphere stroke patients and normal volunteers. These results were confirmed in several studies by Borod and colleagues (see Borod, 2002 for a review) who also found reduced emotional facial expressivity following unilateral damage to the right hemisphere. Furthermore, recent research by Kazandjian et al. (2007) suggests that reductions in facial expressivity are associated with lesions in the right frontal lobes.

In contrast to studies showing reductions in facial expressivity in RHD stroke, Caltagirone et al. (1989) and Mammucari et al. (1988) used the Facial Affect Coding System (FACS; Ekman & Friesen 1978) and failed, in part, to support these findings. However, Mammucari et al. (1988) found that RHD patients did show reduced gaze aversion to an unpleasant movie, suggesting that they failed to process the negative emotions depicted.

Most studies of nonverbal expressivity in neurologic patients used laboratory-based experiments to examine the ability of patients to produce emotional expression. Blonder et al. (1993) examined the effects of unilateral stroke on emotional communication in the natural environment. We compared facial expressivity in RHD stroke patients, LHD stroke patients, and normal controls during videotaped semi-structured interviews with the patient and spouse in their home. Three research assistants rated 120 ten-second segments of videotape per patient on a seven-point expressivity scale. Raters were trained to a criterion reliability of 0.80 using segments of videotape not included in the analysis. Following attainment of this criterion, raters rated the study videotapes. We found that RHD patients showed reduced facial expressivity in comparison to both LHD and normal control subjects during spontaneous conversation. In particular, RHD patients smiled and laughed significantly less than LHD patients and normal controls. These findings were not a general feature of communicative incompetence in RHD patients as discourse production equaled that of normal controls. Reduced facial expressivity and smiling were not a manifestation of dysphoria, as these patients did not report depression.

More recently, Blonder et al (2005) compared spontaneous emotional facial and verbal expressivity in RHD and LHD stroke patients. Nine aprosodic RHD patients and 14 aphasic LHD patients participated in a videotaped interview within a larger treatment protocol. Two naïve raters viewed segments of videotape and rated facial expressivity. Verbal affect production was tabulated using Linguistic Inquiry and Word Count software (Pennebaker et al. 2001). Results indicated that RHD patients smiled and laughed significantly less than did LHD patients. In contrast, RHD patients produced a greater percentage of emotion words relative to total words than did LHD patients. These findings suggest that aprosodia and diminished emotional facial expressivity in RHD patients are not induced by an impaired ability to experience or express emotions verbally. Rather, they likely represent encoding abnormalities specific to nonverbal processing. This interpretation is not supported by the work of Montreys & Borod (1998) however, who found that RHD patients produced less intense facial expressions and reported less intense emotional experiences during storytelling than did LHD and healthy control participants.

Based on the findings of Blonder et al. (1993) and others, Langer, Pettigrew, & Blonder (1998) hypothesized that reduced facial expressivity might cause others to form negative impressions of RHD stroke patients. We asked naïve coders to rate the likeability of unilateral stroke patients in videotaped interviews. Results indicated that when liking judgments were based on facial expressions, RHD stroke patients were liked less than LHD patients and normal controls, suggesting that reduced facial expressivity associated with RHD may negatively impact patients' relationships with others.

In a subsequent study, we hypothesized that the nonverbal impairments typically associated with right hemisphere strokes and the verbal impairments typically associated with left hemisphere strokes would result in patients sending channel-inconsistent messages—in which the verbal and nonverbal elements are not matched in emotional valence (e.g., uttering positive words with a frown; Langer et al. 2000). Eleven RHD, ten LHD, and six normal control participants were videotaped while engaging in social interaction. Observers made judgments about the valence of the patients' (1) words (based on transcripts of the interactions); and (2) facial expressions (based on soundless videos of the interactions). Analysis of word-face difference scores confirmed our hypothesis: messages of RHD patients were judged more positive in verbal content than in facial expression; messages of LHD patients were judged more positive in facial expression than in verbal content, and messages of controls were judged as channel-consistent (similar in valence across facial and verbal channels).

Communication research that supports the nonverbal primacy hypothesisunderscores the significance of these findings. In particular, investigators have found that the message communicated by non-verbal signals is judged to have greater veracity than the message communicated verbally in the event of inconsistency (Hale & Stiff 1990). Channel-inconsistent messages are more difficult to interpret, and if individuals attribute greater significance to nonverbal signals when judging the true meaning of the message, then RHD patients with flat affect will be misunderstood.

In sum, most past work on emotional communication in RHD stroke patients indicates that these patients display loss of ability to express their feelings via facial behavior. These deficits tend to be associated with lesions in the right frontal regions and basal ganglia. Furthermore, loss of facial expressivity in these patients is associated with reduced likeability. Finally, their messages are inconsistent due to perceived differences in valence between verbal and non-verbal components. These impairments place the patients at risk for social isolation and may also affect family members struggling to interpret patients' messages.

In addition to this research showing loss of facial expressivity associated with focal lesions in the right hemisphere, clinicians have long observed that a core feature of idiopathic Parkinson's disease is the expressionless, hypomimic, or "masked" face. Several studies conducted over the last thirty years have used experimental methods to investigate this phenomenon. Buck & Duffy (1980) videotaped Parkinson patients, unilateral left and right hemisphere damaged stroke patients, and normal controls while each participant viewed a set of emotionally evocative slides. Raters then watched the videotapes and rated subjects' emotional expressivity on a seven point scale. Participants with either right hemisphere stroke or Parkinson's disease were rated as significantly less expressive than individuals with left hemisphere stroke or no history of neurologic disease. Scott et al. (1984) found specific deficits in Parkinson patients' ability to produce facial expressions of anger. Katsikitis & Pilowski (1988, 1991) used a microcomputer program to quantify facial expressions of Parkinson patients who had observed a series of amusing slides. They found that patients smiled less frequently than controls did.

Historically, neurologists have distinguished between disorders of volitional facial expression that result from lesions to the motor strip or corticobulbar projections, and those of spontaneous facial expression that result from subcortical lesions, particularly involving the basal ganglia. Although Parkinson patients do not have facial paralysis for volitional movement, there is some controversy as to whether reductions in facial expressivity are limited to spontaneous displays or also involve voluntary or posed expressions of emotion (Borod et al., 1990; Bowers et al., 2006; Jacobs et al., 1995; see Rinn 1984, 2007). Thus it has been observed that PD patients are able to make facial expressions to command, but that resting, spontaneous facial expression tends to be "flat" (Rinn, 1984). Additional studies have found diminished emotional facial expressivity during posed conditions, suggesting that both systems are affected by PD (Borod et al. 1990, Jacobs et al., 1995).

Smith et al. (1996) used the Facial Action Coding system developed by Ekman & Friesen (1978) to analyze both spontaneous and posed facial expressions. They found that Parkinson patients displayed less emotional reactivity to emotionally laden film clips than the normal control group. Furthermore, in those with moderate Parkinson's disease, the intensity of spontaneous smiles was less than the intensity of posed smiles, and the Parkinson group produced fewer true or "felt" smiles than the controls did during the spontaneous condition. These results corroborate those of Pitcairn and collaborators (1990) who found that PD patients produced fewer true or "felt" smiles than the controls during the spontaneous condition. Loss of facial expressivity in PD does not appear to be associated with diminished capacity to experience emotion: Smith et al. (1996) found that patient ratings of subjective emotion experienced in response to the videoclips were comparable, if not more intense, than ratings by controls. The investigators concluded that spontaneous facial expression appears to be selectively affected in Parkinson's disease, whereas posed expression and the ability to experience emotion remain relatively intact. In contrast to these results, Bowers et al. (2006) undertook computerized analysis of facial expressions in Parkinson patients and controls. They found that the patients had reduced facial movement and were significantly slowed in reaching a peak expression during posed conditions. Taken together, these results suggest that Parkinson's disease affects spontaneous expressions and may also affect expressions that are posed.

An unresolved issue in the Parkinson literature is whether loss of facial expressivity is linked to emotional dysfunction (e.g., depression, apathy, or anhedonia) or whether it is but another manifestation of bradykinesia. In the study by Smith et al. (1996) cited above, Parkinson patients with reduced facial expressivity performed normally in ratings of felt emotion. Furthermore, loss of facial expressivity is more prevalent among Parkinson patients than is dysphoria, suggesting that the two disorders may share only partially overlapping brain regions (Rinn, 1984). In two studies of spontaneous facial expressions, investigators failed to find a correlation between depression scores and facial expressivity scores, suggesting that diminished facial expressivity is not necessarily reflective of depressed mood or linked to affective state (Katsikitis & Pilowsky, 1991; Smith et. al., 1996). Alternatively, the masked facies of Parkinson's disease might be related to apathy and frontal lobe dysfunction, both known concomitants of the illness (Isella et al,. 2002; Pluck & Brown, 2002; Starkstein et al., 1992; Zgaljardic et al., 2007). In a recent study of awareness of blunted affect, Mikos et al. (2009) found that PD participants are aware of reduced expressivity, yet report experiencing emotions as intensely as healthy controls.

Pentland et al. (1987) conducted a study of the impact of flattened affect in PD on observers' judgments of these patients. They videotaped PD patients and control patients with ischemic heart disease while they participated in a semi-structured interview. Observers (physiotherapists and occupational therapists) watched silent videorecordings of the interviews and then made judgments about the mood, personality, and intellect of the patients; they also made a judgment about how much they liked the patients. Patients also completed a battery of psychological tests. Both groups showed no abnormalities with respect to affect, personality, and intelligence on these tests; however, the Parkinsonian patients were perceived by the observers as more anxious, hostile, suspicious, unhappy, bored, introverted, and tense than the normal controls. They were also perceived as less intelligent, and were less liked than the normal controls. What this study tells us is that informed perceivers, including physiotherapists and occupational therapists who one might expect to be empathetic toward the patients, in fact formed negative impressions of them.

Facial Affect Processing and Mirror Circuitry

Experimental studies in normal volunteers have identified a phenomenon termed "primitive contagion" or the "chameleon effect," in which humans tend to mimic or synchronize gestures or facial expressions with those of another person (Hatfield et al. 1994, Chartrand & Bargh 1999). This "mirroring" of emotional behavior has been shown to facilitate interpersonal communication and is associated with increased empathy (Chartrand & Bargh 1999). Furthermore, research has demonstrated that when exposed to photographs of emotional faces, individuals respond with distinct facial electromyographic reactions (EMG; Lundqvist 1995, Dimberg et al. 2000). There is evidence that this EMG reactivity pattern is mediated by the right hemisphere (Dimberg & Petterson 2000). Studies by Adelmann & Zajonc (1989) and Levenson et al. (1990) have shown that producing an emotional facial expression through volitional contraction of facial muscles induces the emotional state normally associated with that expression.

More recently, functional neuroimaging studies have identified an action representation system in the human brain that appears to be homologous to a network of "mirror" neurons in the brains of macaque monkeys (Iacoboni et al 1999). This network includes the inferior frontal gyrus, the superior temporal sulcus, and the posterior parietal lobe. In a functional magnetic resonance imaging (fMRI) study in humans, Carr et al. (2003) found activation in these regions plus the premotor face area, the insula, and the amygdala during passive viewing of emotional facial expressions and, to a greater extent, during facial imitation (Carr et al. 2003). These findings lead Carr et al. (2003) to conclude that "action representation mediates the recognition of emotion in others even during simple observation." Subsequently, Leslie et al. (2004) found that passive viewing of emotional faces produced activation in the right ventral premotor area, suggesting a special role for the right hemisphere in unconscious facial mimicry. Furthermore, many imaging studies have implicated mirror neuron regions such as the inferior frontal gyrus, superior temporal sulcus, and/or amygdala in the processing of emotional facial expressions (Baird et al. 1999, Breiter et al. 1996, Glascher et al. 2004, Kesler-West et al. 2001, Phillips et al. 1997, Sato et al. 2004, Sprengelmeyer et al. 1998, Whalen et al. 1998, Williams et al. 2005). Finally, Shamay-Tsoory et al. (2003) conducted lesion analysis examining the neural substrates of empathy and associated functions and found that individuals with right posterior cortical pathology were impaired in empathy and facial affect recognition. Taken together, these studies suggest that facial affect recognition, facial mimicry, and empathy are interdependent functions that share overlapping neural substrates, predominantly located in right hemisphere mirror neuron circuits. This research also provides a mechanism linking disorders of facial affect recognition and expression. If the decoding of affective facial expressions by neurologically intact individuals induces mimicry and empathy that are expressed facially, then damage to mirror circuits by infarcts could explain co-morbid disorders of affective facial expression and recognition. There is considerable evidence in the neurology literature that deficits in the production and recognition of emotional facial expressions reliably co-occur (see Brozgold et al. 1998, Heilman et al. 2003).

Verbal Emotional Expression

Some investigators have found impairments in verbal emotional expression in the speech of RHD patients. For example, Bloom et al. (1990) found that RHD patients were judged to produce words of lower emotional intensity in response to emotionally-laden slides than LHD patients and normal volunteers. In a second study, Bloom et al. (1992) showed that RHD patients produced fewer emotional content elements than visual-spatial or neutral content elements on a picture story task. Cimino et al. (1991) found that RHD patients produced autobiographical memories that were judged as less emotional than those of normal volunteers.

Borod et al. (1996) had raters judge emotionality in monologues produced by RHD, LHD, and normal volunteers. RHD patients' monologues were rated as significantly less emotional than the monologues of normal controls. There was also a trend for RHD patients' monologues to be rated as less emotional than LHD patients. This research suggests that the reductions in affective expression associated with RHD span multiple communicative channels. Montreys & Borod (1998) videotaped unilateral stroke patients and normal controls while recollecting emotional and non-emotional experiences. They found that RHD patients reported less intense emotional experiences than LHD patients and normal volunteers.

Several studies conducted in our laboratory, however, do not support these findings and suggest that disorders of affective communication are specific to non-verbal representations of emotion (Blonder et al. 1991, 2004, Langer et al. 2000, Blonder et al. 2005). For example, in a study of spontaneous expression during videotaped interviews, Langer et al. (2000) showed that the messages of RHD patients were judged to be channel inconsistent; i.e., more positive in verbal content than in facial expression. LHD patients' messages showed the opposite pattern. These results reveal a discrepancy in the emotional content of the verbal versus nonverbal message. As such, they lend support to the hypothesis that affective impairments following RHD may reflect specific disruption of the ability to encode and communicate feelings via non-verbal channels. More recently, we found that RHD stroke patients with aprosodia also had significant reductions in facial expressivity, particularly smiling and laughing, when compared with left hemisphere damaged aphasic stroke patients (Blonder et al. 2005). In contrast, these RHD stroke patients produced a significantly larger proportion of positive and negative emotion words during the interviews than LHD aphasics. These results suggest that RHD disrupts patients' ability to encode or communicate emotions via non-verbal signals but that verbal communication of emotion remains functional. Furthermore, this conclusion is consistent with prior findings that the right hemisphere may house a non-verbal affect lexicon, i.e., an internal representation of non-verbal communicative signals coupled with information regarding the emotional significance of these displays (see Blonder et al. 1991, Bowers et al. 1993). In past research, Blonder et al. (1991) showed that RHD patients lacked the ability to infer the emotion communicated by verbal descriptions of non-verbal expressions (e.g., "he smiled"), but had no difficulty correctly interpreting the emotional message of verbal descriptions of evocative events (e.g. "children tracked dirt over your new white carpet").

In sum, the clinical literature on neural representations of affective communication shows that circuits in the right hemisphere specialize in facial affect expression. The basis for this conclusion largely derives from studies of impairments in patients with focal brain lesions, particularly stroke. Some of the discrepancies in the literature regarding verbal affect production deficits in RHD patients may be due to lack of adequate anatomic data and subsequent inclusion of patients who have undetected bilateral damage. Adolphs et al. (2000) found an association between naming the affect on the face and left frontal opercular damage. In particular, "silent" bilateral lesions could account for inconsistencies in the literature regarding the extent to which right hemisphere networks control the verbal affect lexicon. For example, Rapcsak et al. (1989, 1993) reported two individuals who sustained selective deficits in naming facial emotion following lesions in the middle temporal gyrus of the right hemisphere. However, the two patients both had anomalous cerebral dominance.

There are several unresolved questions that emerge from this literature. First, what is the relationship between facial affect perceptual disorders and impairments in expression among RHD patients? Research by Adolphs et al. (2000) in which right somatosensory cortices were essential in processing affective facial expressions suggests a mechanism whereby perception and expression might be linked. If an individual's prior internal experience of affect and its manifestation on the face is critical feedback in interpreting facial expression, then this region might constitute a center of integration in decoding and encoding emotion on the face. Leventhal et al. (1990) established that voluntary facial activity matching particular emotional expressions produced significant levels of subjective experience of the associated emotion, and that autonomic distinctions among emotions exist both between negative and positive emotions and among negative emotions. If proprioceptive feedback is critical in judging the emotional expression displayed on the face of another, then blunted facial expressivity may contribute to difficulty interpreting facial affect. Similarly, if facial affect recognition disorders associated with stroke are due in part to damage to somatosensory cortices, then the loss of knowledge pairing facial configuration and emotional expression may also influence encoding abilities.

In conclusion, emotional expressivity is a fundamental aspect of human communication. Research on the fractionation and impairment of affective expression in patients with neurologic disease has revealed a considerable amount regarding the neural organization, function, and significance of this behavior. These studies have laid the foundation for fields such as "affective" or "social" neuroscience that tend to use functional neuroimaging rather than the lesion model to study the neural substrates of affective processing. However, as mentioned previously, current imaging modalities are not well suited to examine the neural substrates of expressive behavior, particularly as it occurs in the context of social interaction. Nor would such research reveal the extent of disability in neurologic patients who suffer from such disorders. Future efforts point to a paradigm shift in which the knowledge gained from this research further stimulates translational studies to develop therapeutic interventions that help patients with focal brain injury and neurodegenerative diseases improve communicative competence.

Acknowledgments

The author would like to acknowledge the support of NIMH/NINDS grant R01MH78228.

References

Adelmann, P. K., & Zajonc R. B. (1989). Facial efference and the experience of emotion. *Annual Review of Psychology 40*, 249–280.

Adolphs, R., H. Damasio, D. Tranel, G. Cooper, & A. R. Damasio. (2000). A role for somatosensory cortices in the visual recognition of emotion as revealed by three-dimensional lesion mapping. *Journal of Neuroscience 20*, 2683–2690.

Baird, A. A., S. A. Gruber, D. A. Fein, L. C. Maas, R. J. Steingard, P. F. Renshaw, B. M. Cohen, & D. A. Yurgelun-Todd. (1999). Functional magnetic resonance imaging of facial affect recognition in children and adolescents. *Journal of the American Academy of Child & Adolescent Psychiatry 38*, 195–199.

Blonder, L. X., Gur, R. E., & Gur, R. C. (1989). The effects of right and left hemiparkinsonism on prosody. *Brain and Language 36*, 193–207.

Blonder, L. X., D. Bowers, & K. M. Heilman. (1991). The role of the right hemisphere in emotional communication. *Brain 114*, 1115–1127.

Blonder, L. X., A. F. Burns, D. Bowers, R. W. Moore, & K. M. Heilman. (1993). Right hemisphere facial expressivity during natural conversation. *Brain and Cognition 21*, 44–56.

Blonder, L. X., K. M. Heilman, T. U. Ketterson, J. C. Rosenbek, B. Crosson, S. Raymer, L. Maher, R. Glueckauf, & L. G. Rothi. (2005). Affective facial and lexical expression in aprosodic versus aphasic stroke patients. *Journal of the International Neuropsychological Society 11*, 677–685.

Blonder, L.X., Pickering, J.E., Heath, R.L, Smith, C., & Butler, S. (1995). Prosodic characteristics of speech before and after right hemisphere stroke. *Brain and Language 51*, 318–335.

Bloom, R.L., Borod, J.C., Obler, L.K., & Koff, E. (1990). A preliminary characterization of lexical emotional expression in right and left brain-damaged patients. *International Journal of Neuroscience 55*, 71–80.

Bloom, R., Borod, J. C., Obler, L., & Gerstman, L. (1992). Impact of emotional content on discourse production in patients with unilateral brain damage. *Brain and Language 42*, 153–164.

Borod, J. C., E. Koff, M. P. Lorch, & M. Nicholas. (1986). Channels of emotional expression in patients with unilateral brain damage. *Archives of Neurology 42*, 345–348.

Borod, J. C., E. Koff, M. P. Lorch, & M. Nicholas. (1986). Expression and perception of facial emotion in brain-damaged patients. *Neuropsychologia 24*, 169–180.

Borod, J.C., Rorie, K.D., Haywood, C.S,, Andelman, F., Obler, L.K., Welkowitz, J., Bloom, R.L., & Tweedy, J.R.. (1996). Hemispheric specialization for discourse reports of emotional experiences: relationships to demographic, neurological, and perceptual variables. *Neuropsychologia, 34*:351–359.

Borod, J.C., Welkowitz, Alpert, M., Brozgold, A.C., Martin, C., Peselow, E.& Diller, L. (1990). Parameters of emotional processing in neuropsychiatric disorders: Conceptual issues and a battery of tests. *Journal of Communication Disorders 23*, 247–271.

Borod, J. C., Bloom, R. L. Brickman, A. M. Nakhutina, L. & Curko, E. A. (2002). Emotional processing deficits in individuals with unilateral brain damage. *Applied Neuropsychology 9*, 23–36.

Bowers, D., Miller, K., Bosch, W., Gokcay, D., Pedraza, & O. Springer, U. et al. (2006). Faces of emotion in Parkinson's disease: micro-expressivity and bradykinesia during voluntary facial expressions. *Journal of the International Neuropsychological Society 12*, 765–773.

Bowers, D., Bauer, R. M., & Heilman, K. M. (1993). The nonverbal affect lexicon: Theoretical perspectives from neuropsychological studies of affect perception. *Neuropsychology 7*, 433–444.

Bradvik, B., Dravins, C., Holtas, S., Rosen, I., Ryding, E., & Ingvar, D. H. (1991). Disturbances of speech prosody following right hemisphere infarcts. *Acta Neurologica Scandinavica, 54*, 114–126.

Breiter, H. C., N. L. Etcoff, P. J. Whalen, W. A. Kennedy, S. L. Rauch, R. L. Buckner, M. M. Strauss, S. E. Hyman, & B. R. Rosen. (1996). Response and habituation of the human amygdala during visual processing of facial expression. *Neuron 17*, 875–887.

Brozgold, A.Z., Borod, J.C., Martin. C.C., Pick, L.H., Alpert, M., & Welkowitz, J. (1998). Social functioning and facial emotional expression in neurological and psychiatric disorders. *Applied Neuropsychology 5*, 15–23.

Buck, R., Duffy, R. J. (1980). Nonverbal communication of affect in brain-damaged patients. *Cortex 16*, 351–362.

Caltagirone, C., Ekman, P., Friesen, W., Gainotti, G., Mammucari, A., Pizzamiglio, L., & Zoccolatti, P. (1989). Posed emotional facial expressions in brain damaged patients. *Cortex 25*, 653–663.

Cancelliere, A.E., & Kertesz, A. (1990). Lesion localization in acquired deficits of emotional expression and comprehension. *Brain and Cognition 13*, 133–147.

Canter, G. 1963. Speech characteristics of patients with Parkinson's disease. I. Intensity, pitch, and duration. *Journal of Speech and Hearing Disorders 28*, 221–229.

Carr, L., Iacoboni, M. Dubeau, M. C. Mazziotta, J. C., & Lenzi, G. L. 2003. Neural mechanisms of empathy in humans: a relay from neural systems for imitation to limbic areas. *Proceedings of the National Academy of Sciences of the United States of America 100*, 5497–5502.

Chartrand, T. L., & Bargh, J. A. 1999. The chameleon effect: the perception-behavior link and social interaction. *Journal of Personality and Social Psychology 76*, 893–910.

Cimino CR, Verfaellie M, Bowers D, Heilman KM. 1991. Autobiographical memory: Influence of right hemisphere damage on emotionality and specificity. Brain and Language 15: 106–118.

Cooper, W., Soares, C., Nicol, J., Michelow, D., & Goloskie, S. 1984 Clausal intonation after unilateral brain damage. *Language and Speech 27*, 17–24.

Darley F. L., Aronson A. E., & Brown J. R. 1969. Clusters of deviant speech dimensions in the dysarthrias. *J of Speech and Hearing Research 12*, 462–96.

Dimberg, U., & Petterson, M. 2000. Facial reactions to happy and angry facial expressions: evidence for right hemisphere dominance. *Psychophysiology 37*, 693–696.

Dimberg, U., Thunberg, M. & Elmehed, K. 2000. Unconscious facial reactions to emotional facial expressions. *Psychological Science 11*, 86–89.

Ekman, P., & Friesen, W. V. (1978). *Facial Action Coding System*. Palo Alto, CA: Consulting Psychologists Press.

Glascher J, Tuscher O, Weiler C, Buchel C. Eleveated responses to constant facial emotions in different faces in the human amygdala: an fMRI study of facial identify and expression. BMC Neuroscience 2004 5: 45–54

Hale, J., Stiff, J.B. (1990). Non-verbal primacy in veracity judgments. *Southern Speech Communication Journal 55*, 206–229.

Hatfield, E., Cacioppo, J. T. & Rapson, R. L. (1994). *Emotional contagion*. Cambridge University Press, Cambridge.

Heilman, K.M., Blonder, L.X., Bowers, D. & Valenstein, E. (2003). Emotional Disorders Associated with Neurological Diseases. In K.M. Heilman and E. Valenstein (Eds.), *Clinical Neuropsychology*, Fourth Edition (pp. 447–478). Oxford, UK: Oxford University Press.

Heilman, K.M., Leon, S.A., & Rosenbek, J.C. (2004). Affective aprosodia from a medial frontal stroke. *Brain and Language 89*, 411–416.

Heller, W., Nitschke, J.B., Miller, G.A. (1998). Lateralization in Emotion and Emotional Disorders. Current Directions in Psychological Science. Vol. 7, No. 1, In M. T. Banich and W. Heller *Evolving Perspectives on Lateralization of Function*, (pp. 26–32). Published by Sage on behalf of Association for Psychological Science.

Iacoboni, M., Woods, R. P. Brass, M. Bekkering, H. Mazziotta, J. C. & Rizzolatti, G. (1999). Cortical mechanisms of human imitation. *Science 286*, 2526–2528.

Isella, V., Melzi, P., Grimaldi, M., Iurlaro, S., Piolti, R., Ferrarese, C., & Appollonio, I. (2002). Clinical, neuropsychological, and morphometric correlates of apathy in Parkinson's disease. *Movement Disorders 17*, 366–371.

Jacobs, D.H., Shuren, J., Bowers, D. & Heilman, K.M. 1995. Emotional facial imagery, perception, and expression in Parkinson's disease. *Neurology 45*, 1696–1702.

Katsikitis, M. & Pilowski, I. (1988). A study of facial expression in Parkinson's disease using a novel microcomputer-based method. *Journal of Neurology, Neurosurgery, & Psychiatry 51*, 362–366.

Katsikitis, M. & Pilowsky, I. 1991. A controlled quantitative study of facial expression in Parkinson's disease and depression. *Journal of Nervous and Mental Disease 179*, 683–688.

Kazandjian, S., Borod, J.C., & Brickman, A.M. (2007). Facial expression during emotional monologues in unilateral stroke: an analysis of monologue segments. *Applied Neuropsychology 14*, 235–246.

Kent, R. & Rosenbek, J.C. (1982). Prosodic disturbance and neurologic lesion. *Brain and Language 15*, 259–291.

Kesler-West, M. L., Andersen, A. H. Smith, C. D. Avison, M. J. Davis, C. E. Kryscio, R. J. & Blonder, L. X. 2001. Neural substrates of facial emotion processing using fMRI. *Cognitive Brain Research 11*, 213–226.

Langer, S. L., Pettigrew, L. C. & Blonder, L. X. (1998). Observer liking of unilateral stroke patients. *Neuropsychiatry, Neuropsychology, and Behavioral Neurology 11*, 218–224.

Langer, S. L., Pettigrew, L. C., Wilson, J. F & Blonder, L. X. (2000). Channel-consistency following unilateral stroke: An examination of patient communication across verbal and non-verbal domains. *Neuropsychologia 38*, 337–344.

Leon, S.A., Rosenbek, J.C., Crucian, G.P., Hieber, B., Holiway, B., Rodriguez, A.D., Ketterson, T.U., Ciampitti, M.Z., Freshwater, S., Heilman, K., & Gonzalez-Rothi, L. (2005). Active treatments for aprosodia secondary to right hemisphere stroke. *Journal of Rehabilitation Research and Development 42*, 93–101.

Leslie, K., Johnson-Frey, S. & Grafton, S. 2004. Functional imaging of face and hand imitation: towards a motor theory of empathy. *Neuroimage 21*, 601–607.

Levenson, R. W., Ekman, P., & Friesen, W. V. (1990). Voluntary facial action generates emotion-specific autonomic nervous system activity. *Psychophysiology 27*, 363–384.

Lundqvist, L. O. (1995). Facial EMG reactions to facial expressions: a case of facial emotional contagion? *Scandinavian Journal of Psychology 36*, 130–141.

Mammucari, A., Caltagirone, C., Ekman, P., Friesen, W., Gainotti, G., Pizzamiglio, L., & Zoccolatti, P. (1988). Spontaneous facial expression of emotions in brain damaged patients. *Cortex 24*, 521–533.

Mikos, A.E., Springer, U.S., Nisenzon, A.N., Kellison, I.L., Fernandez, H.H., Okun M.S., & Bowers, D. (2009). Awareness of expressivity deficits in non-demented Parkinson disease. *Clinical Neuropsychology 23*, 805–817.

Möbes, J. , Joppich, G., Stiebritz, F., Dengler, R., & Schröder, C. (2008). Emotional speech in Parkinson's disease. *Movement Disorder 23*, 824–829.

Montreys, C.R. & Borod, J.C. (1998). A preliminary evaluation of emotional experience and expression following unilateral brain damage. *International Journal of Neuroscience 96*, 269–283.

Pell, M. D., & Leonard, C. L. (2005). Facial expression decoding in early Parkinson's disease. *Cognitive Brain Research 23,* 327–340.

Pennebaker, J.W., Francis, M.E., & Booth, R.J. (2001). *Linguistic inquiry and word count software program.* Austin, TX: e LIWC.net.

Pentland, B., Pitcairn, T. K., Gray, J. M. & Riddle, W.J.R. (1987). The effects of reduced expression in Parkinson's disease on impression formation by health professionals. *Clinical Rehabilition 1,* 207–313.

Phillips, M. L., Young, A. W., Senior, C., Brammer, M., Andrew, C., Calder, A. J., Bullmore, E. T., Perrett, D. I., Rowland, D., Williams, S. C., Gray, J. A., & David, A. S. (1997). A specific neural substrate for perceiving facial expressions of disgust. *Nature 389,* 495–508.

Pitcairn, T.K., Clemie, S., Gray, J.M., & Pentland, B. (1990). Non-verbal cues in the self-presentation of Parkinsonian patients. *British Journal of Clinical Psychology, 29,* 177–184.

Pluck, G. C. & Brown, R. G. (2002). Apathy in Parkinson's disease. *Journal of Neurology, Neurosurgery,& Psychiatry 73,* 636–642.

Rapscak, S., Kasniak, A., & Rubins, A. (1989). Anomia for facial expressions: evidence for a category specific visual verbal disconnection. *Neuropsychologia 27,* 1031–1041.

Rapcsak, S. Z., Comer, J. F., & Rubens A. B. (1993). Anomia for facial expressions. neuropsychological mechanisms and anatomical correlates. *Brain and Language 45,* 233–252. 184.

Rinn, W.E. (1984). The neuropsychology of facial expression: a review of the neurological and psychological mechanisms for producing facial expressions. *Psychological Bulletin 95,* 52–77.

Rinn, W. E. (2007). Emotional facial expression in Parkinson's disease: a response to Bowers. *Journal of the International Neuropsychological Society 13,* 721–722.

Rosenbek, J.C., Crucian, G.P., Leon, S.A., Hieber, B., Rodriguez, A.D., Holiway, B., Ketterson, T.U., Ciampitti, M., Heilman, K., & Gonzalez-Rothi, L. (2004). Novel treatments for expressive aprosodia: a phase I investigation of cognitive linguistic and imitative interventions. *Journal of the International Neuropsychological Society 10,* 786–793.

Rosenbek, J.C., Rodriguez, A.D., Hieber, B., Leon, S.A., Crucian, G.P., Ketterson, T.U., Ciampitti, M., Singletary, F., Heilman, K.M., & Gonzalez Rothi, L.J. (2006). Effects of two treatments for aprosodia secondary to acquired brain injury. *Journal of Rehabilitation Research and Development 43,* 379–390.

Ross, E. D. (1981). The aprosodias. Functional-anatomic organization of the affective components of language in the right hemisphere. *Archives of Neurology 38,* 561–569.

Ross, E.D., Edmondson, J.A., Seibert, G.B., & Homan, R.W. (1988) Acoustic analysis of affective prosody during right-sided Wada test: a within-subjects verification of the right hemisphere's role in language. *Brain and Language 33,* 128–145.

Ross, E.D., and Mesulam, M.M. (1979). Dominant language functions of the right hemisphere? Prosody and emotional gesturing. *Archives of Neurology 36,* 144–148.

Ross, E.D., Monnot, M. (2008). Neurology of affective prosody and its functional-anatomic organization in right hemisphere. *Brain and Language 104,* 51–74.

Ross, E.D., Thompson, R.D., Yenkosky, J. (1997). Lateralization of affective prosody in brain and the callosal integration of hemispheric language functions. *Brain and Language 56,* 27–54.

Ryalls, J., Joanette, Y., & Feldman, L. (1987). An acoustic comparison of normal and right hemisphere damaged speech prosody. *Cortex 23,*:685–694.

Sato, W., Kochiyama, T. Yoshikawa, S. Naito, E., & Matsumura, M. (2004). Enhanced neural activity in response to dynamic facial expressions of emotion: an fMRI study. *Cognitive Brain Research 20,* 81–91.

Scott, S., Caird, F. I., & Williams, B. O. (1984). Evidence for an apparent sensory speech disorder in Parkinson's disease. *Journal of Neurology, Neurosurgery, & Psychiatry 47,* 840–843.

Shamay-Tsoory, S.G., Tomer, R. Berger, B.D. & Aharon-Peretz, J. (2003). Characterization of empathy deficits following prefrontal brain damage: the role of the right ventromedial prefrontal cortex. *Journal of Cognitive Neuroscience 15,* 324–37.

Shapiro, B., & Danly, M. (1985). The role of the right hemisphere in the control of speech prosody in prepositional and affective contexts. *Brain and Language 25*, 19–26.
Smith, M.C., Smith, M.K., & Ellgring, H. (1996). Spontaneous and posed facial expression in Parkinson's disease. *Journal of the International Neuropsychological Society 2*, 383–391.
Sprengelmeyer, R., Rausch, M. Eysel, U. T. & Przuntek, H. (1998). Neural structures associated with recognition of facial expressions of basic emotions. *Proceedings of the Royal Society B: Biological Sciences 265*, 1927–1931.
Starkstein, S. E., Mayberg, H. S., Preziosi, T. J., Andrezejewsk, P., Leuguarda, R. & Robinson, R. G. (1992). Reliability, validity, and clinical correlates of apathy in Parkinson's disease. *Journal of Neuropsychiatry & Clinical Neuroscience 4*, 134–139.
Whalen, P. J., Rauch, S. L. Etcoff, N. L McInerney, S. C. Lee, M. B., & Jenike, M. A. (1998). Masked presentations of emotional facial expressions modulate amygdala activity without explicit knowledge. *Journal of Neuroscience 18*, 411–418.
Williams, M. A., McGlone, F. Abbott, D. F., & Mattingley, J. B. (2005). Differential amygdala responses to happy and fearful facial expressions depend on selective attention. *Neuroimage 2*, 417–425.
Zgaljardic, D. J., Borod, J. C., Foldi, N. S., Rocco, M., Mattis, P. J., Gordon, M. F., et al. (2007). Relationship between self-reported apathy and executive dysfunction in nondemented patients with Parkinson disease. *Cognitive Behavioral Neurology 20*, 184–192.

CHAPTER 13

Behavioral and Cognitive Effects of Antiepileptic Drugs

Kimford J. Meador

Case Descriptions

Three cases will be presented followed by a discussion of the literature and descriptions of management for these cases.

Case 1. A 22 year old man has suffered a generalized convulsion. His roommate recalls that on two recent occasions, the patient had episodes of unresponsive staring, sometimes with lip smacking movements. Neurological exam is normal. MRI demonstrates a few small subcortical hyperdensities. EEG reveals intermittent slowing and sharp waves in the right anterior temporal lobe. History includes an automobile accident with severe closed head injury at 17 years old associated with coma for five days. The patient recovered except for an acquired attentional problem, requiring methylphenidate to maintain school performance. A diagnosis of focal epilepsy is made, and antiepileptic drug (AED) therapy is recommended. The patient is concerned about possible cognitive effects of AEDs. What should be included in the discussion of options and risks?

Case 2. A 68 year-old man has had repeated episodes of brief time lapses, which began five months ago and have been increasing. His wife noted that he is unresponsive during these episodes. Previously, he has had three MRIs and three EEGs, all of which were normal. Past medical history is significant for resection of esophageal cancer three years ago followed by radiation and chemotherapy. He has had no recurrence of the cancer, and is otherwise healthy except for well controlled hypertension. In the review of systems, his wife notes that his personally has been different ever since the diagnosis of cancer; she states that he is pessimistic when before he was always optimistic. He does not meet diagnosis of major depression, but has dysphoria. What actions should be recommended, and what options and risks should be included in the informed consent process?

Case 3. A 19-year-old woman has suffered two generalized convulsions in the last month without any obvious precipitants or known risk factors. On questioning, she admits to occasional jerks of her arms in the early morning on first awakening. Neurological examination and MRI are normal. EEG reveals generalized spike wave discharges with frontal predominance. A diagnosis of juvenile myoclonic epilepsy is made. Should AED risks to a possible child in a future pregnancy be discussed at this time and should such risks affect recommendations for choice of AED? If so, what are the known cognitive and behavioral risks for a child exposed *in utero* to AEDs?

Cognitive Deficits in Patients with Epilepsy

A variety of factors can affect cognition in epilepsy patients, including: 1) etiology of epilepsy; 2) cerebral lesions acquired prior to onset of epilepsy; 3) type of seizures; 4) age at seizure onset; 5) seizure frequency; 6) duration and severity of seizures; 7) transient dysfunction from interictal discharges, seizures or postictal effects; 8) structural brain damage from seizures; 9) genetic factors; 10) psychosocial issues; 11) epilepsy surgery; and 12) antiepileptic drugs (AEDs) (Meador, 2009). Cognition is impaired at epilepsy onset (Hermann, et al., 2006; Smith, Craft, Collins, Mattson, & Cramer, 1986) consistent with the etiology of seizures acting as a major factor on cognition (Meador, 2009). The incidence of epilepsy is increased in patients with mental retardation, progressive cerebral degeneration, or focal brain lesions (Dodrill, 1992). Patients with idiopathic epilepsy are more likely to have normal intelligence. Epilepsy is more likely to be refractory in certain conditions (e.g., mental retardation). Patients with multiple generalized convulsions are more likely to have cognitive impairments compared to those with absence seizures or focal seizures without loss of awareness. Earlier age of seizure onset is associated with increased risk of cognitive impairment.

Seizure frequency, duration, and severity can impact cognition (Dikmen & Matthews, 1977). Seizures may alter consciousness, and interictal epileptiform discharges can impair cognition (Shewmon & Erwin, 1988). Todd's paralysis lasts less than 24 hours, but postictal cognitive dysfunction may last several days, including confusion, dysphasia, and impaired memory consolidation (Jokeit, Daamen, Zang, Janszky, & Ebner, 2001). Chronic dysfunction can extend beyond the area of seizure focus. Interictal hypometabolism extends to the lateral temporal cortex in patients with mesial temporal epilepsy (Henry & Votaw, 2004). Repetitive or prolonged seizures may damage the brain via anoxia, lactic acidosis, or excessive excitatory neurotransmitters. Temporal lobe seizures over several decades can cause hippocampal atrophy and reduce cognitive abilities (Helmstaedter, 2002). Memory is impaired in patients with epilepsy, and it is remarkable that the molecular mechanisms of animal models for epilepsy (i.e., kindling) and memory formation (i.e., long term potentiation) are similar (Meador, 2007).

Factors unrelated or indirectly related to epilepsy contribute to cognition. In population studies, maternal intelligence is the most predictive of a child's intelligence (Sattler, 1992). Psychosocial variables such as depression or other environmental factors can affect cognition.

Treatments for seizures may impact cognition. Epilepsy surgery may improve cognition or result in deficits. The remainder of the chapter will focus on the cognitive and behavioral effects of antiepileptic drugs.

Antiepileptic Drugs

AEDs are the major therapeutic modality for seizures and are frequently used for other indications (e.g., pain and psychiatric disorders). Therefore, the behavioral and cognitive effects of AEDs including differences between AEDs and their effects relative to other clinical considerations are important. When AEDs are used within the standard therapeutic ranges, their adverse cognitive effects are generally modest, especially when these effects are modulated by reduced seizures (Meador, 2009). However, the effects may be clinically significant even under these conditions, as evidenced by the highly significant inverse correlation of neurotoxicity symptoms and quality of life, even in the absence of overt toxicity (Gilliam, Carter, & Vahle, 2004). Some AEDs reduce verbal paragraph memory by 15–20 percent (Motamedi & Meador, 2004) and withdrawal of some AEDs can produce an 11–28 percent improvement on neuropsychological tests (Lossius, et al., 2008). The risks of adverse cognitive effects are increased by with polypharmacy and with increasing AED dosages/blood levels, although the risks of polytherapy with newer AEDs are less clear. An individual patient may achieve the best seizure control with the fewest cognitive side effects using polytherapy. Both positive (e.g., mood stabilization) and negative (e.g., depression, irritability/agitation, psychosis) psychotropic effects have been observed for AEDs. Several AEDs are used routinely to treat psychiatric conditions (e.g., carbamazepine, lamotrigine, valproate).

Methodological Issues. Flaws in experimental design, analysis, and interpretation are common in investigations of AED cognitive effects, including subject selection bias, non-equivalence of clinical and of dependent variables, sample size, test–retest effects, neuropsychological tests employed, inappropriate statistics, type I and II errors, non-orthogonal contrasts, and comparison of studies with non-equivalent designs/statistics (Meador, 2009). Statistical findings have to be interpreted taking into account the magnitude of effects, overall risk-to-benefit ratio, and severity of seizure disorder. Although cognitive side effects are primarily monitored in the clinical setting by patient report, subjective perception of cognitive effects is related more to mood than objective performance (Marino, et al., 2009).

Older Antiepileptic Drugs. The greatest and most consistent adverse AED cognitive effects are observed with barbiturates and benzodiazepines (Meador, 2009). Double-blind, randomized, crossover, monotherapy design studies have demonstrated that carbamazepine, phenytoin, and valproate have similar adverse cognitive effects (Dodrill & Troupin, 1991; Meador, Loring, Huh, Gallagher, & King, 1990; Meador, et al., 1995; Prevey, et al., 1996). Other studies have also confirmed these findings (see Table 13.1). (Hessen, Lossius, & Gjerstad, 2009; Meador, et al., 1993; Meador, et al., 1991; Meador, et al., 1990; Meador, et al., 1995; Pulliainen & Jokelainen, 1994).

Newer Antiepileptic Drugs. Some newer AEDs have fewer cognitive side effects than older AEDs. Cognitive effects have not been formally assessed for all AEDs. Thus, the relative cognitive/behavioral effects of the newer AEDs are not fully determined, but pertinent data are described below.

Felbamate. In clinical trials, felbamate had few cognitive side effects, but it is reported anecdotally to be alerting, which can be beneficial or detrimental. No studies with formal cognitive assessments exist.

Gabapentin. Although gabapentin can produce some cognitive side effects, it has a favorable cognitive profile in epilepsy patients. Gabapentin has exhibited less cognitive side effects than carbamazepine (Meador, et al., 1999; Salinsky, et al., 2002). Gabapentin can produce improvements in perceived well-being in epilepsy patients (Dimond, Pande, Lamoreaux, & Pierce, 1996; Wolf, Shinnar, Kang, Gil, & Moshe, 1995), but it can also result in irritability and agitation in children (Wolf, et al., 1995).

Table 13.1 **Cognitive Effects of Older Antiepileptic Drugs**

% of Variables Significantly Different	*Antiepileptic Drugs*
4–10%*	carbamazepine = phenytoin = valproate
32%	phenobarbital worse than phenytoin & valproate
52–55%	older AEDs** worse than no drug

* percent of variables that differed across the three drugs; no consistent differential pattern present.

** carbamazepine, phenytoin, and valproate.

Lamotrigine. No cognitive effects with lamotrigine versus placebo were seen on a limited neuropsychological battery in epilepsy patients (62). Lamotrigine had fewer cognitive side effects compared to carbamazepine, diazepam, phenytoin, placebo, topiramate, and valproate in healthy adults (Aldenkamp, et al., 2002; Cohen, et al., 1985; Meador, et al., 2001; Meador, et al., 2005). In clinical trials, lamotrigine has been better tolerated than carbamazepine and phenytoin (Brodie, Overstall, & Giorgi, 1999; Steiner, et al., 1999). Lamotrigine has shown beneficial effects on perceived quality of life in epilepsy patients compared with placebo or carbamazepine (Brodie, Richens, & Yuen, 1995; Smith, Baker, Davies, Dewey, & Chadwick, 1993), and has positive psychotropic properties in bipolar disorder patients and epilepsy patients. In epilepsy patients, lamotrigine exhibits positive mood effects compared to levetiracetam (Labiner, et al., 2009).

Levetiracetam. The cognitive profile of levetiracetam is favorable in patients, but a few adult and pediatric patients can experience adverse behavioral side effects. Levitiracetam had less adverse cognitive effects than carbamazepine in a double-blind, randomized, healthy volunteer study (Meador, Gevins, et al., 2007).

Oxcarbazepine. Similar cognitive effects were seen for oxcarbazepine and phenytoin in an epilepsy patient study and a healthy volunteer study (Aikia, Kalviainen, Sivenius, Halonen, & Riekkinen, 1992; Salinsky, Spencer, Oken, & Storzbach, 2004).

Rufinamide. No statistically significant cognitive changes were found for rufinamide in a placebo-controlled study (Aldenkamp & Alpherts, 2006).

Tiagabine. No significant cognitive effects were reported in a randomized, double-blind, placebo-controlled study of epilepsy patients (Sveinbjornsdottir, et al., 1994).

Topiramate. Greater adverse cognitive side effects were seen for topiramate than gabapentin and lamotrigine in healthy volunteers (Salinsky, et al., 2005) (Meador, et al., 2005), and lamotrigine in epilepsy patients (Blum, et al., 2006). Two randomized patient studies comparing adjunctive topiramate to valproate reported worse effects for topiramate, but the effects were few after extended treatment (Aldenkamp, et al., 2000; Meador, Loring, Hulihan, Kamin, & Karim, 2003). Verbal fluency, attention, processing speed, and working memory are particularly vulnerable to topiramate. Irritability and psychosis have been reported with topiramate. The risk of cognitive effects from topiramate are increased by faster initial titration, higher dosage, and polytherapy, but some patients experience adverse effects even when these risk factors do not exist.

Vigabatrin. Vigabatrin produced few adverse effects on cognition or quality of life compared to placebo in epilepsy patients (Dodrill, Arnett, Sommerville, & Sussman, 1993, 1995). Drug-induced depression and psychosis have been reported (Ferrie, Robinson, & Panayiotopoulos, 1996).

Table 13.2 **Newer AEDs vs. Placebo**

% Variables Significantly Worse on Placebo	*Antiepileptic Drug*
0%	tiagabine
1–17%	lamotrigine
0–19%	gabapentin
11%	levetiracetam
46%	oxcarbazepine
29–88%	topiramate

Zonisamide. Although limited formal neuropsychological data are available for zonisamide, it impaired cognition in two studies of epilepsy patients (Berent, et al., 1987; Park, et al., 2008).

Tables 13.2 and 13.3 summarize the data presented above. Information on cognitive effects of other new AEDs is inadequate.

EFFECTS OF ANTIEPILEPTIC DRUGS AT AGE EXTREMES

Elderly. Although the elderly have increased risk of epilepsy and increased susceptibility to drug-induced cognitive effects for both pharmacokinetic and pharmacodynamic reasons, there are few studies examining AED cognitive effects in the elderly. Phenytoin and valproate had similar cognitive effects in elderly patients (Craig & Tallis, 1994). Reanalysis of the original VA Cooperative Study demonstrated that elderly patients were more likely to have cognitive side effects

Table 13.3 **Comparative Cognitive Effects of Newer AEDs**

% of Variables Significantly Different	*Antiepileptic Drugs*
26%	carbamazepine worse than gabapentin
48%	carbamazepine worse than lamotrigine
42%	carbamazepine worse than levetiracetam
0%	oxcarbazepine = phenytoin
50%	topiramate worse than gabapentin
80%	topiramate worse than lamotrigine

(Ramsay & Pryor, 2000). The recent VA Cooperative Study in elderly epilepsy patients showed that patients tolerated gabapentin and lamotrigine better than carbamazepine, and that intolerance to carbamazepine was mainly due to adverse side effects on the central nervous system (Rowan, et al., 2005).

Children. Even though adverse cognitive AED effects during neurodevelopment could pose a special risk, investigations in children are fewer than adults. The observed AED effects available for children are similar to the findings in adults. See Table 13.4. Studies of carbamazepine, oxcarbazepine, phenytoin, and valproate in children have demonstrated comparable cognitive effects (Aldenkamp, et al., 1993; Donati, et al., 2007; Forsythe, Butler, Berg, & McGuire, 1991; Forsythe & Sills, 1984; Tonnby, et al., 1994). Phenobarbital has greater adverse cognitive effects compared to valproate and carbamazepine in children with epilepsy (Chen, Chi Chow, & Lee, 2001; Chen, Kang, & So, 1996; Vining, et al., 1987) and compared to placebo in children with febrile seizures (Farwell, et al., 1990). Lamotrigine had no significant effects compared to placebo in children with epilepsy (Pressler, 2006). Carbamazepine had fewer effects than topiramate (Kang, et al., 2007). Additional studies are needed in children not only to define the cognitive effects, but also to define relative effectiveness across AEDs.

Neurodevelopmental Effects of *In Utero* AED Exposure

Neurodevelopmental of children whose mothers have epilepsy may be influenced by AEDs, type and severity of seizures during pregnancy, genetics, maternal age/parity, and socioeconomic status (Meador, 2009). Although data is incomplete, animal and human studies indicate that AEDs play a role.

Animal Studies. AED-induced behavioral teratogenesis (i.e., cognitive/behavioral deficits) has been observed in animals at dosages lower than those required

Table 13.4 **Antiepileptic Drug (AED) Cognition Studies in Children**

Relative AED Cognitive Effects
valproate less than phenobarbital
placebo less than phenobarbital
carbamazepine = phenytoin = valproate
carbamazepine = valproate; both less than phenobarbital
placebo = lamotrigine
carbamazepine = oxcarbazepine = valproate
carbamazepine less than topiramate.

to produce anatomical malformations (Finnell & Dansky, 1991). Prenatal exposure to phenobarbital or phenytoin can alter neurons and result in cognitive and behavioral abnormalities in animals. Similar to alcohol in the third trimester, exposure of the immature neonatal rat brain to clonazepam, diazepam, phenobarbital, phenytoin, vigabatrin, or valproate can result in widespread neuronal apoptosis (Bittigau, et al., 2002; Bittigau, Sifringer, & Ikonomidou, 2003; Stefovska, et al., 2008). This effect occurs at therapeutically relevant blood levels and is dose-dependent. The effect is associated with reduced expression of neurotrophins and levels of protein kinases that promote neuronal growth and survival. Similar apoptotic effects were not seen at therapeutic dosages for carbamazepine, lamotrigine, levetiracetam, or topiramate monotherapy (Glier, et al., 2004; Katz, Kim, Gale, & Kondratyev, 2007; Kim, Kondratyev, & Gale, 2007; Manthey, et al., 2005). However, synergistic effects can produce apoptosis in polytherapy. These observations raise serious concern that AEDs commonly used in women of childbearing potential and in neonate could cause adverse effects in exposed children. Future studies should investigate other AEDs in animals and determine if similar effects occur in humans.

Human Studies. Neurodevelopmental deficits are increased in children of women with epilepsy, but AED risks in humans are only partially delineated (Meador, 2009). Many studies have not been prospective with adequate assessment of confounding factors such as parental IQ and education, etiology of epilepsy, seizure type and frequency, AED dose/blood levels, maternal age/parity, socioeconomic status, and home environment. Formal cognitive assessments in children have not always been blinded to AED exposure.

A population-based study found developmental delay in 19 percent of children exposed *in utero* to AEDs versus 3 percent unexposed (Dean, et al., 2002). The risk of developmental delay is increased higher dose and numbers of AEDs, decreased maternal education, impaired maternal-child relationship, and maternal focal seizure disorder (Meador, 2009; Meador, Baker, Cohen, Gaily, & Westerveld, 2007). Men exposed prenatally to phenobarbital had significantly lower verbal IQ scores (about 7 points) in two retrospective studies from Denmark, and the effect was markedly increase by lower socioeconomic status and "unwanted" pregnancy (Reinisch, Sanders, Mortensen, & Rubin, 1995).

Children exposed *in utero* to valproate monotherapy had increased risk of developmental delay in a cohort less than 6 years old, and reduced verbal IQ (6–15 points) in a second cohort age 6–16 years compared to unexposed and those exposed to other AEDs in a retrospective UK study (Adab, et al., 2004). Verbal IQ was reduced (13–14 points) in children exposed *in utero* to valproate compared to unexposed and to carbamazepine-exposed children in a prospective Finnish study, but the valproate sample size was small and maternal IQ was not measured (Gaily, et al., 2004). These earlier findings were confirmed recently by a large prospective study controlling for multiple confounding factors including maternal

IQ (Meador, et al., 2009; 2013). Children exposed *in utero* to valproate exhibited a 6–9 IQ point reduction at age 3 years and 7–10 IQ point reduction at age 6 years compared to those exposed to carbamazepine, lamotrigine, or phenytoin. The valproate effect was dose dependent. A small study suggests that fetal exposure to levetiracetam has low risk for cognitive deficits (Shallcross, et al., 2011. The behavioral teratogenetic risks for other AEDs remain to be fully delineated.

Conclusions

Cognitive and behavioral effects of AEDs have to be assessed within the context of other factors, which may adversely affect brain function in patients with epilepsy. AED cognitive effects are increased with polypharmacy and with higher dosage/anticonvulsant blood levels. AED cognitive effects can be clinically significant since they can reduce the patient's quality of life. AEDs can impair psychomotor processing speed, sustained attention, memory, and dual processing. Special concern should be directed at patients dependent on these skills for work or school. Further, fetal exposure to some AEDs (e.g., valproate) may have long-lasting neurodevelopment consequences. Some AEDs have positive psychotropic effects (e.g., carbamazepine, lamotrigine, valproate), but these and other AEDs can also produce negative behavioral effects. For an individual patient, the goal is to achieve the best seizure control while producing the fewest side effects. Subjective perception of cognitive side effects may be altered by mood and by habituation of the subjective effects. Clinicians should be aware of the limitations of subjective reports and be alert to increased risk for cognitive side effects posed by specific AEDs and by the circumstances noted above. Further studies are needed to fully delineate the cognitive and behavioral effects for many AEDs.

Management of Cases (Described at Beginning of Chapter)

Case 1. The 22 year old college student with new onset temporal lobe epilepsy and a history of acquired attentional deficit disorder due to head trauma was concerned about possible AED cognitive effects. The informed consent process should include options and risks. Issues to address include AED effectiveness, systemic side effects (e.g., skin rash, osteoporosis), drug interactions, and central nervous system risks (e.g., sedation, slowed cognition, memory problems, depression). The student's concern is well justified as some AEDs can reduce memory acquisition and impact school performance, even in students without pre-existing cognitive problems. Thus, those AEDs with the lowest demonstrated adverse cognitive risks were considered (e.g., lamotrigine, levetiracetam). The patient was started on levetiracetam and titrated up to 500mg twice a day. He became seizure free and maintained good school performance.

Case 2. The 68-year-old man with episodes of loss of awareness was felt to have seizures due to focal epilepsy despite his normal MRIs, EEGs and neurological examinations. His epilepsy risk factors are age and hypertension. It is unlikely that there is any direct relationship to his prior esophageal cancer. A therapeutic AED trial was recommended to confirm the diagnosis and control the spells. Because of increased susceptibility of elderly to AED cognitive effects, those AEDs with the lowest demonstrated adverse cognitive risks were considered. Lamotrigine was recommended given his dysphoria and its positive psychotrophic effects. However, the patient chose phenytoin because he wanted a quick response, a less costly medicine, and was worried about the skin rash with lamotrigine. Once he started an AED, he never had another episode of loss of awareness, confirming his diagnosis. However, he suffered problems with attention and mental speed despite borderline low therapeutic levels of phenytoin and a month of therapy for habituation. He was switched to levetiracetam because he was still concerned about lamotrigine skin rash. Levetiracetam is frequently used in the elderly because of its favorable cognitive profile and lack of pharmacokinetic interactions, which is important in the elderly as they typically are taking multiple medications. Once he was converted to levetiracetam, his cognitive problems resolved, and he remained seizure free. However, his wife noted that he had been become extremely irritable, which is a known side effect in a minority of patients on levetiracetam. Next, he was slowly titrated onto lamotrigine and tapered off levetiracetam. His irritability resolved, and he remained seizure free without cognitive complains. Furthermore, his wife noted that his dysphoria resolved and his premorbid optimistic personality returned.

Case 3. The 19-year-old woman with new onset juvenile myoclonic epilepsy was started on AED therapy to prevent recurrent convulsions. For women of childbearing potential, the informed consent process should include additional issues such as potential AED effects on reproductive function and AED teratogenic effects. These teratogenic risks include not only malformations but also behavioral/cognitive risks to the unborn child. Discussion of teratogenic effects should be included even if there are no immediate plans for pregnancy since almost half of pregnancies are unplanned. Further, juvenile myoclonic epilepsy has a high recurrence rate when AEDs are withdrawn, so that the choice of AED in this case may be lifelong. Although valproate has the best efficacy for idiopathic generalized epilepsies, it has the highest risk for both malformations and reduced cognitive abilities. Further, there are other effective therapies that work for many women. Of the AEDs which are effective in primary generalized epilepsy, the AED with the lowest risks for the fetus based on current information is lamotrigine. Other alternatives might include levetiracetam, topiramate, and zonisamide.

Topiramate has an approximately 4.5 percent risk of major congenital malformations (especially cleft palate). Levetiracetam appears to have a low risk of malformations, and one small study suggests that it has low risk for cognitive deficits. Information on malformation risks for zonisamide is inadequate, and human data on the risks of impaired cognitive development from fetal exposure to topiramate or zonisamide do not exist. The decision was made with the patient to begin her on lamotrigine, and seizures were well controlled.

References

Adab, N., Kini, U., Vinten, J., Ayres, J., Baker, G., Clayton-Smith, J., et al. (2004). The longer term outcome of children born to mothers with epilepsy. *Journal of Neurology, Neurosurgery, & Psychiatry, 75*(11), 1575–1583.

Aikia, M., Kalviainen, R., Sivenius, J., Halonen, T., & Riekkinen, P. J. (1992). Cognitive effects of oxcarbazepine and phenytoin monotherapy in newly diagnosed epilepsy: one year follow-up. *Epilepsy Research, 11*(3), 199–203.

Aldenkamp, A. P., & Alpherts, W. C. (2006). The effect of the new antiepileptic drug rufinamide on cognitive functions. *Epilepsia, 47*(7), 1153–1159.

Aldenkamp, A. P., Alpherts, W. C., Blennow, G., Elmqvist, D., Heijbel, J., Nilsson, H. L., et al. (1993). Withdrawal of antiepileptic medication in children—effects on cognitive function: The Multicenter Holmfrid Study. *Neurology, 43*(1), 41–50.

Aldenkamp, A. P., Arends, J., Bootsma, H. P., Diepman, L., Hulsman, J., Lambrechts, D., et al. (2002). Randomized double-blind parallel-group study comparing cognitive effects of a low-dose lamotrigine with valproate and placebo in healthy volunteers. *Epilepsia, 43*(1), 19–26.

Aldenkamp, A. P., Baker, G., Mulder, O. G., Chadwick, D., Cooper, P., Doelman, J., et al. (2000). A multicenter, randomized clinical study to evaluate the effect on cognitive function of topiramate compared with valproate as add-on therapy to carbamazepine in patients with partial-onset seizures. *Epilepsia, 41*(9), 1167–1178.

Berent, S., Sackellares, J. C., Giordani, B., Wagner, J. G., Donofrio, P. D., & Abou-Khalil, B. (1987). Zonisamide (CI-912) and cognition: results from preliminary study. *Epilepsia, 28*(1), 61–67.

Bittigau, P., Sifringer, M., Genz, K., Reith, E., Pospischil, D., Govindarajalu, S., et al. (2002). Antiepileptic drugs and apoptotic neurodegeneration in the developing brain. *Proceedings of the National Academy of Sciences of the United States of America, 99*(23), 15089–15094.

Bittigau, P., Sifringer, M., & Ikonomidou, C. (2003). Antiepileptic drugs and apoptosis in the developing brain. *Annals of the New York Academy of Sciences, 993*, 103–114; discussion 123-104.

Blum, D., Meador, K., Biton, V., Fakhoury, T., Shneker, B., Chung, S., et al. (2006). Cognitive effects of lamotrigine compared with topiramate in patients with epilepsy. *Neurology, 67*(3), 400–406.

Brodie, M. J., Overstall, P. W., & Giorgi, L. (1999). Multicentre, double-blind, randomised comparison between lamotrigine and carbamazepine in elderly patients with newly diagnosed epilepsy. The UK Lamotrigine Elderly Study Group. *Epilepsy Research, 37*(1), 81–87.

Brodie, M. J., Richens, A., & Yuen, A. W. (1995). Double-blind comparison of lamotrigine and carbamazepine in newly diagnosed epilepsy. UK Lamotrigine/Carbamazepine Monotherapy Trial Group. *Lancet, 345*(8948), 476–479.

Chen, Y., Chi Chow, J., & Lee, I. (2001). Comparison the cognitive effect of anti-epileptic drugs in seizure-free children with epilepsy before and after drug withdrawal. *Epilepsy Research, 44*(1), 65–70.

Chen, Y. J., Kang, W. M., & So, W. C. (1996). Comparison of antiepileptic drugs on cognitive function in newly diagnosed epileptic children: a psychometric and neurophysiological study. *Epilepsia, 37*(1), 81–86.

Cohen, A. F., Ashby, L., Crowley, D., Land, G., Peck, A. W., & Miller, A. A. (1985). Lamotrigine (BW430C), a potential anticonvulsant. Effects on the central nervous system in comparison with phenytoin and diazepam. *British Jourmal of Clinical Pharmacology, 20*(6), 619–629.

Craig, I., & Tallis, R. (1994). Impact of valproate and phenytoin on cognitive function in elderly patients: results of a single-blind randomized comparative study. *Epilepsia, 35*(2), 381–390.

Dean, J. C., Hailey, H., Moore, S. J., Lloyd, D. J., Turnpenny, P. D., & Little, J. (2002). Long term health and neurodevelopment in children exposed to antiepileptic drugs before birth. *Journal of Medical Genetics, 39*(4), 251–259.

Dikmen, S., & Matthews, C. G. (1977). Effect of major motor seizure frequency upon cognitive-intellectual functions in adults. *Epilepsia, 18*(1), 21–29.

Dimond, K. R., Pande, A. C., Lamoreaux, L., & Pierce, M. W. (1996). Effect of gabapentin (Neurontin) [corrected] on mood and well-being in patients with epilepsy. *Progress in Neuropsychopharmacology and Biological Psychiatry, 20*(3), 407–417.

Dodrill, C. B. (1992). Neuropsychological aspects of epilepsy. *Psychiatric Clinics of North America, 15*(2), 383–394.

Dodrill, C. B., Arnett, J. L., Sommerville, K. W., & Sussman, N. M. (1993). Evaluation of the effects of vigabatrin on cognitive abilities and quality of life in epilepsy. *Neurology, 43*(12), 2501–2507.

Dodrill, C. B., Arnett, J. L., Sommerville, K. W., & Sussman, N. M. (1995). Effects of differing dosages of vigabatrin (Sabril) on cognitive abilities and quality of life in epilepsy. *Epilepsia, 36*(2), 164–173.

Dodrill, C. B., & Troupin, A. S. (1991). Neuropsychological effects of carbamazepine and phenytoin: a reanalysis. *Neurology, 41*(1), 141–143.

Donati, F., Gobbi, G., Campistol, J., Rapatz, G., Daehler, M., Sturm, Y., et al. (2007). The cognitive effects of oxcarbazepine versus carbamazepine or valproate in newly diagnosed children with partial seizures. *Seizure, 16*(8), 670–679.

Farwell, J. R., Lee, Y. J., Hirtz, D. G., Sulzbacher, S. I., Ellenberg, J. H., & Nelson, K. B. (1990). Phenobarbital for febrile seizures—effects on intelligence and on seizure recurrence. *New England Journal of Medicine, 322*(6), 364–369.

Ferrie, C. D., Robinson, R. O., & Panayiotopoulos, C. P. (1996). Psychotic and severe behavioural reactions with vigabatrin: a review. *Acta Neurologica Scandinavica, 93*(1), 1–8.

Finnell, R. H., & Dansky, L. V. (1991). Parental epilepsy, anticonvulsant drugs, and reproductive outcome: epidemiologic and experimental findings spanning three decades; 1: animal studies. *Reproductive Toxicology, 5*, 281–299.

Forsythe, I., Butler, R., Berg, I., & McGuire, R. (1991). Cognitive impairment in new cases of epilepsy randomly assigned to carbamazepine, phenytoin and sodium valproate. *Developmental Medicine and Child Neurology, 33*(6), 524–534.

Forsythe, W. I., & Sills, M. A. (1984). One drug for childhood grand mal: medical audit for three-year remissions. *Developmental Medicine and Child Neurology, 26*(6), 742–748.

Gaily, E., Kantola-Sorsa, E., Hiilesmaa, V., Isoaho, M., Matila, R., Kotila, M., et al. (2004). Normal intelligence in children with prenatal exposure to carbamazepine. *Neurology, 62*(1), 28–32.

Gilliam, F., Carter, J., & Vahle, V. (2004). Tolerability of antiseizure medications: implications for health outcomes. *Neurology, 63*(10 Suppl 4), S9–S12.

Glier, C., Dzietko, M., Bittigau, P., Jarosz, B., Korobowicz, E., & Ikonomidou, C. (2004). Therapeutic doses of topiramate are not toxic to the developing rat brain. *Experimental Neurology, 187*(2), 403–409.

Helmstaedter, C. (2002). Effects of chronic epilepsy on declarative memory systems. *Progress in Brain Res, 135*, 439–453.

Henry, T. R., & Votaw, J. R. (2004). The role of positron emission tomography with [18F]fluorodeoxyglucose in the evaluation of the epilepsies. *Neuroimaging Clinics of North America, 14*(3), 517–535, ix.

Hermann, B., Jones, J., Sheth, R., Dow, C., Koehn, M., & Seidenberg, M. (2006). Children with new-onset epilepsy: neuropsychological status, and brain structure. *Brain, 129*(Pt 10), 2609–2619.

Hessen, E., Lossius, M. I., & Gjerstad, L. (2009). Antiepileptic monotherapy significantly impairs normative scores on common tests of executive functions. *Acta Neurologica Scandinavica, 119*(3), 194–198.

Jokeit, H., Daamen, M., Zang, H., Janszky, J., & Ebner, A. (2001). Seizures accelerate forgetting in patients with left-sided temporal lobe epilepsy. *Neurology, 57*(1), 125–126.

Kang, H. C., Eun, B. L., Wu Lee, C., Ku Moon, H., Kim, J. S., Wook Kim, D., et al. (2007). The effects on cognitive function and behavioral problems of topiramate compared to carbamazepine as monotherapy for children with benign rolandic epilepsy. *Epilepsia, 48*(9), 1716–1723.

Katz, I., Kim, J., Gale, K., & Kondratyev, A. (2007). Effects of lamotrigine alone and in combination with MK-801, phenobarbital, or phenytoin on cell death in the neonatal rat brain. *Journal of Pharmacology and Experimental Therapeutics, 322*(2), 494–500.

Kim, J., Kondratyev, A., & Gale, K. (2007). Antiepileptic drug-induced neuronal cell death in the immature brain: effects of carbamazepine, topiramate, and levetiracetam as monotherapy versus polytherapy. *Journal of Pharmacology and Experimental Therapeutics, 323*(1), 165–173.

Labiner, D. M., Ettinger, A. B., Fakhoury, T. A., Chung, S. S., Shneker, B., Tatum Iv, W. O., et al. (2009). Effects of lamotrigine compared with levetiracetam on anger, hostility, and total mood in patients with partial epilepsy. *Epilepsia, 50*(3), 434–442.

Lossius, M. I., Hessen, E., Mowinckel, P., Stavem, K., Erikssen, J., Gulbrandsen, P., et al. (2008). Consequences of antiepileptic drug withdrawal: a randomized, double-blind study (Akershus Study). *Epilepsia, 49*(3), 455–463.

Manthey, D., Asimiadou, S., Stefovska, V., Kaindl, A. M., Fassbender, J., Ikonomidou, C., et al. (2005). Sulthiame but not levetiracetam exerts neurotoxic effect in the developing rat brain. *Experimental Neurology, 193*(2), 497–503.

Marino, S. E., Meador, K. J., Loring, D. W., Okun, M. S., Fernandez, H. H., Fessler, A. J., et al. (2009). Subjective perception of cognition is related to mood and not performance. *Epilepsy & Behavior, 14*(3), 459–464.

Meador, K. J. (2007). The basic science of memory as it applies to epilepsy. *Epilepsia, 48 Suppl 9*, 23–25.

Meador, K. J. (2011). Cognitive effects of epilepsy and of antiepileptic medications. In E. Wyllie, G. Cascino, B. Gidal & H. Goodkin (Eds.), *The Treatment of Epilepsy: Principles & Practice* (5th ed., pp. 1028–1036). Philadelphia: Lippincott Williams & Wilkins.

Meador, K. J., Baker, G., Cohen, M. J., Gaily, E., & Westerveld, M. (2007). Cognitive/behavioral teratogenetic effects of antiepileptic drugs. *Epilepsy &Behavior, 11*(3), 292–302.

Meador, K. J., Baker, G. A., Browning, N., Clayton-Smith, J., Combs-Cantrell, D. T., Cohen, M., et al. (2009). Cognitive function at 3 years of age after fetal exposure to antiepileptic drugs. *New England Journal of Medicine, 360*(16), 1597–1605.

Meador, K. J., Baker, G. A., Browning, N., Cohen, M. J., Bromley, R. L., Clayton-Smith, J., . . . , NEAD Study Group. (2013). Fetal antiepileptic drug exposure and cognitive outcomes at age 6 years: a prospective observational study. *Lancet Neurology, 12*(3), 244–252.

Meador, K. J., Gevins, A., Loring, D. W., McEvoy, L. K., Ray, P. G., Smith, M. E., et al. (2007). Neuropsychological and neurophysiologic effects of carbamazepine and levetiracetam. *Neurology, 69*(22), 2076–2084.

Meador, K. J., Loring, D. W., Abney, O. L., Allen, M. E., Moore, E. E., Zamrini, E. Y., et al. (1993). Effects of carbamazepine and phenytoin on EEG and memory in healthy adults. *Epilepsia, 34*(1), 153–157.

Meador, K. J., Loring, D. W., Allen, M. E., Zamrini, E. Y., Moore, E. E., Abney, O. L., et al. (1991). Comparative cognitive effects of carbamazepine and phenytoin in healthy adults. *Neurology, 41*(10), 1537–1540.

Meador, K. J., Loring, D. W., Huh, K., Gallagher, B. B., & King, D. W. (1990). Comparative cognitive effects of anticonvulsants. *Neurology, 40*(3 Pt 1), 391–394.

Meador, K. J., Loring, D. W., Hulihan, J. F., Kamin, M., & Karim, R. (2003). Differential cognitive and behavioral effects of topiramate and valproate. *Neurology, 60*(9), 1483–1488.

Meador, K. J., Loring, D. W., Moore, E. E., Thompson, W. O., Nichols, M. E., Oberzan, R. E., et al. (1995). Comparative cognitive effects of phenobarbital, phenytoin, and valproate in healthy adults. *Neurology, 45*(8), 1494–1499.

Meador, K. J., Loring, D. W., Ray, P. G., Murro, A. M., King, D. W., Nichols, M. E., et al. (1999). Differential cognitive effects of carbamazepine and gabapentin. *Epilepsia, 40*(9), 1279–1285.

Meador, K. J., Loring, D. W., Ray, P. G., Murro, A. M., King, D. W., Perrine, K. R., et al. (2001). Differential cognitive and behavioral effects of carbamazepine and lamotrigine. *Neurology, 56*(9), 1177–1182.

Meador, K. J., Loring, D. W., Vahle, V. J., Ray, P. G., Werz, M. A., Fessler, A. J., et al. (2005). Cognitive and behavioral effects of lamotrigine and topiramate in healthy volunteers. *Neurology, 64*(12), 2108–2114.

Motamedi, G. K., & Meador, K. J. (2004). Antiepileptic drugs and memory. *Epilepsy & Behavior, 5*(4), 435–439.

Park, S. P., Hwang, Y. H., Lee, H. W., Suh, C. K., Kwon, S. H., & Lee, B. I. (2008). Long-term cognitive and mood effects of zonisamide monotherapy in epilepsy patients. *Epilepsy Behav, 12*(1), 102–108.

Pressler, R. M., Binnie, C. D., Coleshill, S. G., Chorley, G. A., & Robinson, R. O. (2006). Effect of lamotrigine on cognition in children with epilepsy. *Neurology, 66*, 1495–1499.

Prevey, M. L., Delaney, R. C., Cramer, J. A., Cattanach, L., Collins, J. F., & Mattson, R. H. (1996). Effect of valproate on cognitive functioning. Comparison with carbamazepine. The Department of Veterans Affairs Epilepsy Cooperative Study 264 Group. *Archives of Neurology, 53*(10), 1008–1016.

Pulliainen, V., & Jokelainen, M. (1994). Effects of phenytoin and carbamazepine on cognitive functions in newly diagnosed epileptic patients. *Acta Neurologica Scandinavica, 89*(2), 81–86.

Ramsay, R. E., & Pryor, F. (2000). Epilepsy in the elderly. *Neurology, 55*(5 Suppl 1), S9–14; discussion S54-18.

Reinisch, J. M., Sanders, S. A., Mortensen, E. L., & Rubin, D. B. (1995). In utero exposure to phenobarbital and intelligence deficits in adult men. *Journal of the American Medical Association, 274*(19), 1518–1525.

Rowan, A. J., Ramsay, R. E., Collins, J. F., Pryor, F., Boardman, K. D., Uthman, B. M., et al. (2005). New onset geriatric epilepsy: A randomized study of gabapentin, lamotrigine, and carbamazepine. *Neurology, 64*(11), 1868–1873.

Salinsky, M. C., Binder, L. M., Oken, B. S., Storzbach, D., Aron, C. R., & Dodrill, C. B. (2002). Effects of gabapentin and carbamazepine on the EEG and cognition in healthy volunteers. *Epilepsia, 43*(5), 482–490.

Salinsky, M. C., Spencer, D. C., Oken, B. S., & Storzbach, D. (2004). Effects of oxcarbazepine and phenytoin on the EEG and cognition in healthy volunteers. *Epilepsy & Behavior, 5*(6), 894–902.

Salinsky, M. C., Storzbach, D., Spencer, D. C., Oken, B. S., Landry, T., & Dodrill, C. B. (2005). Effects of topiramate and gabapentin on cognitive abilities in healthy volunteers. *Neurology, 64*(5), 792–798.

Sattler, J. M. (1992). *Assessment of Children* (3rd ed.). San Diego: Jerome M. Sattler Pub., Inc.

Shallcross, R., Bromley, R. L., Irwin, B., Bonnett, L. J., Morrow, J., Baker, G. A. (2011). Liverpool Manchester Neurodevelopment Group; UK Epilepsy and Pregnancy Register. Child development following in utero exposure: levetiracetam vs. sodium valproate. *Neurology, 76*, 383–399.

Shewmon, D. A., & Erwin, R. J. (1988). The effect of focal interictal spikes on perception and reaction time. I. General considerations. *Electroencephalography and Clinical Neurophysiology, 69*(4), 319–337.

Smith, D., Baker, G., Davies, G., Dewey, M., & Chadwick, D. W. (1993). Outcomes of add-on treatment with lamotrigine in partial epilepsy. *Epilepsia, 34*(2), 312–322.

Smith, D. B., Craft, B. R., Collins, J., Mattson, R. H., & Cramer, J. A. (1986). Behavioral characteristics of epilepsy patients compared with normal controls. *Epilepsia, 27*(6), 760–768.

Stefovska, V. G., Uckermann, O., Czuczwar, M., Smitka, M., Czuczwar, P., Kis, J., et al. (2008). Sedative and anticonvulsant drugs suppress postnatal neurogenesis. *Annals of Neurology, 64*(4), 434–445.

Steiner, T. J., Dellaportas, C. I., Findley, L. J., Gross, M., Gibberd, F. B., Perkin, G. D., et al. (1999). Lamotrigine monotherapy in newly diagnosed untreated epilepsy: a double-blind comparison with phenytoin. *Epilepsia, 40*(5), 601–607.

Sveinbjornsdottir, S., Sander, J. W., Patsalos, P. N., Upton, D., Thompson, P. J., & Duncan, J. S. (1994). Neuropsychological effects of tiagabine, a potential new antiepileptic drug. *Seizure, 3*(1), 29–35.

Tonnby, B., Nilsson, H. L., Aldenkamp, A. P., Alpherts, W. C., Blennow, G., Elmqvist, D., et al. (1994). Withdrawal of antiepileptic medication in children. Correlation of cognitive function and plasma concentration--the multicentre "Holmfrid" study. *Epilepsy Research, 19*(2), 141–152.

Vining, E. P., Mellitis, E. D., Dorsen, M. M., Cataldo, M. F., Quaskey, S. A., Spielberg, S. P., et al. (1987). Psychologic and behavioral effects of antiepileptic drugs in children: a double-blind comparison between phenobarbital and valproic acid. *Pediatrics, 80*(2), 165–174.

Wolf, S. M., Shinnar, S., Kang, H., Gil, K. B., & Moshe, S. L. (1995). Gabapentin toxicity in children manifesting as behavioral changes. *Epilepsia, 36*(12), 1203–1205.

CHAPTER 14

Neuropsychopharmacology and Cognition

David Q. Beversdorf

Introduction

In behavioral neurology and neuropsychology, one typically thinks of localization studies involving focal lesions of the brain or functional neuroimaging. One also thinks of the understanding of the brain obtained from the neuropsychological effects of a specific neurological condition. However, another critical part of the puzzle is revealed by examining the role of neurotransmitter systems in how the brain relates to behavior. The importance of the major neurotransmitter systems will be examined in the context of specific cases descriptions.

Case 1: A 19-year-old male college student without a history of any neurological or psychiatric conditions presents with progressive difficulty with taking tests. In high school, most of the classes were not terribly challenging for him, and he did not experience any problems with taking the tests on this material. However, when he took his Scholastic Aptitude Test (SAT) he became very anxious and reports that he did not do as well as he expected. His high school counselor agreed that his performance on the SAT was below what would be predicted based upon the rest of his academic performance. Upon entering college, he did not initially encounter any difficulties, but during finals week of each semester, he would become extremely anxious while preparing for and taking his examinations, and would perform at a level somewhat below his performance during the rest of the semester. As he was seriously considering applying to competitive graduate programs in psychology to prepare for a career in neuropsychology, or applying to medical school with the goal of training in behavioral neurology, he was very concerned about this problem. He was beginning his second year during which he was to take a full load with several challenging psychology and required pre-medical courses, and he needed to get grades that would allow him to pursue these goals. After consultation with a physician, he was given several tablets of a low dose of propranolol, a central and peripherally active nonselective beta-adrenergic antagonist, to take before each anxiety-inducing exam. The patient complied with these recommendations, and reported significant improvement in his anxiety during these exams, and his performance on final exams improved to within the range expected based on his performance during the rest of the semester on those classes.

Noradrenergic Effects on Cognition

Performance anxiety and test anxiety have long been suspected to be due to activation of the noradrenergic system, leading to the development of treatment limiting the adrenergic activating effects of stress. Propranolol has been used to mitigate stress-induced impairment in performance on tasks including public speaking in anxiety-prone individuals (Lader, 1998; Laverdue and Boulenger, 1991). This practice supports a role of the noradrenergic system in the impact of stress on performance. Furthermore, research involving healthy adolescents with a history of stress-induced cognitive impairment during exams has demonstrated that treatment with the beta-adrenergic antagonist propranolol significantly improved scores on the SAT (Faigel, 1991). However, the effects of stress and the noradrenergic system on cognition are not limited to patients with stress-induced cognitive impairment. Stress has been known to impair performance on tasks requiring "creativity" (Martindale & Greenough, 1973), and stress also increases activity of the noradrenergic system (Ward et al., 1983; Kvetnansky et al., 1988). Therefore, one might expect that in the patient described above, the stress of examination increased activity in the noradrenergic system, which contributed to impairments in performance on the challenging task of taking a test on difficult material. Presumably, propranolol reversed the impairing effects of this stress response by blocking the action of the noradrenergic system. Future understanding of who is most susceptible to stress-induced cognitive impairment will be clinically important. We found that in individuals without any history of anxiety-related disorders, that a well characterized social stressor characterized by public speaking and mental arithmetic (Kirschbaum et al., 1993) resulted in impaired performance on a tasks requiring flexibility of access to lexical, semantic, and associative networks. This impairment was reversed by propranolol (Alexander et al., 2007). Therefore, the pharmacological and stress effects on cognition in this setting appear to represent a fundamental aspect of the brain-behavior relationship, not requiring the presence of an anxiety-related disorder or a dysregulated noradrenergic system. However, the effect of propranolol in this study does not exclusively implicate the noradrenergic system, since propranolol also blocks the corticosterone-induced impairment of working memory (Roozendaal et al., 2004).

The locus coeruleus contains the majority of noradrenergic neurons in the central nervous system, sending efferents throughout the brain (Barnes & Pompeiano, 1991) (Figure 14.1). The effects of the noradrenergic system outside the setting of stress are subtle. In our previous work, performance on the anagram task was better after administration of the centrally and peripherally acting beta-adrenergic antagonist propranolol than after the noradrenergic agonist ephedrine (Beversdorf et al., 1999; Heilman et al., 2003). Performance on the anagram task was also better after administration of propranolol than after the peripheral-only beta-adrenergic antagonist nadolol (Beversdorf et al., 2002), suggesting that the effect of propranolol on this aspect of cognition is mediated centrally rather than as a result of peripheral feedback. A central mechanism would be predicted by the effect of norepinephrine on the signal-to-noise ratio of neuronal activity within the cerebral cortex, where increased norepinephrine results in greater sensitivity to the dominant signal input in recordings taken from neurons in cortical sections, and decreased norepinephrine results in greater noise from remote inputs (Hasselmo et al., 1997). As further support of a central mechanism, the electronic coupling of noradrenergic neurons in the monkey cortex is correlated with the proportions of goal-directed versus exploratory

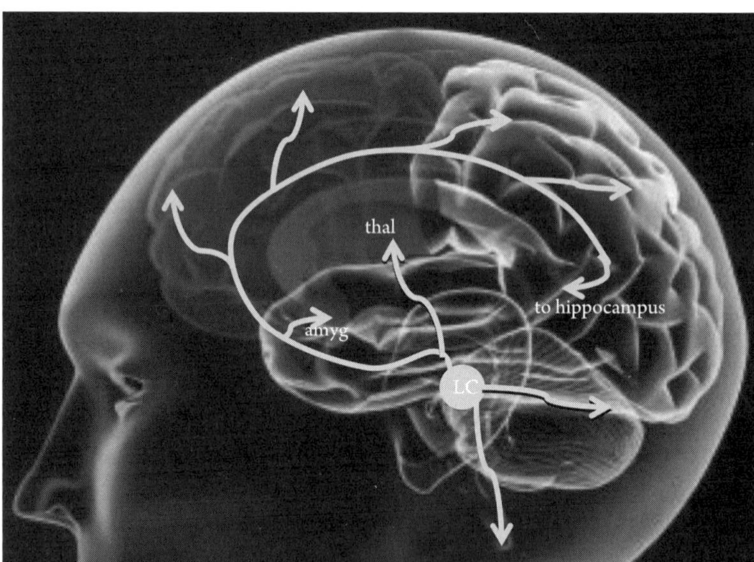

Figure 14.1 Noradrenergic pathways. The locus coeruleus (LC) projects posteriorly to the cerebellum and up to the thalamus (thal) and amygdala (amyg), as well as throughout the neocortex along a pericingular tract, also terminating posteriorly at the hippocampus (Heimer, 1995). The descending fibers to the spinal cord are also shown. Not shown is the lateral tegmental noradrenergic system which also projects to the amygdala and down to the spinal cord (see color insert).

behavior in these animals (Usher et al., 1999). However, in the anagram studies, whereas performance on propranolol was better than on ephedrine or nadolol, it did not significantly differ from placebo (Beversdorf et al., 1999; Beversdorf et al., 2002). In order to better understand the effect of propranolol, subsequent research examined how task difficulty might relate to the drug's effect, as this drug might be expected to benefit a broad search of a network due to increased sensitivity to remote inputs resulting from blockade of noradrenergic receptors, with the aforementioned effects of norepinephrine on signal-to-noise. Therefore, propranolol might be expected to yield a greater beneficial effect when problems are more challenging, requiring greater access to remote inputs. Consistent with this, propranolol helped for a range of verbal problem-solving tasks requiring network flexibility, where access to more remote inputs is necessary, when the subject was struggling, and did not help and, in some cases, hurt performance when the subject was solving problems without difficulty (Campbell et al., 2008). The benefit was seen both for the subjects who had the greatest difficulty solving the problems, and for the most difficult problems across all subjects (Campbell et al., 2008). However, propranolol can benefit performance on such language tasks for the easiest problems in situations where there is upregulated activity of the noradrenergic system due to cocaine withdrawal (Kelley et al., 2005; Kelley et al., 2007) and psychosocial stress (Alexander et al., 2007), or where there are anatomic alterations of the language network due to conditions such as autism, with decreased interaction between language regions in the brain (Beversdorf et al., 2007a; Beversdorf et al., 2008), and Broca's aphasia due to stroke, due to anatomical damage to the language areas (Beversdorf et al., 2007b).

The variability in effect of noradrenergic drugs between individuals, as observed in cocaine withdrawal, autism, and aphasia, may also be important for attention deficit disorder. Early theories proposed that arousal and optimal performance might be related on inverted U shaped curve (Yerkes & Dodson, 1908). Therefore, whereas markedly increased arousal or noradrenergic tone might result in hyperarousal and an inability to perform a task in most individuals, a person with attention deficit disorder might at baseline be in a suboptimal point on the inverted U shaped curve and require stimulants to perform optimally. Animal data suggest that the locus coeruleus has an optimal point of tonic activity that supports the emergence of phasic activity, which in single unit studies in animals has been shown to be associated with optimal performance on tasks requiring focused or selective attention (Aston-Jones et al., 1999; Aston-Jones and Cohen, 2005). Noradrenergic transmission is known to be genetically weaker, due to presence of genetic variants that reduce catecholaminergic transmission to suboptimal levels, in some patients with attention deficit disorder (Arnsten, 2007).

In addition to variation in response between patient groups, performance on verbal problem solving tasks is also affected by alterations in noradrenergic tone due to changes in posture (Lipnicki and Byrne, 2005), sleep phase (Stickgold et al., 2001), and vagal nerve stimulation (Ghacibeh et al., 2006). Such cognitive effects do not appear to occur with non-adrenergic anxiolytics (Silver et al., 2004).

However, data are only beginning to emerge regarding how propranolol might affect network performance. As described above, evidence from models derived from activity in brain slice preparations support an effect of norepinephrine on the signal-to-noise ratio of neuronal activity within the cerebral cortex, with greater sensitivity in responding to dominant inputs with higher levels of norepinephrine, but less sensitivity to dominant inputs and greater sensitivity to noise with lower levels of norepinephrine (Hasselmo et al., 1997). Presumably, propranolol increases access to "noise," which in this case would be represented by increased associational input that might be adaptive for solving more difficult problems, where the most immediate response is not optimal (Alexander et al., 2007). In one population characterized by decreased flexibility of network access (Beversdorf et al., 2007a), a potential imaging marker is observed. Decreased functional connectivity on functional magnetic resonance imaging (fMRI), or a decrease in the synchrony of activation between activated brain regions, is observed in autism (Just et al., 2004; Just et al., 2007) and is believed to be related to the underconnectivity between distant cortical regions in autism (Belmonte et al., 2004). Recent evidence suggests that propranolol increases functional connectivity on fMRI in autism, lending some support to the proposed mechanism of action of propranolol on access to more remote inputs in a network (Narayanan et al., 2010).

It is not clear, though, whether the noradrenergic system is dysregulated in autism. Increased reactivity to clinical procedures such as blood drawing and urine collection in autism may have led to the earlier atypical findings in studies assessing noradrenergic activity in autism (Minderaa et al., 1994). Pathology is also not found in the volume, cell counts, or cell density in postmortem tissue from the locus coeruleus in autism (Martchek et al., 2006). However, others have proposed that the behavioral effects of fever in autism (Curran et al., 2007) may be related to normalization of a developmentally dysregulated noradrenergic system in autism (Mehler & Purpura, 2009). Regardless of the ambient activity of the noradrenergic system in autism, network rigidity in autism (Beversdorf et al., 2007a) and the suggested effect or propranolol on access to more remote inputs in a network (Campbell et al., 2008) suggest a potential for benefit from noradrenergic blockade in ASD. Furthermore, case series have suggested a benefit in both social and language domains in autism with beta-adrenergic antagonists (Ratey et al., 1987).

The role of the noradrenergic system in behavior is, of course, not limited to effects on networks as is detailed above. The noradrenergic system is critical in arousal (Smith & Nutt, 1996; Coull et al., 1997; Coull et al., 2004).

Furthermore, the prefrontal cortex, important in a range of types of cognitive flexibility (Vikki et al., 1992; Karnath & Wallesch, 1992; Eslinger & Grattan, 1993; Duncan et al., 1995; Robbins, 2007), has afferent projections to the locus coeruleus in primates (Arnsten & Goldman-Rakic, 1984). The locus coeruleus is the region containing the majority of noradrenergic neurons in the central nervous system and sending efferents throughout the brain (Barnes & Pompeiano, 1991), as described above. The verbal problem solving tasks such as anagrams on the compound remote associates task (where the participant must produce a word that forms a compound with tree presented words, example: presented words- cone+ apple+ tree, solution- pine) (Bowden & Jung-Beeman, 2003), which involve a search through a wide network in order to identify a solution ("unconstrained flexibility", where the number of potential solutions is not limited), appear to be modulated by the noradrenergic system as described above. For such tasks, performance generally improves with decreased noradrenergic activity. However, other cognitive flexibility tasks such as the Wisconsin Cart Sort Test (Heaton, 1981) involve set-shifting between a limited range of options ("constrained flexibility", where the solution is one of a limited set of options), which may not be modulated by the noradrenergic system in the same manner, and may even benefit from increased noradrenergic activity (Usher et al., 1999; Aston-Jones & Cohen, 2005). Evidence suggests that decreased noradrenergic activity appears to benefit tasks such as anagrams when subjects are struggling or challenged by stressors (Alexander et al., 2007, Campbell et al., 2008), whereas increased set switching on a two alternative forced choice tasks is associated with increased noradrenergic tone in primate studies (Usher et al., 1999; Aston-Jones & Cohen, 2005). "Constrained" flexibility can be further subdivided into intradimensional and extradimensional set-shifting (Robbins, 2007). Intradimensional set shift requires a shift to responding to new cues from within the same stimulus modality (the subject is still responding to odor, but there are two new odors). Extradimensional Set Shift involves a shift to responding to new cues from a different stimulus modality (switching from responding to odor to responding to texture). The dopaminergic system appears to affect intradimensional set-shifting (Robbins, 2007), while the noradrenergic system, specifically by action on the alpha-1 receptor, appears to modulate performance on extradimensional set-shifting (Lapiz & Morilak, 2006; Robbins, 2007). The beta adrenergic receptors in the noradrenergic system, though, appear to modulate the "unconstrained" flexibility (Beversdorf et al., 1999; Beversdorf et al., 2002; Alexander et al., 2007). Noradrenergic agents are also known to have a range of other cognitive effects, including effects on motor learning (Foster et al., 2006), response inhibition (Chamberlain et al., 2006b), working memory and emotional memory (Chamberlain et al., 2006a).

The role of the noradrenergic system in emotional memory deserves particular comment, due to a potentially important clinical role. Centrally acting beta-adrenergic receptor antagonists are known to reduce the enhancement of memory resulting from emotional arousal (Cahill et al., 1994; van Stegeren et al., 1998). The enhancement may contribute to the development of intrusive memories in clinical conditions such as posttraumatic stress disorder (Ehlers et al., 2002; Ehlers et al., 2004; Smith & Beversdorf, 2008). Propranolol may help prevent the development of posttraumatic stress disorder, by interfering with reconsolidation, the process of reinforcement of a memory trace that results after reactivation of that previously consolidated memory trace (Pitman et al., 2002; Vaiva et al., 2003). Alpha-1 antagonists have similar benefits in patients with posttraumatic stress disorder (Arnsten, 2007).

In the periphery, alpha-2 adrenergic agonists inhibit release of norepinephrine presynaptically, which might make one consider that they would have a similar effect as the postsynaptic beta-adrenergic antagonists. However, alpha-2 agonists have distinct effects. High-dose clonidine, an alpha-2 agonist, improves immediate spatial memory in monkeys (Arnsten et al., 1988; Arnsten et al', 1991) (Franowicz and Arnsten, 1999). This effect is believed to be mediated by action at the prefrontal cortex (Li et al., 1999). Lower doses of clonidine, those typically utilized clinically in humans, demonstrate varying results at different doses, including impaired visual working memory, impulsive responses on planning tasks, and varying effects on spatial working memory (Coull et al., 1995; Jäkälä et al., 1999). Pharmacological stimulation of postsynaptic alpha-2A adrenoreceptors decreases noise and results in beneficial effects for attention deficit disorder patients (Brennan& Arnsten, 2008). However, alpha-2 agonists do not appear to have the effect on verbal problem solving that beta-adrenergic antagonists do (Choi et al., 2006).

Less is known about the specific cognitive effects of beta-1 and beta-2 adrenergic receptors. However, in one animal study, endogenous beta-1 selective activation impaired working memory (Ramos et al., 2005). Subsequent study demonstrated that beta-2 selective agonists enhance working memory in aging animals (Ramos et al., 2008), suggesting opposing effects between beta-1 and beta-2 receptors on working memory, explaining the lack of effect of propranolol on working memory in previous research (Li and Mei, 1994; Arnsten and Goldman-Rakic, 1985). Further research will be necessary to better understand the specific cognitive effects on selective beta receptors.

Case 2: A 65 year-old male with a fifteen-year history of Parkinson's disease reports a new complaint. His parkinsonian motor signs have slowly progressed over the years, and he now has a moderate degree of rigidity and resting pill-rolling tremor. He has observed that whenever he is working on one task, he has a much more difficult time shifting his attention to another task. He is unable to describe the effect of his dopaminergic agents on this symptom, as it is only observed on those occasions when he is very focused on a task. However, it has become challenging for him to keep up with activities around the house.

Dopaminergic Effects on Cognition

The majority of dopaminergic neurons originate in the substantia nigra, projecting to the striatum, critical for motor control, and in the ventral tegmentum, projecting to the limbic system and the cortex, that is thought to be important in the reward pathway. The predominant cortical target of the dopaminergic projecting fibers is the prefrontal cortex (Hall et al., 1994; Lidow et al., 1991) (Figure 14.2).

One early window on the effects of the dopaminergic system on cognition was revealed in priming studies. Kischka et al (1996) showed in a priming experiment that in healthy individuals, word recognition occurs more rapidly when presented 700 ms after exposure to another directly related or indirectly related word. After administration of L-dopa, the precursor for dopamine, only words presented after directly related words are recognized quickly. This finding was interpreted as a dopaminergic restriction of the semantic network in priming, since the spreading activation of either a directly or indirectly related word facilitated word recognition without L-dopa, but only the directly related word facilitated word recognition with L-dopa. This effect is sensitive to the time between the initial and target stimuli, likely a reflection of the timing of spreading activation. Angwin et al (2004) found that L-dopa affected both direct and indirect

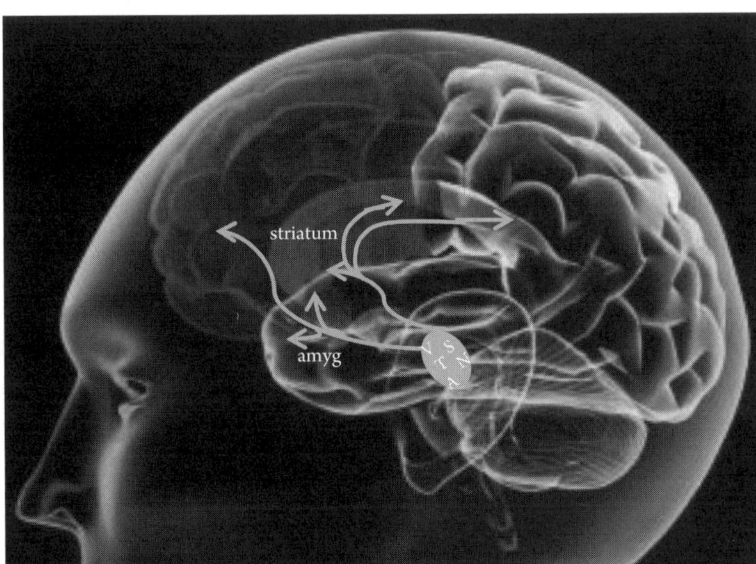

Figure 14.2 Dopaminergic pathways. Projections from the substantia nigra (SN) to the striatum are demonstrated, as are projections from the ventral tegmental area (VTA) to the amygdala (amyg), ventral striatum, and frontal cortex (Heimer, 1995). Not shown are the tuberoinfundibular and posterior hypothalamic dopaminergic systems (see color insert).

priming with an interstimulus interval of 500 ms, but had no effect at 250 ms. However, since L-dopa is a dopamine precursor, it remained unclear as to which specific dopamine receptors were responsible for the priming effect. Studies in healthy volunteers (Roesch-Ely et al., 2006), in addition to work in our lab in patients with Parkinson's disease (Pederzolli et al., 2008), suggest that the priming effect is mediated by the D1 receptor. L-dopa, though, is also a precursor to norepinephrine. Therefore, further study was then required to disentangle the potential dopaminergic and noradrenergic roles in priming and "unconstrained" cognitive flexibility in problem solving, both of which are known to be sensitive to catecholaminergic agents (dopamine and norepinephrine) acting on semantic networks (Kischka et al., 1996; Campbell et al., 2008). Dopaminergic agonists did not have effects on "unconstrained" cognitive flexibility in problem solving (Smyth & Beversdorf, 2007), and noradrenergic agents did not affect priming in the manner observed with dopaminergic agents (Cios et al., 2009). In order to determine how dopaminergic agents might exhibit an effect on semantic network, the effect of L-dopa on functional connectivity was examined during a non-priming language task. An isolated increase in connectivity was observed with L-dopa between the left fusiform and the receptive language areas, with no other region pairs affected (Tivarus et al., 2008). Because the Visual Word Form Area is thought to be located in the left fusiform gyrus (Beversdorf et al., 1997), this would appear to fit with the effects on priming as an interaction between this fusiform area and Wernicke's area. However, as the predominant target among cortical areas for dopaminergic projecting fibers is the frontal lobe (Hall et al., 1994; Lidow et al., 1991), such an effect of L-dopa on posterior regions seems unexpected. Evidence from our lab using independent component analysis of fMRI data during language tasks suggests that the posterior effects of L-dopa may be mediated indirectly by the fronto-thalamic connections from the areas containing the frontal projections of the dopaminergic fibers (Kim et al., 2010). A more recent fMRI study examining the effect of L-dopa on priming reported activation with drug in the dorsal prefrontal cortex, anterior cingulate, left rolandic operculum, and left middle temporal gyrus (Copland et al., 2009). This activation pattern may suggest an indirect frontal-posterior interaction.

The dopaminergic system has a range of other cognitive effects, in addition to the well known effects on the motor system. Animal studies demonstrate varying effects of dopaminergic agents on set shifting tasks, depending on the receptor subtype sensitivity for each agent (Floresco et al., 2005). This effect is appears to be specific to intradimensional set-shifting (Robbins, 2007). Whereas agonists for both D1 and D2 receptors did not affect set shifting, D2 antagonists impaired set shifting in rodents (Stefani & Moghaddam, 2005; Floresco et al., 2006) and humans (Mehta et al., 2004). This may explain the difficulties with attentional shifting reported in the patient with Parkinson disease described above. Ability to maintain and flexibly alter cognitive representations in response to environmental demands is impaired in Parkinson disease (Cools, 2006). Computational models propose that phasic stimulation of D2 receptors in the striatum drives flexible adaptation of cognitive representation which are maintained by the prefrontal cortex, such as the updating of working memory (Cohen et al., 2002), which contrasts with the effect on priming which appears to be mediated by D1 receptors (Roesch-Ely et al., 2006; Pederzolli et al., 2008). Regarding the effect of dopamine in patient populations, though, the interaction between dopaminergic agonists and Parkinson disease and their effect on cognition is a complex relationship for set shifting and working memory (Cools, 2006).

In healthy subjects, individuals with lower working memory capacity tend to be the ones that benefit from increased prefrontal function with dopaminergic stimulation (Gibbs & D'Esposito, 2005; Kimberg et al., 1997). This effect is probably because dopamine synthesis in the striatum is related to working memory capacity. Diminished working memory capacity is associated with less dopamine production, and therefore benefit from dopaminegic stimulation (Cools et al., 2008). In animal models, this effect on working memory is mediated at the D1 receptor (Arnsten et al., 1994; Sawaguchi & Goldman-Rakic, 1991; Williams & Goldman-Rakic, 1995). Dopamine also appears to be critical for a range of other aspects of cognition involving frontal-subcortical circuits, including the temporal coupling of deliberation and execution during decision-making. As evidence of this, dopamine replacement reverses the delay specific to decision-related hesitations, independent of motor slowing, in situations requiring decision-making in uncertainty in patients with Parkinson disease (Pessiglione et al., 2005). Furthermore, recent positron emission tomography (PET)/fMRI comparison studies have investigated the role of the dopaminergic system in activation of the amygdala, demonstrating a relationship between PET D1 receptor binding correlating with amygdala signal change in response to fearful faces as assessed by fMRI, a relationship not observed for PET D2 receptor binding (Takahashi et al., 2010).

Another critical role of dopamine has recently become apparent with the development of pathological gambling in the setting of treatment with dopaminergic agonists (Dodd et al., 2005; Gallagher et al., 2007). This has contributed to a greater understanding of the roles of dopamine in decision making, revealing that dopamine neurons encode the difference between expected and received rewards, and interact with other neurotransmitter systems to regulate such decision-making (Nakamura et al., 2008).

Case 3: A 67 year-old female presented to clinic while spending the winter in Florida with a one-year history of difficulty with memory. The family acknowledged her slight slowing in ambulation. In the previous couple of months, the patient reported seeing little children running around the room, when none were there. The patient's symptoms also showed a high degree of day-to-day variability, and she had some difficulty sleeping. Her husband reported that she would thrash around a lot in her sleep. Examination confirmed memory impairment and visuospatial processing difficulties, and difficulty with frontal systems tasks, including response inhibition and motor programming. She had mild masked facies, mild bradykinesia, and some cogwheel rigidity. She was diagnosed with dementia with Lewy bodies and started on cholinesterase inhibitors. The cognitive symptoms showed marked improvement. She returned home for the summer in New Jersey, where she saw her physician. He assessed her, and found her cognitive performance on his screening assessment to be normal, and told her to stop taking the cholinesterase inhibitor. Within a few weeks, she exhibited cognitive decline, and began to see animals running around her room. This prompted a visit to the emergency room, where neuroleptics were started. The patient rapidly became rigid and poorly responsive. This prompted a call to her memory specialists in Florida, at which point the neuroleptics were discontinued and the cholinesterase inhibitors restarted. The patient improved, but not quite back to her previous baseline.

Cholinergic Effects on Cognition

Neurons in the nucleus basalis, medial septal nucleus, and the diagonal band of Broca in the basal forebrain are the main sources of cholinergic projection throughout the neocortex and hippocampus (Figure 14.3). The cholinergic system is another neurotransmitter system involved in modulating the signal-to-noise ratio within the cortex by suppressing background intrinsic cortical activity (Hasselmo & Bower, 1992), thus modulating efficiency of cortical processing of sensory or associational information (Sarter and Bruno, 1997). Acetylcholine is particularly important for attention (Sarter & Bruno, 2001). Studies in rodents demonstrate that acetylcholine is critical for both top-down and bottom-up processing of stimuli, mediated by action on the prefrontal cortex (Gill et a., 2000; Newman & McGaughy, 2008). Cholinergic dysfunction has been used as a model for Alzheimer's disease (Whitehouse et al., 1982), due to the significant degeneration of the cholinergic neurons in these patients. Among the two main subtypes of acetylcholine receptors, muscarinic receptors have been clearly demonstrated to interfere with encoding of new information with less of an effect on previously stored information (Hasselmo & Wyble, 1997). Blockade of nicotinic receptors has significant effects on memory in an age-dependent manner (Newhouse et al., 1992; Newhouse et al., 1994). However, despite clear effects on signal-to-noise ratio in the cortex as well as memory effects, neither muscarinic nor nicotinic blockade affected performance on the unconstrained cognitive flexibility tasks as previously described that are affected by blockade ofthe noradrenergic system (Smyth & Beversdorf, in preparation).

Whereas cholinesterase inhibitor treatment to increase the availability of acetylcholine in the synapse is a mainstay of treatment for Alzheimer's disease

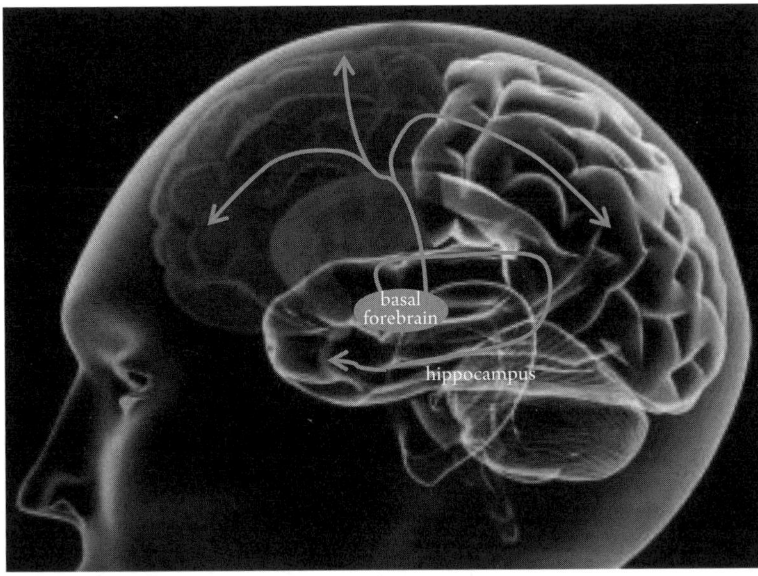

Figure 14.3 Cholinergic pathways. Cortical projections from the basal forebrain are demonstrated to the cingulate, and pericingulate cortex, as well as the mesial frontal cortex along a mesial pericingular tract, and laterally through the external capsule and claustrum to the capsular region and lateral neocortex (Selden et al., 1998) (see color insert).

(Doody et al., 2001), evidence suggests that patients with dementia with Lewy bodies, such as the one described above, have a greater impairment of cholinergic activity than is observed in Alzheimer disease (Perry et al., 1994). In fact, in the original cholinesterase inhibitor trials for Alzheimer's disease, many of the best responders were subsequently found to have Lewy body dementia on postmortem examination (Levy et al., 1994; Perry et al., 1994). Subsequent studies have revealed a robust effect of cholinesterase inhibitors in Lewy body dementia to further support this (McKeith et al., 2000; Beversdorf et al., 2004). This may explain the high degree of sensitivity to cholinesterase inhibitors in the patient described above. Perception, attention, and working memory are particularly impaired in Lewy body dementia (Calderon et al., 2001). Sleep and balance disturbances are also common in Lewy body dementia, and the cognitive impairment can fluctuate markedly over time (McKeith et al., 2004). Many of these feature were observed in the aforementioned patient. Furthermore, REM behavior disorder is particularly common in these patients (Boeve et al., 2001), which is the most likely etiology of the "thrashing around a lot in her sleep" reported in the described patient. Finally, due to the prominence of both cholinergic and dopaminergic dysfunction, these patients are extremely sensitive to anticholinergic and antidopaminergic agents (McKeith et al., 2004). Unfortunately, antidopaminergic agents are often attempted for the hallucinations, as was the case in the patient described above, or anticholinergic agents for sleep, possible incontinence, and occasionally presumed vertigo, resulting in significant decline.

Other Neurotransmitters and Other Considerations

Our understanding of the role of individual neurotransmitter systems in cognition has significantly progressed over the past 20 years. However, these systems do not act in isolation. Complex interactions occur between them, which are only beginning to be understood. For example, action at D2 dopaminergic receptors and at NMDA receptors appear to interact in their effects on set-shifting (Floresco et al., 2005; Floresco et al., 2006; Stefani & Moghaddam, 2005). Also, as described above, the dopaminergic system appears to affect intradimensional set-shifting (Robbins, 2007), while the noradrenergic system, specifically by action on the alpha-1 adrenergic receptor, appears to modulate performance on extradimensional set-shifting (Lapiz & Morilak, 2006; Robbins, 2007). Noradrenergic innervation of dopaminergic neurons, specifically by action on alpha 1 adrenergic receptors, is known to directly inhibit the activity of the dopaminergic neurons (Paladini & Williams, 2004). In addition, the effects of drugs on cognition also depend on location of action, when isolated brain regions are studied (Cools & Robbins, 2004). Also, the mechanism by which the regulatory neurotransmitters is beginning to be more fully understood, with potential treatment options including targeting of second messenger systems, which are the intermediaries inside of neurons through which action on a neurotransmitter receptor is transmitted, allowing communication of the receptor binding with the neurotransmitter to impact the functioning of the neuron (Arnsten, 2007; Arnsten, 2009).

The serotonergic system has neurons in the dorsal raphe nucleus projecting throughout the forebrain and neocortex (Figure 14.4). This system has effects on mood and affect. However, recent research reveals that the serotonergic system and its interaction with other neurotransmitter systems serve important cognitive roles as well. The balance between the serotonergic and dopaminergic systems appears to be critical for processing of reward and punishment (Krantz et al., 2010). The firing of midbrain dopamine neurons show a firing pattern that reflects the magnitude and probability of rewards (Schultz, 2007; Roesch et al., 2007), while tryptophan depletion enhances punishment prediction but does not affect reward prediction (Cools et al., 2008), but serotonergic neurons do appear to signal reward value (Nakamura et al., 2008). Furthermore, prefrontal serotonin depletion affects reversal learning, but not set shifting (Clarke et al., 2005).

The role of neuropeptides is also beginning to be elucidated. For example, oxytocin has been found to play an important role in social approach and engagement

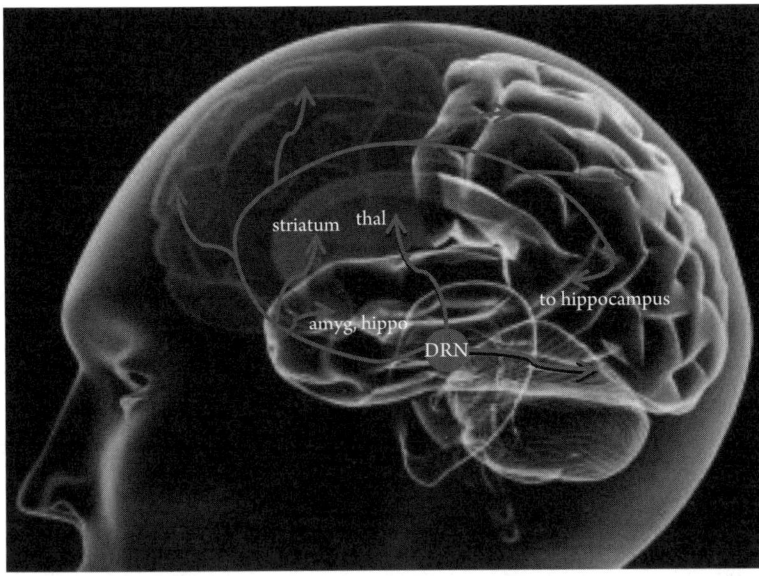

Figure 14.4 Serotonergic pathways. The dorsal raphe nuclei (DRN) project posteriorly to the cerebellum and intracerebellar nuclei, and up to the thalamus (thal), with projections also to the amygdala (amyg), hippocampus (hippo), hypothalamus, olfactory and entorhinal cortices, then to the ventral striatum as well as throughout the neocortex along a pericingular tract, also terminating posteriorly at the hippocampus (Heimer, 1995). Not shown is the caudal raphe nuclei, which also project to the cerebellum and intracerebellar nuclei, and down to the spinal cord (see color insert).

behavior (Kosfeld et al., 2005; Carter, 1998), which may have implications for clinical populations such as autism (Andari et al., 2010). Continued understanding of the roles of neurotransmitter interactions, localized effects, and other types of neurotransmitters will be needed to fully understand the how cognitive processes are carried out in the brain. Further understanding of this will result in clinical benefits for patients with a wide variety of clinical syndromes.

References

Alexander, J.K., Hillier, A., Smith, R.M., Tivarus, M.E., Beversdorf, D.Q. (2007). Noradrenergic modulation of cognitive flexibility during stress. *Journal of Cognitive Neuroscience, 19*:468–478.

Andari, E., Duhamel, J-R., Zalla, T., Herbrecht, E., Leboyer, M., Sirigu, A. (2010). Promoting social behavior with oxytocin in high-functioning autism spectrum disorders. *Proceedings of the National Academy of Sciences of the United States of America, 107*:4389–4394.

Angwin, A.J., Chenery, H.J., Copland, D.A., Arnott, W.L., Murdoch, B.E., Silburn, P.A. (2004). Dopamine and Semantic Activation: An Investigation of Masked Direct and Indirect Priming. *Journal of the International Neuropsychological Society, 10*:15–25.

Arnsten, A.F.T. (2007) Catecholamine and second messenger influences on prefrontal cortical networks of "representational knowledge": a rational bridge between genetics and the symptoms of mental illness. *Cerebral Cortex 17*:i6–i15.

Arnsten, A.F.T. (2009) Ameliorating prefrontal cortical dysfunction in mental illness: inhibition of phosphotidyl inositol-protein kinase C signaling. *Psychopharmacology 202*:445–455.

Arnsten, A.F., Goldman-Rakic, P.S. (1984) Selective prefrontal cortical projections to the region of the locus coeruleus and raphe nuclei in the rhesus monkey. *Brain Research. 306*:9–18.

Arnsten, A.F., Goldman-Rakic, P.S. (1985) Alpha-2 adrenergic mechanisms in prefrontal cortex associated with cognitive decline in aged non-human primates. *Science 230*:1273–1276.

Arnsten, A.F.T., Cai, J.X., Goldman-Rakic, P.S. (1988) The alpha-2 adrenergic agonist guanfacine improves memory in aged monkeys without sedative or hypotensive side effects: evidence for alpha-2 receptor subtypes. *Journal of Neuroscience 8*:4287–4298.

Arnsten, A.F., Cai, J.X., Murphy, B.L., Goldman-Rakic, P.S. (1994) Dopamine D1 receptor mechanisms in the cognitive performance of young adult and aged monkeys. *Psychopharmacology* (Berl) *116*:143–151.

Arnsten, A.F.T., Leslie, F.M. (1991) Behavioral and receptor binding analysis of the alpha-2 adrenergic agonist, 5-bromo-6 [2-imidazoline-2-yl amino] quinoxaline (uk-14304): evidence for cognitive enhancement at an alpha-2-adrenoreceptor subtype. *Neuropharmacology 30*:1279–1289.

Aston-Jones, G., Cohen, J.D. (2005) An integrative theory of locus coeruleus-norpeinephrine function: adaptive gain and optimal performance. *Annual Review of Neuroscience 28*:403–450.

Aston-Jones, G., Rajkowski, J., Cohen, J. (1999) Role of locus coeruleus in attention and behavioral flexibility. *Biological Psychiatry 46*:1309–1320.

Barnes, C.A., Pompeiano, M. (1991) Neurobiology of the locus coeruleus. *Progress in Brain Research 88*:307–321.

Belmonte, M.K., Allen, G., Beckel-Mitchener, A., Boulanger, L.M., Carper, R.A., Webb, S.J. (2004) Autism and abnormal development of brain connectivity. *Journal of Neuroscience 24*:9228–9231.

Beversdorf, D.Q., Carpenter, A.L., Miller, R.F., Cios, J.S., Hillier, A. (2008) Effect of propranolol on verbal problem solving in autism spectrum disorder. *Neurocase 14*:378–383.

Beversdorf, D.Q., Hughes, J.H., Steinberg, B.A., Lewis, L.D., Heilman, K.M. (1999) Noradrenergic modulation of cognitive flexibility in problem solving. *NeuroReport 10*:2763–2767.

Beversdorf, D.Q., Narayanan, A., Hillier, A., Hughes, J.D. (2007a) Network model of decreased context utilization in autism spectrum disorder. *Journal of Autism and Developmental Disorders 37*:1040–1048.

Beversdorf, D.Q., Ratcliffe, N.R., Rhodes, C.H., Reeves, A.G. (1997). Pure alexia: clinical-pathologic evidence for a lateralized visual language association cortex. *Clinical Neuropathology, 16*:328–331.

Beversdorf, D.Q., Sharma, U.K., Phillips, N.N., Notestine, M.A., Slivka, A.P., Friedman, N.M., Schneider, S.L., Nagaraja, H.N., Hillier, A. (2007b) Effect of propranolol on naming in chronic Broca's aphasia with anomia. *Neurocase 13*:256–259.

Beversdorf, D.Q., Warner, J.L., Davis, R.A., Sharma, U.K., Nagaraja, H.N., Scharre, D.W. (2004) Donepezil in the treatment of dementia with Lewy bodies. *American Journal of Geriatric Psychiatry 12*:542–544.

Beversdorf, D.Q., White, D.M., Cheever, D.C., Hughes, J.D., Bornstein, R.A. (2002) Central beta-adrenergic blockers modulation of cognitive flexibility. *NeuroReport 13*:2505–2507.

Boeve, B., Silber, M., Ferman, T., Lucas, J., Parisi, J. (2001) Association of REM sleep behavior disorder and neurodegenerative disease may reflect an underlying synucleinopathy. *Movement Disorders 16*:622–630.

Bowden, E.M., Jung-Beeman, M. (2003) Normative data for 144 compound remote associate problems. *Behavior Research Methods, Instruments, & Computers, 35*:634–639.

Brennan, A.R., Arnsten, A.F.T. (2008) Neuronal mechanisms underlying attention deficit hyperactivity disorder: the influence of arousal on prefrontal cortical function. *Annals of the New York Academy of Sciences 1129*:236–245.

Cahill, L., Prins, B., Weber, M., McGaugh, J.L. (1994). β-Adrenergic activation and memory for emotional events. *Nature 371*:702–704.

Calderon, J., Perry, R.J., Erzinclioglu, S.W., Berrios, G.E., Dening, T.R., Hodges, J.R. (2001) Perception, attention, and working memory are disproportionately impaired in dementia with Lewy bodies compared with Alzheimer's disease *Journal of Neurology, Neurosurgery, & Psychiatry 70*:157–164.

Campbell, H.L., Tivarus, M.E., Hillier, A., Beversdorf, D.Q. (2008) Increased task difficulty results in greater impact of noradrenergic modulation of cognitive flexibility. *Pharmacology, Biochemistry, and Behavior 88*:222–229.

Carter, C.S. (1998) Neuroendocrine perspectives on social attachment and love. *Psychoneuroendocrinology 23*:779–818.

Chamberlain, S.R., Müller, U., Blackwell, A.D., Clark, L., Robbins, T.W., Sahakian, B. (2006) Neurochemical modulation of response inhibition and probabilistic learning in humans. *Science 311*:861–863.

Chamberlain, S.R., Müller, U., Blackwell, A.D., Robbins, T.W., Sahakian, B. (2006) Noradrenergic modulation of working memory and emotional memory in humans. *Psychopharmacology 188*:397–407.

Choi, Y., Novak, J., Hillier, A., Votolato, N.A., Beversdorf, D.Q. (2006). The effect of α-2 adrenergic agonists on memory and cognitive flexibility *Cognitive and Behavioral Neurology 19*:204–207.

Cios, J.S., Miller, R.F., Hillier, A., Tivarus, M.E., Beversdorf, D.Q. (2009). Lack of noradrenergic modulation of indirect semantic priming. *Behavioral Neurology 21*:137–143.

Clarke, H.F., Walker, S.C., Crofts, H.S., Dalley, J.W., Robbins, T.W., Roberts, A.C. (2005). Prefrontal serotonin depletion affects reversal learning but not attentional set shifting. *Journal of Neuroscience 25*:532–538.

Cohen, J.D., Braver, T.S., Brown, J.W. (2002) Computational perspectives in dopamine function in prefrontal cortex. *Current Opinion in Neurobiology 12*: 223–229.

Cools, R. (2006) Dopaminergic modulation of cognitive function-implications for L-DOPA treatment in Parkinson's disease. *Neuroscience & Biobehavioral Reviews 30*: 1–23.

Cools, R., Gibbs, S.E., Miyakawa, A., Jagust, W., D'Esposito, M. (2008) Working memory capacity predicts dopamine synthesis capacity in the human striatum. *Journal of Neuroscience 28*:1208–1212.

Cools, R., Robbins, R.W. (2004). Chemistry of the adaptive mind. *Philosophical Transactions of the Royal Society of London A 362*:2871–2888.

Cools, R., Robinson, O.J., Sahakian, B. (2008). Acute tryptophan depletion in healthy volunteers enhances punishment prediction but does not affect reward prediction. *Neuropsychopharmacology 33*:2291–2299.

Copland, D.A., McMahon, K.L., Silburn, P.A., de Zubicaray. G.I. (2009) Dopaminergic neruomodulation of semantic priming: a 4T fMRI study with levodopa. *Cerebral Cortex 19*:2651–2658.

Coull, J.T., Frith, C.D., Dolan, R.J., Frackowiak, R.S.J., Grasby, P.M. (1997) The neural correlates of the noradrenergic modulation of human attention, arousal and learning. *European Journal of Neuroscience 9*:589–598.

Coull, J.T., Jones, M.E.P., Egan, T.D., Frith, C.D., Maze, M. (2004) Attentional effects of noradrenaline vary with arousal level: selective activation of thalamic pulvinar in humans. *NeuroImage 22*:315–322.

Coull, J.T., Middleton, H.C., Robbins, T.W., Sahakian, B.J. (1995) Contrasting effects of clonidine and diazepam on tests of working memory and planning. *Psychopharmacology 120*:311–321.

Curran, L.K., Newschaffer, C.J., Lee, L., Crawford, S.O., Johnston, M.V., Zimmerman, A.W. (2007). Behaviors associated with fever in children with autism spectrum disorders. *Pediatrics 120*:e1386–e1392.

Dodd, M.L., Klos, K.J., Bower, J.H., Geda, Y.E., Josephs, K.A., Ahlskog, J.E. (2005) Pathological gambling caused by drugs used to treat Parkinson disease. *Archives of Neurology 62*:1377–1381.

Doody, R.S., Stevens, J.C., Beck, C., Dubinsky, R.M., Kaye, J.A., Gwyther, L., Mohs, R.C., Thal, L.J., Whitehouse, P.J., DeKosky, S.T., Cummings, J.L. (2001) Practice parameter: management of dementia (an evidence based review). Report of the Quality Standards Subcommittee of the American Academy of Neurology. *Neurology 56*:1154–1166.

Duncan, J., Burgess, P., Emslie, H. (1995) Fluid intelligence after frontal lobe lesions. *Neuropsychologia 33*:261–268.

Ehlers, A., Hackmann, A., Michael, T. (2004). Intrusive re-experiencing in post-traumatic stress disorder: Phenomenology, theory, and therapy. *Memory 12*:403–415.

Ehlers, A., Hackmann, A., Steil, R., Clohessy, S., Wenninger, K., Winter, H. (2002). The nature of intrusive memories after trauma: the warning signal hypothesis. *Behaviour Research and Therapy 40*: 995–1002.

Eslinger, P.J., Grattan, L.M. (1993) Frontal lobe and frontal-striatal substrates for different forms of human cognitive flexibility. *Neuropsychologia 31*:17–28.

Faigel, H.C. (1991) The effect of beta blockade on stress-induced cognitive dysfunction in adolescents. *Clinical Pediatrics 30*:441–445.

Floresco, S.B., Ghods-Sharifi, S., Vexelman, C., Magyar, O. (2006) Dissociable roles for the nucleus accumbens core and shell in regulating set shifting. *Journal of Neuroscience 26*: 2449–2457.

Floresco, S.B., Magyar, O., Ghods-Sharifi, S., Vexelman, C., Tse, M.T.L. (2005) Multiple dopamine receptor subtypes in the medial prefrontal cortex of the rat regulate set-shifting. *Neuropsychopharmacology 31*: 297–309.

Foster, D.J., Good, D.C., Fowlkes, A., Sawaki, L. (2006) Atomoxetine enhances a short-term model of plasticity in humans. *Archives of Physical Medicine and Rehabilitation 87*:216–221.

Franowicz, J.S., Arnsten, A.F.T. (1999) Treatment with the noradrenergic alpha-2 agonist clonidine, but not diazepam, improves spatial working memory in normal rhesus monkeys. *Neuropsychopharmacology 21*:611–621.

Gallagher, D.A., O'Sullivan, S.S., Evans, A.H., Lees. A.L., Schrag, A. (2007) Pathological gambling in Parkinson's disease: risk factors and differences from dopaminergic dysregulation. An analysis of published case series. *Movement Disorders 22*:1757–1763.

Ghacibeh, G.A., Shenker, J.I,, Shenal, B., Uthman, B.M., Heilman, K.M. (2006) Effect of vagus nerve stimulation on creativity and cognitive flexibility. *Epilepsy & Behavior 8*:720–725.

Gibbs, S.E., D'Esposito, M. (2005) Individual capacity differences predict working memory performance and prefrontal activity following dopamine receptor stimulation. *Cognitive, Affective, & Behavioral Neuroscience 5*:212–221.

Gill, T.M., Sarter, M., Givens, B. (2000) Sustained visual attention performance-associated prefrontal neuronal activity evidence for cholinergic modulation. *Journal of Neuroscience 20*:4745–4757.

Hall, H., Sedvall, G., Magnusson, O., Kopp, J., Halldin, C., Farde, L. (1994) Distribution of D1- and D2-dopamine receptors, and dopamine and its metabolites in the human brain. *Neuropsychopharmacology 11*:245–256.

Hasselmo, M.E., Bower, J.M. (1992) Cholinergic suppression specific to intrinsic not afferent fiber synapses in rat piriform (olfactory) cortex. *Trends in Neurosciences 67*: 1222–1229.

Hasselmo, M.E., Linster, C., Patil, M., Ma, D., Cecik, M. (1997) Noradrenergic suppression of synaptic transmission may influence cortical signal-to-noise ratio. *Journal of Neurophysiology 77*: 3326–3339.

Hasselmo, M.E., Wyble, B.P. (1997) Simulation of the effects of scopolamine on free recall and recognition in a network model of the hippocampus. *Behavioural Brain Research 89*:1–34.

Heaton, R.K. (1981) *Wisconsin Card Sort Test Manual.* Odessa, FL: Psychological Assessment Resources.
Heilman, K.M., Nadeau, S.E., Beversdorf, D.Q. (2003). Creative innovation: possible brain mechanisms. *Neurocase, 9*:369–379.
Heimer, L. (1995). *The Human Brain and Spinal Cord,* 2nd Edition. New York, Berlin: Springer-Verlag.
Jäkälä, P., Riekkinen, M., Sirvi, J, Koivisto, E., Kejonen, K., Vanhanen, M., Riekkinen, P. Jr (1999) Guanfacine, but not clonidine, improves planning and working memory performance in humans. *Neuropsychopharmacology 20*:460–470.
Just, M.A., Cherkassky, V.L., Keller, T.A., Kana, R.K., Minshew, N.J. (2007) Functional and anatomical cortical underconnectivity in autism: evidence from an fMRI study of an executive function task and corpus callosum morphometry. *Cerebral Cortex 17*:951–961.
Just, M.A., Cherkassky, V.L., Keller, T.A., Minshew, N.J. (2004) Cortical activation and synchronization during sentence comprehension in high-functioning autism: evidence of underconnectivity. *Brain 127*:1811–1821.
Karnath, H.O., Wallesch, C.W. (1992) Inflexibility of mental planning: a characteristic disorder with prefrontal lobe lesions. *Neuropsychologia 30*:1011–1016.
Kelley, B.J., Yeager, K.R., Pepper, T.H., Beversdorf, D.Q. (2005). Cognitive impairment in acute cocaine withdrawal. *Cognitive and Behavioral Neurology, 18*:108–112.
Kelley, B.J., Yeager, K.R., Pepper, T.H., Bornstein R.A., Beversdorf, D.Q (2007) The effect of propranolol on cognitive flexibility and memory in acute cocaine withdrawal. *Neurocase 13*:320–327.
Kim, N., Goel, P.K., Tivarus, M.E., Hillier, A., Beversdorf, D.Q. (2010) Independent component analysis of the effect of L-dopa on fMRI of language processing. *PLoS ONE 5*: e11933. doi:10.1371/journal.pone.0011933
Kimberg, D.Y., D'Esposito, M., Farah, M.J. (1997) Effects of bromocriptine on human subjects depend on working memory capacity. *Neuroreport 8*:3581–3585.
Kirschbaum, C., Pirke, K.M., Hellhammer, D.H. (1993). The "Trier Social Stress Test"—a tool for investigating psychobiological stress responses in a laboratory setting. *Neuropsychobiology, 28*:76–81.
Kischka, U., Kammer, T.H., Maier, S., Weisbord, M., Thimm, M., Spitzer, M. (1996). Dopaminergic Modulation of Semantic Network Activation. *Neuropsychologia, 34*:1107–1113.
Kosfeld, M., Heinrichs, M., Zak, P.J., Fischbacher, U., Fehr, E. (2005). Oxytocin increases trust in humans. *Nature 435*:673–676.
Krantz, G.S., Kasper, S., Lanzenberger, R. (2010). Reward and the serotonergic system. *Neuroscience 166*:1023–1035.
Kvetnansky, R., Pacak, K., Sabban, E.L., Kopin, I.J., Goldstein, D.S. (1998) Stressor specificity of peripheral catecholaminergic activation. *Advances in Pharmacology 42*:556–560.
Lader, M. (1988) Beta-adrenergic antagonists in neuropsychiatry: an update. *Journal of Clinical Psychiatry 49*:213–223.
Lapiz, M.D.S., Morilak, D.A. (2006) Noradrenergic modulation of cognitive function in rat medial prefrontal cortex as measured by attentional set shifting capability. *Neuroscience 137*:1039–1049.
Laverdue, B., Boulenger, J.P. (1991) Medications beta-bloquantes et anxiete. Un interet therapeutique certain. [Beta-blocking drugs and anxiety. A proven therapeutic value.] *L'Encephale 17*:481–492.
Levy, R., Eagger, S., Griffiths, M, Perry, E., Honavar, M., Dean, A., Lanots, P. (1994) Lewy bodies and response to tacrine in Alzheimer's disease. *Lancet 343*:176.
Li, B-M., Mao, Z.M., Wang, M., Mei, Z-T. (1999) Alpha-2 adrenergic modulation of prefrontal cortical neuronal activity related to spatial working memory in monkeys. *Neuropsychopharmacology 21*:601–610.

Li, B-M., Mei, Z-T. (1994) Delayed response deficit induced by local injection of the alpha-2 adrenergic antagonist yohimbine into the dosolateral prefrontal cortex in young adult monkeys. *Behavioral and Neural Biology 62*:134–139.

Lidow, M., Goldman-Rakic, P., Gallager, D., Rakic, P. (1991) Distribution of dopaminergic receptors in the primate cerebral cortex: Quantitative autoradiographic analysis using (H3) raclopide, (H3) spiperone and (H3) SCH23390. *Neuroscience 40*:657–671.

Lipnicki, D.M., Byrne, D.G. (2005) Thinking on your back: solving anagrams faster when supine than when standing. *Cognitive Brain Research 24*:719–722.

Martchek, M., Thevarkunnel, S., Bauman, M., Blatt, G., Kemper, T. (2006) Lack of evidence of neuropathology in the locus coeruleus in autism. *Acta Neuropathologica 111*:497–499.

Martindale, C., Greenough, J. (1973) The differential effect of increased arousal on creative and intellectual performance. *Journal of Genetic Psychology 123*:329–335.

McKeith, I., del Ser, T., Spano, P.F., Emre, M., Wesnes, K., Anand, R., Cicin-Sain, A., Ferrara, R., Spiegel, R. (2000) Efficacy of rivastigmine in dementia with Lewy bodies: a randomized, double-blind, placebo-controlled international study. *Lancet 356*:2031–2036.

McKeith, I., Mintzer, J., Aarsland, D., Burn, D., Chiu, H., Cohen-Mansfield, J., Dickson, D., Dubois, B., Duda, J.E., Feldman, H., Gauthier, S., Halliday, G., Lawlor, B., Lippa, C., Lopez. O.L., Machado, J.C., O'Brien, J., Playfer, J., Reid, W., on behalf of the International Psychogeriatric Association Expert Meeting on DLB (2004) Dementia with Lewy bodies. *Lancet Neurology* 3:19–28.

Mehler, M.F., Purpura, D.P. (2009) Autism, fever, epigenetics and the locus coeruleus. *Brain Research Reviews, 59*:388–392.

Mehta, M.A., Manes, F.F., Magnolfi, G., Sahakian, B.J., Robbins, T.W. (2004) Impaired set-shifting and dissociable effects on tests of spatial working memory following the dopamine D2 receptor antagonist sulpiride in human volunteers. *Psychopharmacology 176*: 331–342.

Minderaa, R.B., Anderson, G.M., Volkmar, F.R., Akkerhuis, G.W., Cohen, D.J. (1994) Noradrenergic and adrenergic functioning in autism. *Biological Psychiatry 36*:237–241.

Nakamura, K., Matsumoto, M., Hikosaka, O. (2008) Reward-dependent modulation of neural activity in the primate dorsal raphe nucleus. *Journal of Neuroscience 28*:5331–5343.

Narayanan, A., White, C.A., Saklayen, S., Scaduto, M.J., Carpenter, A.L., Abduljalil, A., Schmalbrock, P., Beversdorf, D.Q. (2010) Effect of propranolol on functional connectivity in autism spectrum disorder-a pilot study. *Brain Imaging and Behavior 4*:189–197.

Newhouse, P.A., Potter, A., Corwin, J., Lenox, R. (1992) Acute nicotinic blockade produces cognitive impairment in normal humans. *Psychopharmacology 108*:480–484.

Newhouse, P.A., Potter, A., Corwin, J., Lenox, R. (1994) Age-Related effects of the nicotinic antagonist mecamylamine on cognition and behavior. *Neuropsychopharmacology 10*:93–107.

Newman, L.A., McGaughy, J. (2008) Cholinergic deafferentation of prefrontal cortex increases sensitivity to cross-modal distractors during a sustained attention task. *Journal of Neuroscience 28*:2642–2650.

Paladini, C.A., Williams, J.T. (2004) Noradrenergic inhibition of midbrain dopamine neurons. *Journal of Neuroscience 24*:4568–4575.

Pederzolli, A.S., Tivarus, M.E., Agrawal, P., Kostyk, S.K., Thomas, K.M., Beversdorf, D.Q. (2008). Dopaminergic modulation of semantic priming in Parkinson disease. *Cognitive and Behavioral Neurology 21*:134–137.

Perry, E.K., Haroutunian, V., Davis, K.L., Levy, R., Lantos, P., Eagger, S., Honavar, M., Dean, A., Griffiths, M., McKeith, I.G., Perry, R.H. (1994) Neocortical cholinergic activities differentiate Lewy body dementia from classical Alzheimer's disease. *NeuroReport 5*:747–749.

Pessiglione, M., Czernecki, V., Pillon, B., Dubois, B., Schüpback, M., Agid, Y., Tremblay, L. (2005) An effect of dopamine depletion on decision-making: the temporal coupling of deliberation and execution. *Journal of Cognitive Neuroscience 17*:1886–1896.

Pitman, R.K., Sanders, K.M., Zusman, R.M., Healy, A.R., Cheema, F., Lasko, N.B., Cahill, L., Orr, S.P. (2002) Pilot study of secondary prevention of posttraumatic stress disorder with propranolol. *Biological Psychiatry 51*:189–192.

Ramos, B.P., Colgan, L.A., Nou, E., Arnsten, A.F.T. (2008) β2 adrenergic agonist, clenbuterol, enhances working memory performance in aging animals. *Neurobiology of Aging 29*:1060–1069.

Ramos, B.P., Colgan, L., Nou, E., Ovaria, S., Wilson, S.R., Arnsten, A.F.T. (2005) The beta-1 adrenergic antagonist, betaxolol, improves working memory performance in rats and monkeys. *Biological Psychiatry 58*:894–900.

Ratey, J.J., Bemporad, J., Sorgi, P., Bick, P., Polakoff, S., O'Driscoll, G., Mikkelsen, E. (1987) Brief report: open trial effects of beta-blockers on speech and social behaviors in 8 autistic adults. *Journal of Autism & Developmental Disorders 17*:439–446.

Robbins, T.W. (2007) Shifting and stopping: fronto-striatal substrates, neurochemical modulation and clinical implications. *Philosophical Transactions of the Royal Society B: Biological Sciences 362*:917–932.

Roesch, M.R., Calu, D.J., Schoenbaum, G. (2007). Dopamine neurons encode the better option in rats between deciding between differently delayed or sized rewards. *Nature Neuroscience 10*:1615–1624.

Roesch-Ely, D., Weiland, S., Scheffel, H., Schwaninger, M., Hundemer, H-P., Kolter, T., Weisbrod, M. (2006). Dopaminergic modulation of semantic priming in healthy volunteers. *Biological Psychiatry 60*:604–611.

Roozendaal, B., McReynolds, J.R., McGaugh, J.L. (2004). The basolateral amygdala interacts with the medial prefrontal cortex in regulating glucocorticoid effects on working memory impairment. *Journal of Neuroscience 24*:1385–1392.

Sarter, M., Bruno, J.P. (1997) Cognitive functions of cortical acetylcholine: toward a unifying hypothesis. *Brain Research Reviews 23*:28–46.

Sarter, M., Bruno, J.P. (2001) The cognitive neuroscience of sustained attention: where top-down meets bottom-up. *Brain Research Reviews 35*:146–160.

Sawaguchi, T., Goldman-Rakic, P.S. (1991) D1 dopamine receptors in prefrontal cortex: Involvement in working memory. *Science 251*:947–950.

Schultz, W. (2007). Multiple dopamine functions at different time courses. *Annual Review of Neuroscience 30*:259–288.

Selden, N.R., Gitelman, D.R., Salamon-Murayama, N., Parrish, T.B., Mesulam, M-M. (1998). Trajectories of cholinergic pathways within the cerebral hemispheres of the brain. *Brain 121*:2249–2257.

Silver, J.A., Hughes, J.D., Bornstein, R.A., Beversdorf, D.Q. (2004) Effect of anxiolytics on cognitive flexibility in problem solving. *Cognitive and Behavioral Neurology 17*:93–97.

Smith, A., Nutt, D. (1996) Noradrenaline and attention lapses. *Nature 380*:291.

Smith, R.M., Beversdorf, D.Q. (2008) Effects of semantic relatedness on recall of stimuli preceding emotional oddballs. *Journal of the International Neuropsychological Society 14*:620–628.

Smyth, S.F., Beversdorf, D.Q. (2007). Lack of dopaminergic modulation of cognitive flexibility. *Cognitive and Behavioral Neurology 20*:225–229.

Smyth, S.F., Beversdorf, D.Q. (in preparation) Muscarinic and nicotinic modulation of memory but not cognitive flexibility.

Stefani, M.R., Moghaddam, B. (2005) Systemic and prefrontal cortical NMDA receptor blockade differentially affect discrimination learning and set-shift ability in rats. *Behavioral Neuroscience 119*: 420–428.

Stickgold, R., Hobson, J.A., Fosse, R., Fosse, M. (2001) Sleep, learning, and dreams: off-line memory reprocessing. *Science 294*:1052–1057.

Takahashi, H., Takano, H., Kodaka, F., Arakawa, R., Yamada, M., Otsuka, T., Hirano, Y., Kikyo, H., Okubo, Y., Kato, M., Obata, T., Ito, H., Suhara, T. (2010) Contribution of dopamine D1 and D2 receptors to amygdala activity in humans. *Journal of Neuroscience 30*:3043–3047.

Tivarus, M.E., Hillier, A., Schmalbrock, P., Beversdorf, D.Q. (2008). Functional connectivity in an fMRI study of semantic and phonological processes and the effect of L-dopa. *Brain and Language 104*:42–50.

Usher, M., Cohen, J.D., Servan-Schreiber, D., Rajkowski, J., Aston-Jones, G. (1999) The role of locus coeruleus in the regulation of cognitive performance. *Science 283*:549–554.

Vaiva, G,, Ducrocq, F., Jezequel, K., Averland, B., Lestavel, P., Brunet, A., Marmar, C.R. (2003) Immediate treatment with propranolol decreases posttraumatic stress disorder two months after trauma. *Biological Psychiatry 54*:947–949.

van Stegeren, A.H., Everaerd, W., Cahill, L., McGaugh, J.L., Gooren, L.J.G. (1998). Memory for emotional events: differential effects of centrally versus peripherally acting β-blocking agents. *Psychopharmacology 138*:305–310.

Vikki, J. (1992) Cognitive flexibility and mental programming after closed head injuries and anterior and posterior cerebral excisions. *Neuropsychologia 30*:807–814.

Ward, M.M., Metford, I.N., Parker, S.D., Chesney, M.A., Taylor, C.B., Keegan, D.L., Barchas, J.D. (1983) Epinephrine and norepinephrine responses in continuously collected human plasma to a series of stressors. *Psychosomatic Medicine 45*:471–486.

Whitehouse, P.J., Price, D.L., Strubble, R.G., Clark, A.W., Coyle, J.T., DeLong, M.R. (1982) Alzheimer's disease and senile dementia—loss of neurons in the basal forebrain. *Science 215*: 1237–1239.

Williams, G., Goldman-Rakic, P. (1995) Modulation of memory fields by dopamine D1 receptors in prefrontal cortex. *Nature 376*:549–550.

Yerkes, R.M., Dodson, J.D. (1908) The relation of strength of stimulus to rapidity of habit-formation. *Journal of Comparative Neurology and Psychology 18*:458–482.

CHAPTER 15

Attractor Basins: A Neural Basis for the Conformation of Knowledge

A UNIFIED ACCOUNT OF PATTERNS OF LINGUISTIC IMPAIRMENT, MAGNITUDE ESTIMATION, AND HEMISPATIAL NEGLECT

Stephen E. Nadeau

Norman Geschwind (1965), in his landmark paper "Disconnexion syndromes in animals and man," demonstrated the power of knowledge of neuroanatomy in enabling us to understand the complex behavioral syndromes described by behavioral neurologists over the prior 100 years. This paper and his other work provided a major contribution to the astonishing cognitive neuroscience renaissance we have observed since. Since then, knowledge of neuroanatomy and neural systems has continued to advance, but not sufficiently rapidly to keep up with the blistering pace of advances in cognitive neuroscience borne of behavioral studies. In fact, knowledge of neural systems now lags so far behind that it now provides but a weak and uneven source of hypothesis generation in behavioral studies. For decades, behavioral studies have been driven either by substantially heuristic models (e.g., information processing models) or theoretical models developed without neuroscientific considerations (e.g., linguistics). Functional imaging studies have sought to fill this void, with only occasional success.

This chapter incorporates a field of science, parallel distributed processing (PDP)(McClelland, Rumelhart, & PDP Research Group, 1986), that is fully capable of filling this void. PDP can enable us to understand how complex behaviors can emerge from neural networks. PDP is a branch of the mathematics of chaotic systems (Gleick, 1987). Chaotic systems are systems in which order emerges from the interactions of large numbers of relatively simple units, each constrained only by its own relatively simple operational constraints. Most of the order we witness in the world is chaotic order, not deterministic order, whether it be in cloud patters, the function of ant colonies, the shape and organization of our organs, including our brains, or the evolution of species. In PDP, the units serve as counterparts to neurons or cortical neural micro-columns, and the constraints governing individual unit behavior are limited to the mathematics governing the generation and spread of unit activity and the modification of unit interconnectivity. With knowledge of neural systems now vastly expanded by the rapid growth of PDP science, we now have a renewed capacity for establishing a full dialectic between human subject studies and theory. A principal aim of this chapter will be to show how this is possible.

I will begin this chapter with some further elaboration of PDP models in general. This will be followed by discussion of a simple computational model that will provide the basis for understanding how concepts might be supported by neural structure. I will then expand on this in discussion of semantic memory, taking full advantage of what we have learned from research on semantic dementia. It will then be possible to understand how the broad principles delineated can be applied to other domains of language function, to be discussed, and indeed, to a broad array of knowledge domains. The latter sections of this chapter will use this background to consider psychophysical phenomena subsumed under Steven's power law of magnitude estimation and hemispatial neglect. One key underlying principle will bring unity to this diversity of knowledge and the behaviors related to it: the computational properties of the activation function of neural networks characterized by autoassociator structure, properties that yield attractor basins and attractor trenches. These concepts will be detailed in later sections.

This chapter will not be a simple review of the PDP-behavioral study dialectic in a number of different cognitive domains. Rather, it will focus on a paradox: on the one hand, the PDP properties of neural networks enable us to miraculously acquire large and apparently seamless domains of knowledge from a series of individual experiences; on the other hand, knowledge acquired in such a way comes with intrinsic limitations, limitations reflected in empirical findings involving broad array of cognitive processes.

The effect of genes on the knowledge stored in the brain appears to lie largely in their influence on the genesis of the neural scaffold upon which knowledge is accumulated. Knowledge itself is acquiredlargely through experience, as modifications of strengths of synaptic connections. In many ways, that knowledge is not veridical. For example, neural networks, in and of themselves, cannot reliably discriminate fact from inference—hence the phenomenon of false memories (Beversdorf et al., 2000).Information is far more likely to be encoded if it is consistent with existing mental models. Its recall, therefore, involves substantially revisionist processes. These phenomena reflect mechanisms that influence the correctness of individual memories. This chapter, however, will focus on limitations and distortions imposed by the neural representation of entire domains of knowledge. A prevailing theme will be that what we know is what we have experienced. Because of this, perceptions and concepts that fall at the margins of our direct experience, or beyond, may be processed differently than perceptions and concepts that are familiar to us. Furthermore, not all that we know is processed equally because all our knowledge is influenced by the frequency of our experience with it, the age at which we acquired it, and our familiarity with it—attributes that are also realized in the relative strength of the neural connections that instantiate the knowledge.

Parallel Distributed Processing

PDP models are neural-like in that they incorporate large arrays of simple units that are heavily interconnected with each other, like neurons in the brain. A PDP model that fully emulates neural network principles constitutes a hypothesis not just about the organization of cognitive processes, but also about neural organization. That hypothesis can then be tested in normal and brain-injured human subjects. The processing sophistication of PDP models stems from the simultaneous interaction of large numbers of units (hundreds or even thousands). The instantiation of short-term (working) memory (as patterns of unit activity) and long-term memory (as unit interconnection strengths) in the same neural nets that are responsible for processing further emulates brain function. PDP models are particularly appealing in the context of language processing because they involve simultaneous processing at a number of levels and locations, apparently mimicking what is going on in the brain. Finally, pure PDP models (models without incorporated digital devices) implicitly learn the rules governing the data they process in the course of their experience with that data (e.g., Plaut, McClelland, Seidenberg, & Patterson, 1996). Thus, in a pure PDP model of phonology, there is no need to build in specific structures to account for specific phonological phenomena. The structure of the model is defined entirely in terms of the domains of information accessible to it and the topographic relationship of these domains to each other. The absence of specific, ad hoc devices motivated by models (e.g., linguistic) designed to account for particular phonological phenomena in an orderly fashion is also crucial to the maintenance of neurological plausibility. In humans, as in PDP models, the phonological phenomena we observe reflect entirely the emergent behavior of the networks and the statistical regularities in the knowledge encoded within them.

PDP models incorporate explicitly defined assumptions that are "wired" into them in the mathematical details of their computer implementation. They produce large numbers of predictions that can be (and have been) empirically tested through observations of normal subjects and brain-damaged individuals. They have been remarkably successful in emulating the behavior of these subjects, and systematic analysis of the internal structure of these models has helped us to understand the network basis for behavior. PDP models exhibit properties of *graceful degradation* and probabilistic selection, that is, when damaged or fed noisy input, they do not produce novel or bizarre output unachievable by an intact network with good input; rather, they tend to produce output that is not so reliably correct but is rule-bound.

A Simple Computational Model of a Knowledge Domain

The nature of concept representations can be best illustrated by a particular model developed by David Rumelhart and his colleagues (Rumelhart, Smolensky, McClelland, & Hinton, 1986). This "rooms in a house" model was comprised of 40 "feature" units, each corresponding to an article typically found in particular rooms or an aspect of particular rooms. Each unit was connected with all the other units in the network—an attribute that defines the model as an *autoassociator network*. Autoassociator networks have the capacity for "settling" into particular states that define representations—states corresponding to *attractorbasins*. Connection strengths were defined by the likelihood that any two features might appear together in a typical house. When one or more units were clamped into the "on" state (as if the network had been shown these particular features or articles), activation spread throughout the model and the model eventually settled into a steady state, an attractor basin, that implicitly defined a particular room in a house. Thus, clamping "oven" ultimately resulted in activation of all the items one would expect to find in a kitchen and thereby *implicitly* defined, via a *distributed representation*, the concept of a kitchen. No kitchen unit *per se* was turned on. Rather, kitchen was defined by the pattern of feature units that were activated. Alternatively, we can say that the kitchen concept was population encoded. The network contained the knowledge, in the totality of its connections, that enabled this representation to be generated. The 40 unit model actually had the capability of generating distributed (population encoded) representations of a number of different rooms in a house (e.g., bathroom, bedroom, living room, study), sub-components of rooms (e.g., easy chair and floor lamp, desk and desk chair, window and drapes) and blends of rooms that were not anticipated in the programming of the model (e.g., clamping both bed and sofa led to a distributed representation of a large, fancy bedroom replete with a fireplace, television, and sofa).

This autoassociator model, simple though it is, has the essential attributes of a network that might be capable of generating the distributed representations of meaning underlying semantics. The brain's semantic autoassociator obviously is comprised of vastly more that 40 features, and enables an enormous repertoire of distributed representations corresponding to the vast number of concepts we are capable of representing—the topic of the next section.

Semantic Memory

Perhaps the best place to start in extrapolating the simple model of the previous section to the neural instantiation of semantic memory is with a dementing process that represents nearly a pure lesion of cortices supporting world knowledge: semantic dementia (Rogers, Ivanoiu, Patterson, & Hodges, 2006). Semantic dementia is associated with pathology that is maximal in the temporal poles but also involves lateral and inferior temporal cortices through much of their extent (Desgranges et al., 2007; Diehl et al., 2004; Grossman & Ash, 2004), albeit usually sparing the most posterior portions of temporal cortex (Lambon Ralph, Graham, & Patterson, 1999) associated with object gnosis, visual perceptual processes, and matching object images reflecting different views (Hovius, Kellenbach, Graham, Hodges, & Patterson, 2003; Rogers, et al., 2006). The regions of the brain that are most severely involved in semantic dementia are visual and auditory association cortices. Temporal polar cortex also provides a major associative link to the amygdala, a core structure of the limbic system. Both hemispheres are affected, but classically left hemisphere pathology is more severe. Semantic dementia is characterized by selective impairment in semantic memory with impoverished knowledge of objects and people, impaired semantic sorting, severe anomia in spontaneous language and naming to confrontation, severely reduced category fluency, and impaired spoken and written word comprehension (Hodges, Patterson, Oxbury, & Funnell, 1992; Rogers, et al., 2006). Perceptual skills and nonverbal problem solving skills are relatively spared, as are grammatic and phonologic function. Because so much of human knowledge of the world is based substantially upon visual and limbic attributes, the impact of semantic dementia on knowledge is pervasive. There may be some involvement of the perirhinal and anterior entorhinal cortex and the hippocampus in semantic dementia, but episodic memory and biographic knowledge are relatively preserved until late in the disease course.

Knowledge of objects and people is *implicitly* hierarchically organized. A broad superordinate category such as *animals* include many exemplars, of which *dogs* is one, and each exemplar may include a number of subordinate types: in the case of dogs, Labradors, German shepherds, poodles, etc. The items in each level of the hierarchy are defined by their characteristic features, and the lower the hierarchical level, the more features are required to define an item and the fewer the items that have the additional, more finely discriminating features. Thus, the category *animals* is for the most part defined by moderate size, four legs, head, eyes, ears, nose, and eating and sexual behavior. To define *dogs*, one must add features of warm blooded, carnivorous, furry, and complex social behavior. To define *Labrador*, one must add further features of black color, medium length hair, weight of 50—80 pounds, and retriever instincts—features shared by relatively few exemplars. The strength with which knowledge of objects and people is instantiated in the brain reflects frequency of exposure, age of knowledge acquisition, and familiarity effects. The resilience of knowledge in the face of disease processes reflects these factors interacting with the number of exemplars possessing a given feature.

Semantic dementia provides a *prima facie* case for neural representation of knowledge in terms of features because the degree to which knowledge of an item is attenuated is: 1) proportional to the number of features required to define that item, which in turn is dependent on the quantity of remaining connections in affected association cortices; and 2) inversely proportional to the strength of the connections between particular features, which is related to the number of concepts that share these features and the frequency with which these concepts are used (Devlin, Gonnerman, Andersen, & Seidenberg, 1998; Harm & Seidenberg, 2004; McClelland & Rumelhart, 1985; McRae, De Sa, & Seidenberg, 1997; Randall, Moss, Rodd, Greer, & Tyler, 2004). Items defined by relatively distinctive features, shared by fewer other items, and used less frequently (with accordingly less redundant interconnectivity) are more susceptible to the effects of pathology. Thus, knowledge supporting superordinate categories is relatively preserved, along with naming, comprehension of, and ability to sort items into these categories, whereas knowledge of subordinate categories is most severely affected (Hodges, Graham, & Patterson, 1995; Hodges, et al., 1992; Rogers et al., 2004; Woollams, Cooper-Pye, Hodges, & Patterson, 2008). Naming errors are either within category substitutions (e.g., hippopotamus for rhinoceros) or superordinate substitutions (e.g., animal for rhinoceros). Superordinate errors or prototype errors (e.g., "horse" for all large animals) become more common as the disease progresses (Hodges, et al., 1995). Low frequency exemplars are much more severely affected than high frequency exemplars (Hodges, et al., 1995; Hodges, et al., 1992), reflecting the relationship between frequency of occurrence in experience and the degree of redundancy with which knowledge borne of experience is encoded. Subjects with semantic dementia are often able to provide broad superordinate information about an object (e.g., an elephant is an animal) but are unable to answer more specific questions, e.g., about an elephant's habitat, size, peculiar features, or disposition (Hodges, et al., 1995). The performance of subjects with semantic dementia on animal drawing tasks is revealing (Bozeat et al., 2003) (see also see also subjectsstatus post herpes simplex encephalitis; Sartori & Job, 1988). Subjects with semantic dementia are very likely to omit features in their drawings in proportion to the severity of their dementia, and they are most likely to omit highly distinctive features, characterizing only one or a few exemplars. They are most likely to *add*features common to the domain. For example, when asked to draw a rhinoceros, the production typically resembles a pig, the distinctive horns and armor having been omitted because the underlying knowledge has been lost. When asked to draw a duck, the production may be a reasonable facsimile of a duck—except that it has four legs. Thus, as knowledge underlying discriminating features is lost, there is a tendency for all items at a given level of the knowledge hierarchy to assume the features of the prototype. Eventually, even knowledge of the prototype may be lost, relegating the subject to reliance on knowledge supporting the next higher level of the knowledge hierarchy.

The pattern of breakdown of semantic knowledge in PDP models precisely recapitulates the behavior of subjects with semantic dementia (Rogers, Lambon Ralph, Garrard, et al., 2004). The rooms in a house model of Rumelhart et al. (1986) was based on an autoassociator network comprised of 40 features. The activation function of an autoassociator neural network supporting semantic knowledge would be based on N features and be expressed in an N-dimensional hyperspace. By taking a 3-dimensional "slab" of the activity function, we can achieve some insight into its operation (Woollams, et al., 2008). Let us take the slab pertaining to animal knowledge. Because we are dealing with an autoassociator network, network activity corresponding to animals will tend to settle into a broad basin—an attractor basin, the central, lowest point of which corresponds to the "centroid" of animal knowledge—the representation of a creature that best defines our sense of animalness. Within the animal basin there are innumerable attractor sub-basins corresponding to specific animals. Very close to the centroid are sub-basins corresponding to animals likely to be very close to the centroid representation, e.g., dogs, cats, cows, horses, etc. Distant from the centroid are sub-basins corresponding to animals that are quite atypical, e.g., platypuses, sea gooseberries, and narwhales. Distance from the centroid is defined by the degree of atypicality (see also Kiran, 2007; Patterson, 2007; Woollams, et al., 2008). Within any given sub-basin, there may be sub-sub basins, e.g., corresponding to types of dogs. Within these sub-sub-basins may be sub-sub-sub-basins corresponding to types within types, or perhaps the Labrador that was our pet and generic Labradors. The depth of a basin, relative to that of its sub-basins, reflects the degree to which features are shared by the sub-basins within that basin. For example, the animal basin is deeper than the tool basin because animals, by and large, share many more features than tools.

The location of the various attractor basins within the semantic field reflects regularities in the knowledge of the relationships between concepts (which are defined by empirical associations between features), acquired through experience, hence the effects of frequency and age of acquisition. Similarities between items reflect the number of features they share. Frequency and age of acquisition also define the depth of sub-basins, simple (corresponding to single entities), and complex (corresponding to quasi-regular domains[1]), regardless of location. Semantic priming occurs to the extent that a stimulus engages features of a concept representation. The more superordinate a concept representation, the greater the number of subordinate representations it shares features with, and the larger the number of subordinate representations that will prime it.

The effect of lesions (focal or diffuse) will be to produce graceful degradation of network performance (Hodges, et al., 1992; Shallice, 1988; Warrington, 1975; Warrington & Shallice, 1984). Deep basins will become shallower and sub-basins, particularly those that are shallower and more distant from the centroid—corresponding to more atypical exemplars—will disappear (Woollams, et al., 2008). The deeper and therefore more resilient basins are defined by knowledge that is represented in neural connectivity with the greatest degree of redundancy, as a result of stronger connection strengths, which reflect frequency, age of acquisition, and familiarity effects (Hinton & Shallice, 1991; Hodges, et al., 1995; Rogers, Lambon Ralph, Garrard, et al., 2004). As sub-basins become shallow or disappear, responses will reflect the settling of the network into surviving neighbors located nearer the centroid—neighbors of higher typicality (yielding coordinate errors, e.g., horse in lieu of donkey); the parent basin (yielding superordinate errors, e.g., animal in lieu of donkey); or failure to settle at all, yielding omission errors (particularly likely to occur with more atypical exemplars that lack near neighbors). This is precisely what has been observed in semantic dementia (Woollams, et al., 2008).

Thus, it is apparent that two major factors impact the probability of retrieving semantic knowledge and the delay in retrieving it: atypicality and frequency. As Patterson (Patterson, 2007)has pointed out, the more atypical the exemplar—that is, the more distant it is from the attractor basin centroid—the less likely it is to be retrievable and the longer it will take to retrieve it. Generally, this atypicality effect dominates, but it can sometimes be mitigated by the presence of deep sub-basins, however atypical, corresponding to single entities or to quasi-regular domains of high frequency. For example, even though whales are atypical animals, because of their compelling features, not the least their size, intelligence, sociability, and history of interaction with man, they are frequently mentioned in discourse. For this reason, features of whales define a quasi-regular domain that provides the basis for a large deep sub-basin within the animal basin that is located rather far from the animal basin centroid. Variable atypicality, frequency, and age of acquisition, the majorfactors influencing sub-basin location and depth, characterize all domains of knowledge. These knowledge attributes, reflected in the attractor basin landscape, will provide the unifying threads in the discussions to follow.

In order to lay further groundwork for sections to follow, I will extend the attractor basin metaphor to pattern associator networks as the *attractor trench*. A pattern associator network is one that translates a representation in one domain, e.g., orthographic, into a representation in another domain, e.g., phonological. The PDP reading model developed by Plaut and colleagues is illustrative(Plaut, et al., 1996; Seidenberg & McClelland, 1989). The model was composed of three layers: 1) an input layer of 105 grapheme units grouped into clusters, the first cluster including all possibilities for the one or more consonants of the onset, the second cluster including all the possible vowels in the nucleus, and the third cluster including all possibilities for the one or more consonants in the coda; 2) a hidden unit layer of 100 units; and 3) an output layer of 61 phoneme units grouped into clusters, including all the possibilities for onset, nucleus, and coda, respectively (as for the graphemes). Local representations were used for the graphemes and phonemes. There were one-way connections from each of the grapheme input units to each of the hidden units, and two-way connections between each of the hidden units and each of the phoneme output units. Every output unit was connected to every other output unit, providing the network the autoassociator capability for "settling into" the best solution (as opposed to its own approximate solution). The model was trained using a mathematical algorithm (back propagation) that incrementally alters the strengths of connections in proportion to their contribution to the error, which is computed as the difference between the actual output of the network and the desired output. The orthographic representations of 3000 English single syllable words and their corresponding phonological forms were presented, one pair at a time, cycling repeatedly through the entire corpus. In this way, the model ultimately learned to produce the correct pronunciation of all the words it had read. One of the most striking things about the trained model is that it also was able to produce correct pronunciations of plausible English nonwords (i.e., orthographic sequences it had never encountered before). How was this possible?

One might have inferred that the model was simply learning the pronunciation of all the words by rote. If this had been the case, however, the model would have been incapable of applying what it had learned to novel words. In fact, what the model learned was the relationships between *sequences* of graphemes and *sequences* of phonemes that are characteristic of the English language. To the extent that there is a limited repertoire of sequence types, the model was able to learn it and then apply that knowledge to novel forms that incorporated some of the sequential relationships in this repertoire. The information the model acquired through its long experience with English orthographic-phonological sequential relationships went considerably beyond this, however, fully reflecting the statistical regularities in its experience. Certain sequences, those most commonly found in English single syllable words, were more thoroughly etched in network connectivity. Thus, the model was very fast with high frequency words. It was also very fast with words with an absolutely consistent orthographic-phonologic sequence relationship, e.g., words ending in *ust*, which are always pronounced /ʌst/ (*must, bust, trust, lust, crust,* etc.). The model encountered difficulty, reflected in prolonged reading latency, only with low frequency words (for which frequency cannot trump atypicality), and only to the extent that it had learned different, competing pronunciations of the same orthographic sequence. Thus, it was slow to read *pint* because in every case but *pint*, the sequence *int* is pronounced /Int/ (e.g., *mint, tint, flint, lint*). It was also slow, though not quite so slow, to read words like *shown* because there are two equally frequent alternatives to the pronunciation of *own* (*gown, down, town* versus *shown, blown, flown*). It was very slow with words that are unique in their orthographic-phonologic sequence relationship, e.g.,*aisle, guide* and *fugue*—i.e., highly atypical words. These behaviors precisely recapitulate the behavior of normal human subjects given reading tasks.

The knowledge the model acquires reflects competing effects of type frequency and token frequency. If a single word is sufficiently common (high token frequency), the model acquires enough experience with it that competing orthographic-phonologic sequential relationships have a negligible impact on naming latency. However, if a word is relatively uncommon (e.g., *pint*), its naming latency will be significantly affected by the knowledge of other words that, though equally uncommon, together belong to a competing type (e.g., *mint, flint, tint, sprint*).

The implicit knowledge of various sequence regularities captured by the model (and the brain), through experience, defines quasi-regular domains (precisely as with dogs or whales in semantic knowledge). For example, in the case of words ending in *own*, orthographic-phonologic regularity exists but it is only quasi-regular because there is not one but two alternatives (*shown* versus *gown*), a particular alternative being determined by the onset cluster. Quasi-regular domains may be composed of more or less equally competing subdomains, each corresponding to a regularity, as in the case of *own* words, or a domain that is regular but for a single member (e.g., *mint, tint, splint*, etc. versus *pint*). In some cases they may be fully regular (e.g., the *ust* words). The higher the frequency of a word and the stronger the connectivity between units involved in its production, the less its production is influenced by similarity to neighbors, and the more it approaches a regular domain that has only one member. Whether or not linguistic forms belong to particular quasi-regular domains depends upon the particular regularities that the network is endowed to capture through experience. When a neural network supporting a quasi-regular domain settles into the wrong state (the wrong sub-basin or sub-trench), the result is a paraphasic error: phonemic, verbal or semantic, but also morphologic (paragrammatic) or syntactic, depending on the network.

A pattern associator network linking two networks with autoassociator properties that supports sequence representations provides the basis for an attractor trench, which constitutes a translation pathway between the two autoassociator domains. Given a particular input pattern of activity (e.g., the orthographic representation), the pattern associator network will tend to settle into a trench, at the other end of which is the correct output pattern of activity (e.g., the corresponding phonological representation). Even a pattern associator network that incorporates knowledge of as many regularities as exist between English orthography and phonology yields an attractor trench landscape that is pretty drab—more like a plane riddled by gullies—compared with the complex sub-sub-basins within sub-basins within basins lunar crater-scape of semantics. Nevertheless, the same two major factors impact the probability of retrieving knowledge and the delay in retrieving it: atypicality (corresponding to distance from the centroid) and frequency (corresponding to trench/basin depth). For example, within the *int* trench, which corresponds to a quasi-regular domain, the sub-trench corresponding to */Int/* is both more typical and deeper because it provides the phonology for most English single syllable *int* words, whereas the sub-trench corresponding to */aint/* is atypical and shallow, corresponding to a single outlier *pint*.

Knowledge Underlying Other Domains of Language

WRITTEN FORCED CHOICE LEXICAL DECISION

Whether or not lexical decision depends upon access to semantics remains a subject of considerable debate. Rogers and colleagues (Patterson et al., 2006; Rogers, Lambon Ralph, Hodges, & Patterson, 2004) sought to address this question, and a related issue central to this chapter—the impact of atypicality on lexical decision—in an ingenious experiment. They created 72 stimulus pairs, each consisting of a word and a possible pseudo-homophone. For half of these pairs, the bigram and trigram frequency of the word was greater (e.g., cheese/cheize). For the other half, the bigram and trigram frequency of the nonword was greater (e.g., seize/seese)—that is, the orthography of the real word was atypical. Normal control subjects performed at ceiling and thus their performance could not address the question of what knowledge, orthographic or semantic, was being recruited to make the lexical decision. Subjects with semantic dementia performed nearly normally when the word representation was more orthographically typical than the nonword—that is, when their response could be guided by the most orthographically typical exemplar. However, when nonwords were more typical than words—that is, sub-basins corresponding to orthographic representations of words were substantially attenuated by disease because of their atypicality, their lexical decision performance fell and it was below chance among the most severely affected subjects for low frequency words/nonwords (there were significant atypicality and frequency effects and a significant atypicality by frequency interaction). The results of this experiment tell us that visual lexical decision can be made on the basis of orthographic representations and that, when these representations are damaged, as they are likely to be in semantic dementia because these networks are located in the inferior temporal lobes, atypicality effects (distance from the centroid of the attractor basin) and frequency effects (depth of attractor basins and sub-basins) become evident.

An alternative explanation, favored by Rogers et al. (Patterson, et al., 2006; Rogers, Lambon Ralph, Hodges, et al., 2004),is that normal attractor basins corresponding to atypical orthographic exemplars are insufficient to support lexical decision, particularly when the exemplars are low frequency, in which case the full extent of meaning representations must be accessed. In subjects with semantic dementia, these extended meaning representations are of course defective, impairing lexical decision. It was thought that because subjects with semantic dementia could read regular words as well as controls, and because the most clear-cut abnormalities on anatomic and functional imaging studies are in more anterior temporal lobe, their orthographic representations must have been intact. Importantly, whichever interpretation is correct, the results provide clear-cut evidence of atypicality, frequency, and atypicality by frequency interaction effects.

READING, SPELLING, AND VERB PAST TENSE PRODUCTION

Patterson and colleagues (Patterson, 2007; Patterson, et al., 2006) reported a pattern of performance by subjects with semantic dementia on three other tasks, reading, spelling, and verb past-tense production, that precisely recapitulates the pattern reported above with visual lexical decision. In all three of these domains, subjects demonstrated atypicality, frequency, and atypicality by frequency interaction effects.

Although performance in all three domains correlated highly with semantic performance, all three domains correspond to attractor trenches, rather than basins. Thus, in all three domains, performance with atypical exemplars, infrequent exemplars, and most particularly, atypical low frequency exemplars, corresponding to the shallowest attractor sub-trenches lying the farthest from the trench centroid, was most affected and in many cases, performance was at worse than chance levels. Furthermore, most errors represented slips into attractor sub-trenches closer to the centroid.

Reading aloud, spelling, and verb past-tense production can be accomplished without recourse to semantic representations, and indeed, it is only in these non-semantic routes that there exist quasi-regular domains containing both typical sub-domains near the trench centroid and atypical sub-domains corresponding to shallower sub-trenches distal from the centroid.Reading by the semantic route engages a pattern associator network that instantiates very few regularities (which define trenches and substrenches) because there is little relationship between orthography and phonology on the one hand, and word meaning on the other. Only reading by the phonologic route provides the opportunity to engage the complex attractor trench landscape of orthographic-phonologic regularities. The evidence suggests that the pathology of semantic dementia attenuates the shallow distal attractor sub-trenches, just as it does the shallow distal sub-basins. Notably, reading, spelling, and verb past-tense production all depend, at least in part, on temporal lobe networks that are at risk for the pathology underlying semantic dementia.

For reading, spelling, and verb past-tense production, low frequency *irregular* exemplarsare supported by both direct phonological pattern associator networks and pattern associator networks that include semantics. However, these low frequency irregular exemplars differentially rely on the semantic route, and therefore are differentially susceptible to degradation of semantic networks, because they do not derive benefit from the sequence regularities encoded in phonological pattern associator networks(Harm & Seidenberg, 2004; Nadeau, 2001; Plaut, et al., 1996; Rapcsak & Beeson, 2000; Seidenberg & McClelland, 1989; Woollams, Lambon Ralph, Plaut, & Patterson, 2007). To the extent that degradation of semantic networks occurs, it will produce a pseudo-atypicality/frequency effect—pseudo because the effect has nothing to do with the topography of attractor trenches supporting the quasi-regular domains of the phonological routes, but rather, owes to dissolution of semantic processing routes. However, direct, non-semantic routes also support processing of all words, regular and irregular, so even accepting the impact of disease on semantic route function, the results reviewed still provide evidence of atypicality, frequency, and atypicality by frequency interaction effects. The combined effects of attractor trench landscape and attenuation of the substrate for semantics provides the basis for the regularization errors observed in subjects with semantic dementia.

Patterson et. al. (2006) argued that because of the very high correlation between semantic impairment on the one hand and reading, spelling, and verb past-tense deficits on the other, the latter deficits were rooted in the semantic deficit. However, their argument seems to be undermined by the absence of quasi-regular domains in semantic reading, spelling, and verb-past tense production routes, as well as by a number of reported dissociations between reading, spelling, and verb past-tense production on the one hand, and semantic impairment on the other (reviewed in their paper).

These scientific issues remain incompletely resolved. However, whichever hypothesis is correct, these data provide strong evidence that atypicality and frequency define the attractor trench topography of reading, spelling, and verb past tense production. Output corresponding to distal, shallow sub-trenches may be defective, either because of attenuation of these sub-trenches, or because noisy, imprecise input generated from degraded semantic representations interferes with the settling of network activity into distal shallow trenches (Woollams, et al., 2007). Instead, the "ball" of network activity tends to tumble down the slope to deep parts of the trench, closer to the centroid.

The Conformation of Linguistic Knowledge

If linguistic knowledge, whether reflected in the attractor basins of semantic memory, or the attractor trenches underlying translation between forms via pattern associator networks, were represented in the brain in veridical fashion, all items of knowledge would be equally accessible. Thus, reaction time (RT) would be a constant, reflecting only generic processing speeds:

$$RT = k$$

and the probability of accessing an exemplar would be equal for all exemplars:

$$P(A) = q$$

However, we know from the foregoing that this is not correct. Reaction times, e.g., word reading times, are longer for normal subjects for highly atypical words (e.g., *aisle*), and they are prolonged when there are competing attractor sub-trenches/sub-basins within basins corresponding to quasiregular domains (e.g., *pint*versus*lint, tint, mint,* and *stint*) (Plaut, et al., 1996; Seidenberg & McClelland, 1989), for which the centroid of the trench lies closer to *lint* than to *pint*, rendering *pint* more atypical. Probability of a correct response declines with increasing atypicality and falling frequency, a phenomenon most apparent in disease states.

Rather, RT and P(A) are likely to be defined by equations of the following general form:

$$RT = \alpha e^{\beta(\text{atypicality/frequency})}$$

$$P(A) = \gamma e^{-\delta(\text{atypicality/frequency})}$$

Where α, β, γ, and δ are scaling factors, and atypicality and frequency ranges are such that β(atyp/frequency) and δ(atyp/frequency) are always ≥ 0. Equation 1 indicates that for exemplars that are low in atypicality and high in frequency, the exponent approaches 0, and because $e^0 = 1$, RT approaches its minimum, α. The higher the atypicality, the longer the RT, unless atypically is mitigated by frequency. By analogy, for low atypicality and high frequency, P(A) reduces to γ. P(A) drops with increasing atypicality, mitigated by frequency.

Although these equations may capture the general relationships of reaction time and probability of access to atypicality and frequency, they nevertheless represent an oversimplification, for a number of reasons:

1) To the extent that an attractor basin or trench is occupied by sub-basins and subtrenches, exemplars may be additionally susceptible to the atypicality/frequency trade-offs of these subregions in activity space.
2) Age of acquisition effects are also a factor with a degree of influence that is inversely proportional to the extent of regularities encoded in the domain (e.g., low in domains with substantial regularity, such as the orthographic-phonologic pattern associator, and high in domains that encode largely arbitrary relationships, e.g., the pattern associator linking word meaning to word sound (Lambon Ralph & Ehsan, 2006)).

3) Measuring the properties of a domain, e.g., semantics, may be confounded by the properties of networks that enable input to or output from that domain. An outstanding example is the basic level effect, which reflects the impact of experience and expertise on our choice of name for a given entity (Rogers & McClelland, 2004).Many people, on seeing a dog, would call it a *dog*. However, many would more often produce the name of the type of dog, e.g., *poodle* or *German shepherd*.Very few would respond *animal*. Basic level names, e.g., *dog* or *poodle,* do not bear a consistent relationship to frequency in word databases, though more often than not they are more frequent than more general or more specific terms. This is because they are substantially defined by personal experience and expertise. The basic level terms employed by a veterinarian might involve, for example, specific types of poodles. Basic level effects are also strongly reflective of age of acquisition (see above). Basic level effects interact with the properties of the semantic system. Because atypical exemplars (e.g., platypus)derive less benefit from semantic attractor basin effects, successful production of the name is more likely to reflect basic level effects. On the other hand, with semantic network damage, superordinate categories (e.g., animals) will have an advantage and will be preserved even as subcategories corresponding to basic level exemplars are lost. Basic level effects also reflect, in part, properties of the semantic system. Expertise affects not just frequency of use of particular terms, but also degree of differentiation in semantic networks.

The pattern of knowledge representation and its attractor basin/attractor trench counterpart detailed here for language characterize a broad range of knowledge domains and can be regarded as a unifying principle for understanding not just cognitive butmany psychophysical functions. This will be the subject of the next section.

Psychophysics and Stevens' Power Law

INTRODUCTION

Perception is defined by the interaction of afferent sensory input and existing knowledge represented as neural connection strengths in sensory association cortices. Knowledge reflects what has been deemed important by the nervous system. Kilgard and Merzenich (1998) provided a dramatic demonstration of this in an ingenious experiment. Microstimulation electrodes were implanted in the nucleus basalis of rats. The nucleus basalis provides the entire cholinergic projection to the cortex. Its extensive afferent input from the limbic system (Sarter & Bruno, 1997), which defines subjective value,translates into cholinergic bursts to the cortex that signal which neural activity is important and should lead to modification of neural connectivity—the instantiation of knowledge. Acetylcholine delays the closing of a potassium channel, thereby prolonging the influx of calcium through NMDA voltage gated sodium/calcium channels, and it acts at a metabotropic receptor to release calcium from intracellular stores. The resultant transient increases in intracellular calcium enable the molecular biologic processes that alter synaptic connection strengths. During the training period, all of the rats were exposed daily to a frequently repeated sound stimulus, e.g., a 9 kHz tone, of no intrinsic behavioral importance. In half the rats, the tone was accompanied by brief stimulation of nucleus basalis, which, by transiently increasing cortical extracellular acetylcholine and hence intracellular calcium, assured that the tone was learned. At the conclusion of the training period, the tonotopic organization of the primary auditory cortex was mapped. In the rats that *did not* receive nucleus basalis stimulation, primary auditory cortex was characterized by the normal systematic array of tonal responsivity ranging from 1 kHz to 64 kHz—there had been no alteration in pre-existing cortical auditory knowledge. In the rats that *did* receive nucleus basalis micro-stimulation, the organization of the primary auditory cortex had been profoundly altered such that it exhibited tonal responses solely to frequencies in the 9±4 kHz range, that is, to the narrow range of frequencies that had been designated important by nucleus basalis stimulation. Thus, even in the domain of auditory perception, which involves a primary sensory cortex that one might have thought would be hard-wired, the knowledge represented had been transformed to reflect the regularities of experience and the value attached to that experience.

Absent such ingenious contrivances as the Kilgard and Merzenich experiment, knowledge constraining perception reflects the experiences of daily life accumulated over a lifetime. Typicality corresponds to perceptual dimensions that are most shared by the entities we have lived with.[2] This knowledge, derived of experience, is instantiated in cortical connectivity in various sensory domains andis the basis for network activity functions characterized by attractor basin properties. Stimuli near the centroids of these basins are likely to be perceived in nearly veridical fashion. Stimuli at the high end (e.g., high pitch, loud sounds, long lines) are likely to be perceived as falling at or near the highest magnitude stimulus ever experienced, characteristic of few, if any, of the entities we have lived with, leaving a substantial probability that these stimuli will be underestimated. Stimuli at the very low end (low pitch, quiet sounds, very short lines) are likely to be perceived as falling at or near the lowest end ever experienced, also characteristic of few entities we have lived with, leaving a substantial probability that they will be overestimated. This has been shown in line length judgment tasks (Hollingworth, 1909; Mennemeier et al., 2005; Tegnér & Levander, 1991; Worth & Poppel, 1988).In attractor basin terms, stimuli falling at or beyond the margins of experience are likely to elicit representations closer to the centroid of the basin.

This qualitative conceptualization corresponds directly to well-studied principles of psychophysics. In a series of influential papers, Stevens (1957, 1970) argued that magnitude estimation in a wide variety of domains can be characterized by a function of the form:

$$\Psi = kS^n$$

where Ψ is the perceived magnitude, S is the actual magnitude, n an exponent that varies from domain to domain, and to a lesser degree, from individual to individual, and k is a scaling factor. If $n = 1$,

$$\Psi = kS$$

and all stimuli are perceived with equal accuracy, modified only by the "skewing" factor, k, which impacts perception at the extremes precisely as it impacts perception in the heavily experienced middle (see below for possible implications). If $n < 1$, the equation yields progressively greater underestimation at the high end. For example, if $n = 0.5$ and $k = 1$,

for $S=1$, $\Psi = 1$
for $S=2$, $\Psi = 1.414$, a 29.3% underestimate,
and for $S = 10$, $\Psi = 3.162$, a 68.4% underestimate.

The attractor basin slope at the low end need not obey the same function as the slope at the high end. However, if the units of measurement are chosen such that the value of S at the centroid is 1, then we can see that the equation above defines the perceptual attractor basin properties discussed above—overestimation at the low end as well as underestimation at the high end. Thus, for $n = 0.5$ and $k = 1$,

for $S = 0.5$, $\Psi = 0.707$, a 41% overestimate,
and for $S = 0.1$, $\Psi = 0.316$, a 316% overestimate, whereas
for $S = 1$, $\Psi =1$ and perception is veridical.

The discussion here has focused on magnitude estimation. However, there are other methods of probing the role of atypicality in perception, most notably reaction time as a function of stimulus intensity (Neumann & Niepel, 2004).

The tendencies to overestimation at the low end and underestimation at the high end might be, and have been, construed as representing merely regression to the mean: because statistically, low-end stimuli occur exclusively in the context of higher/larger stimuli, they are likely to be overestimated, and by the same token, high-end stimuli are likely to be underestimated. Regression to the mean may indeed be an experimental factor but this explanation has difficulty accounting for the variability in the shape of attractor basins governing magnitude estimation, which vary enormously from one sensory domain to another (see below).

Stevens simply accepted the regression effect as a ubiquitous factor that led to underestimation of the exponent of the magnitude estimation power functions (Stevens, 1970). In fact, the impact of the regression effect on the exponent is quite small (Algom & Marks, 1990).

QUALIFICATIONS

Our goal so far has been to establish a plausible, principled relationship between the psychophysical phenomena of magnitude estimation and cortical network structure and function. Psychophysics is now a vast and complicated field, substantially dominated by the work of mathematical psychologists (e.g., Stevens) who have sought to define mathematical models that accurately account for empirical observations. With rare exceptions, however, these models have not been informed by knowledge of neural structure. Consequently, there has not been a neural network theory-behavioral study dialectic: neither the models nor the experiments have been able to benefit from knowledge of neural networks, nor have the models and experiments served to inform us about neural network mechanisms. The ideas proposed here may serve as a beginning of a solution to this problem. However, the neural model proposed above is far too simple to have a chance of accounting for the vast range of psychophysical phenomenology, even in the field of magnitude estimation. In the following, I will briefly discuss some of the most important qualifying factors.

The Exponent

Stevens (1970)estimated the exponent of the power function defining magnitude estimation in a variety of stimulus domains (Table 15.1). Notably, for a number of domains the value of the exponent is >1. The attractor basin model cannot account for exponents >1 because this would mean that the magnitude of response to atypical stimuli would be greater than that for typical stimuli. Four hypotheses can be offered to account for this:

1) Sub-basin effects (see below).
2) Context effects (see below).
3) Effects of interactions of two or more cortical domains engaged in the estimation process.
4) Effects of cortical, subcortical, brainstem, spinal cord, or peripheral receptor processes that serve to magnify response to stimuli at the extremes (e.g., the disproportionate responses to edges by the visual system).

There is no reason to presume that any given magnitude estimation power function is the product of the properties of a single sensory transducer or neural system, and in fact, the evidence is to the contrary. The exponents (some positive and some

Table 15.1 **Magnitude estimation power function exponents (Stevens, 1970)**

Sensory Domain	*Exponent*
Loudness	0.67
Brightness	0.33–0.5
Smell	0.6
Taste	1.3–1.4
Temperature	1.0–1.5
Vibration	0.6–0.95
Visual length	1.0
Visual area	0.7
Duration	1.1
Finger span	1.3
Pressure on palm	1.1
Heaviness	1.45
Force of handgrip	1.7
Vocal effort	1.1
Electric shock	3.5
Tactual roughness	1.5
Tactual hardness	0.8
Angular acceleration	1.41

negative, adding and subtracting) reflect the multiple sequential and interacting stages of neural processing that occur in every sensory modality (see Stevens, 1970). The point to be made here is that, whatever the peripheral, subcortical, and primary cortical processing, components of perception taking place in association cortices, which are likely constrained by attractor basin dynamics and hence characterized by an exponent <1, may provide useful insight into many experimental results, including magnitude estimation, but also hemispatial neglect, which is overwhelmingly associated with cortical lesions, to be discussed in the next section.

Sub-Basin Effects

Attractor basin dynamics defined by cortical networks supporting magnitude estimation are just as likely to be influenced by sub-basin effects as are those associated with semantic function. Line length can be taken as a useful example. All of us have particularly extensive experiences with line lengths characteristic of objects in peripersonal space. Thus, we are likely to have an attractor sub-basin corresponding to this subdomain of experience and the knowledge acquired from it. All of us also have substantial experience with a range of longer lines encountered in our experience within our homes and offices—the basis for another attractor sub-basin. Some people, possibly pilots, may have extensive experience of very long lines, defining yet another attractor sub-basin, but also illustrating a potential source of individual variability in magnitude estimation.

Context Effects

To this point, I have dealt with attractor basins as if the neural network structure (the knowledge base) underling them were static. This is unlikely to be the case, even though underlying knowledge must exert powerful constraining forces. Context effects might act to alter the boundaries of attractor basins, to shift the centroid, or to alter the location of sub-basins relative to the centroid. There are at least four possible ways by which the neural networks defining attractor basins might be at least transiently altered in experimentally important ways:

1) Learning: Even though the human brain and experimental neural networks exhibit age of acquisition effects, without question the knowledge stored in neural network connectivity can be significantly altered at any age by intensive atypical experience. Connectivity within cortical networks can be directly altered in this way, or it can be indirectly altered through changes in multi-synaptic cortical-hippocampal–cortical loops instantiating episodic memory (Alvarez & Squire, 1994; McClelland, McNaughton, & O'Reilly, 1995; Rolls & Treves, 1998; Squire & Zola-Morgan, 1991).Experiential effects may also occur through procedural learning (practice effects), which is instantiated independently of hippocampal systems. Atypical experience may occur over long periods of time or quite acutely (everything sounds quiet on leaving a rock concert). Acute experience may include experience of the experimental paradigm itself.
2) Implicit memory: recent experience leaves temporary traces in network connectivity that define implicit memory—memory that is not consciously accessible but is revealed as "guilty knowledge" in appropriately constructed experiments (Bauer, Grande, & Valenstein, 2003).
3) Working memory: any stimulus automatically leads to a briefly sustained pattern of network activity or network bias that defines working memory. Furthermore, certain experimental paradigms may lead to characteristic patterns of volitional engagement of selected networks, instantiating working memory, which may be prolonged. This phenomenon may account for expectancy and top-down processing effects. Episodic memory, implicit memory, and working memory can potentially account for the effects of response to one stimulus on response to a subsequent stimulus.

4) Concurrent stimuli or their absence. Neural network activity reflects the response of the network, with its incorporated knowledge, to a particular stimulus. However, that activity pattern may be different if there is a concurrent stimulus in the same domain, or in different domains when there is synesthesia. What we know about particular sensory stimuli is typically acquired in variously noisy environments. Exposure to a particular stimulus in the context of a different environment (e.g., a carefully controlled lab) may elicit a somewhat different response.

These four mechanisms have the effect of transiently distorting attractor basins. To illustrate this effect, taking an example from grammar, consider the sentence "the cute bunny attacked the vicious pit bulls." Although we all have a trenchant idea of what cute bunnies are, and this idea will not receive any long term alteration by having read this sentence, for a brief period of time, our cute bunny attractor basin will reflect engagement of features we do not normally associate with cute bunnies. Recent or concurrent stimuli will have an analogous distorting effect on attractor basins related to magnitude estimation. Attractor basin distortion effects on magnitude estimation should be within stimulus modality except to the extent that the ancillary stimulus may have synesthetic effects (e.g., the impact of loud/soft or high/low pitched noise; soft/sharp or hot/cold somatosensory stimulation; or sweet/bitter taste on line length estimation).

Given the number of neural mechanisms that potentially influence magnitude estimation, it is hardly surprising that the study of magnitude estimation has proven to be extraordinarily challenging. The mechanisms discussed potentially provide the basis for context effects that have been the focus of particular interest among psychophysicists (e.g.,Sarris, 2004). It is to be hoped that explicit consideration of these mechanisms may lead us beyond purely empirical approaches to psychophysical modeling, and in turn empower psychophysical modeling to further inform us of specific brain mechanisms. More generally, these considerations serve to emphasize the somewhat ephemeral and non-veridical nature of much of what we "know."

Hemispatial Neglect

Hemispatial neglect is defined by the failure to attend to, orient towards, or respond to stimuli in the contralesional hemispace (Heilman, Watson, & Valenstein, 2003). There may be underlying attentional or intentional deficits (Na et al., 1998). The focus here will be on attention. Attention is the process of focusing sensory resources upon one single stimulus. It involves selective engagement of neural networks in relevant sensory association cortices. Normal individuals exhibit a subtle left-right gradient in attention, as revealed, for example, in a tendency to bisect lines very slightly off center, usually to the left (Milner, Brechman, & Pagliarini, 1992), although not all studies agree (Mennemeier, et al., 2005).In subjects with hemispatial neglect, this gradient is much steeper, leading to behavior that is clearly different in the two horizontal hemispaces, but also to a gradient within each hemispace (Butter, Mark, & Heilman, 1989).

The behavioral consequences of a horizontal gradient in attention can usefully be considered in the attractor basin terms that have been the focus of this paper, and corresponding mathematic interpretation in terms of a power law. In this conceptualization, impaired attention corresponds to a reduction in the depth of attractor basins instantiating perception. Because all representations are affected equally, representations of atypical exemplars (at the high and low extremes) are lost entirely and the breadth of attractor basins is reduced as well. As previously noted, normal subjects overestimate short lines and underestimate long lines, consistent with attractor basin dynamics. Reduction in attractor basin breadth as a result of the attentional impairment associated with hemispatial neglect would be expected to exaggerate this tendency. This has been shown (Mennemeier, Vezey, Lamar, & Jewell, 2002; Tegnér & Levander, 1991). The effect of attenuation of attention should impact attractor basins associated with all cognitive and perceptual processes. As evidence of this, Chatterjee (1995) found that subjects with hemispatial neglect and neglect dyslexia tended to read long letter strings, words or nonwords, as shorter than their objective length and short letter strings as longer than their objective length.

With reduced attention in the left hemispace (as in typical hemispatial neglect), long lines to the left of midline will be differentially underestimated, leading to rightward line bisection errors. Furthermore, as discussed above for magnitude estimation, short lines will be overestimated, with the result that at some point, as lines to be bisected become shorter and shorter, the overestimation should lead to a cross-over effect, in which the line is bisected to the left of center. This, a repeatedly observed but somewhat mysterious phenomenon (Tegnér & Levander, 1991), has also been demonstrated in a test of center estimation in rectangular spaces (Mennemeier, Rapcsak, Dillon, & Vezey, 1998). It depends only upon there being some degree of hemispheric asymmetry in spatial attention. Because normal subjects typically exhibit a subtle asymmetry, usually favoring the left, it could be anticipated that they would demonstrate a crossover effect in which at some point, with very short lines, they should bisect to the right of center. This has now been demonstrated empirically (Jewell & McCourt, 1999; McCourt & Jewell, 1999; Mennemeier, et al., 2005). Expectably, subjects with left hemisphere lesions also demonstrate a crossover effect, but in a direction opposite to that seen in subjects with right hemisphere lesions (Mennemeier, et al., 2002). Because line length estimation and line bisection are driven by the same basic mechanisms, errors on line length estimation are strongly correlated with bisection errors (Mennemeier, et al., 2002). Because attentional impairment and its effects on attractor basin characteristics are greater in subjects with right hemisphere lesions and hemispatial neglect than in subjects with left hemisphere lesions and neglect, both line estimation errors and bisection errors are greater in subjects with left hemispatial neglect (Mennemeier, et al., 2002). Because alterations in attractor basins are at the heart of the line bisection behavior exhibited by subjects with hemispatial neglect, one might expect to see comparable behavior in other domains of perception involving magnitude estimation. This has been borne out in a study by Chatterjee, Ricci, & Calhoun (2000), in which subjects with hemispatial neglect exhibited both a tendency to underestimate the weight of objects held in the left hand relative to objects held simultaneously in the right hand, and a crossover effect.

The position of lines in egocentric space would be expected to have complex effects on long-line bisection behavior in subjects with hemispatial neglect. This is because, added to attractor basin effects, there are two attentional gradient effects: 1) a right-to-left declining gradient of attention related to neglect; and 2) a near midline-to-far-from-midline declining gradient corresponding to reduced attention to stimuli and portions of lines in the periphery (Werth 1988, cited in Werth & Pöppel, (1988). In the left hemispace, both gradients favor rightward bisection errors for long lines, plus the attenuation of attention related to neglect is greatest in left hemispace. In the right hemispace, the neglect-related attentional gradient is less, favoring less extreme rightward bisection errors, and the peripheral attentional reduction favors leftward bisection errors. This has been born out in empirical studies (Mennemeier, Rapcsak, Pierce, & Vezey, 2001). Because most normal subjects tend to bisect lines slightly to the left of center (Milner, et al., 1992), reflecting a subtle declining left to right attentional gradient, one would expect a tendency to behavior opposite to that observed in subjects with left hemispatial neglect, albeit with smaller deviations due to the more subtle right-left attentional gradient. This too has been substantially borne out (Mennemeier, et al., 2001). The magnitude of peripheral attenuation of attention, particularly on very long lines, relatively little studied, is a source of uncertainty.

Simple reduction in attractor basin depth due to impaired attention should correspond to a reduction in the constant, k, of the power law equation. In fact, on average k is slightly elevated in subjects with hemispatial neglect (Chatterjee, Mennemeier, & Heilman, 1994). However, reconsideration of the power function in logarithmic terms:

$$\text{Log}\,\Psi = n \log S + \log k$$

reveals that k is entirely an artifact of the units chosen to represent S—that is, in practice it truly is merely a scaling constant. If S were scaled such that S=1 corresponded to the centroid of the attractor basin (the "optimal stimulus" of Mennemeier and colleagues (Mennemeier, et al., 1998)), as discussed above, k would be related to the depth of the attractor basin. It is uncertain to what extent damage to visuospatial representations themselves in subjects with hemispatial neglect contributes to alteration of the scaling constant and the exponent. If attentional impairment differentially affects atypical stimuli (stimuli peripheral to the centroid of the attractor basin), perhaps by reducing signal-to-noise ratio, then one would expect reduction in the exponent of the power law, which has been reported (Chatterjee, et al., 1994; Mennemeier, et al., 2005; Mennemeier, et al., 2002). The theory propounded here is fundamentally congruent with the orientation/estimation hypothesis of Mennemeier, Chatterjee and colleagues (Mennemeier, et al., 2005). It differs only in its attempt to relate behavior not just to posited neuropsychological mechanisms but to underlying neural network function.

As discussed in the section on psychophysics and Stevens' Power Law, attractor basins may be altered in various ways by context effects. Marshall, Lazar, Krakauer, & Sharma (1998)performed an interesting experiment on context effects on line bisection by subjects with neglect that rather directly tests the central tenets of the theory proposed here. They had subjects bisect lines of various lengths alone and subsequently admixed with an equal number of "reference lines" of a single length. Bisection of an isolated line is guided solely by knowledge acquired through experience (which defines the attractor basin dimensions and location of the centroid), perverted of course by the impact of the attentional gradient. However, recent or concurrent experience can transiently alter the dimensions of a basin. The voice of a soft-spoken companion may seem barely audible during or immediately after the rock concert but overloud in the confines of a quiet apartment. Repeated recent experience with a shorter line would tend to push the longer bisection target to the long side of the centroid and potentiate rightward bisection errors. Repeated recent experience with a longer line should shift a short bisection target to the short side of the centroid, reduce rightward bisection errors, and potentiate crossover. This is exactly what Marshall and colleagues observed.Ricci & Chatterjee (2001) replicated these results. They also showed that the crossover effect is not purely a context effect—it is seen only with absolutely short lines and not simply relatively short lines. This finding fully accords with the theory developed here: the crossover effect is founded in attractor basin properties, which reflect a lifetime of knowledge gained of experience, and therefore is only somewhat susceptible to the effects of recent experience.

Cueing, e.g., by having subjects place the pencil point at one end of a line before bisecting it, would be expected to reduce the attentional gradient (e.g., left cueing in subjects with left hemispatial neglect) or increase the attentional gradient (e.g., right cueing in subjects with left hemispatial neglect). If this effect is multiplicative, the impact of cueing would be expected to be substantial in subjects with large baseline gradients and small in those with minimal gradients (e.g., normal subjects). Both hypotheses have been supported (Mennemeier, et al., 2005). Similar effects were seen on the magnitude of the crossover effect in subjects with left hemispatial neglect. In experiments in which subjects observe a line for a period of time and then bisect an imaginary line of similar length starting at the left or the right end, the impact of attentional gradients on performance should be attenuated and performance should become predominantly a function of magnitude estimation biases. All subjects should overestimate short lines, leading to rightward errors when starting from the left and leftward errors when starting from the right. All subjects should underestimate long lines (leading to leftward errors when starting from the left and rightward errors when staring from the right. These effects should be exaggerated in subjects with reduced attractor basin breadth, e.g., those with left hemispatial neglect. These predictions have also been substantially born out in empirical studies (Mennemeier, et al., 2005).

Conclusion

Concept representations likely have a major influence on all processes involving the cerebral cortex, whether they involve traditional knowledge domains such as semantics, or domains perhaps viewed heretofore as entirely perceptual and/or attentional, such as magnitude estimation and line bisection. Research on PDP models over the past 30 years has revolutionized our understanding of the neural network basis of concept representations. Wedding this research to cognitive neuropsychological studies of subjects with language disorders has been instrumental to our current understanding of the key role played by autoassociator networks and associated attractor basin and attractor trench dynamics, and most particularly, to appreciation of the particular importance of atypicality and frequency in defining robustness of knowledge and the patterns of performance breakdown in normal and brain-injured subjects. The fundamentally PDP nature of neural networks confers the enormous power to assemble continuous knowledge domains from series of individual experiences, but this comes at a cost: knowledge around the edges (high atypicality, low frequency) is fragile and susceptible to systematic distortions. In this chapter, I have tried to show that the approach taken here, inspired by discoveries involving language, has considerable explanatory value in relating magnitude estimation and hemispatial neglect to neural network behavior and considerable power to explain the results of empirical studies. The results provide substantial evidence that this approach has broad applicability to processes based in association cortices and offers a powerful means for strengthening the dialectic between behavioral studies and principles of neural network function.

Notes

1. A quasi-regular domain is a domain that corresponds to two or more closely related entities. Dogs constitute a quasi-regular domain because, while we would all agree on what a dog is, there is enormous variability in the range of characteristics that define different breeds of dogs. In contrast, for most of us, zebras constitute a regular domain.

2. This definition of typicality might seem to be dangerously close to frequency, and certainly typicality and frequency are correlated. However, typicality, when it comes to perceptual domains, is better understood as commonality. Just as atypicality and frequency can be uncoupled in semantics, as in the case of whales, typicality and frequency can be uncoupled in perception, as in the case of white noise, which characterizes nothing we live with (i.e., is atypical), but is a familiar and instantly recognized irritation generated by radios and televisions without a signal (i.e., is frequent).

References

Algom, D., & Marks, L. E. (1990). Range and regression, loudness scales, and loudness processing: toward a context-bound psychophysics. *Journal of Experimental Psychology: Human Perception and Human Performance, 16,* 706–727.

Alvarez, P., & Squire, L. R. (1994). Memory consolidation and the medial temporal lobe: a simple network model. *Proceedings of the National Academy of Sciences, 91,* 7041–7045.

Bauer, R. M., Grande, L., & Valenstein, E. (2003). Amnesic disorders. In K. M. Heilman & E. Valenstein (Eds.), *Clinical Neuropsychology* (pp. 495–573). New York: Oxford University Press.

Beversdorf, D. Q., Smith, B. W., Crucian, G., Anderson, J., Keillor, J., Barrett, A., et al. (2000). Increased discrimination of "false memories" in autism spectrum disorder. *Proceedings of the National Academy of Sciences, 97,* 8734–8737.

Bozeat, S., Lambon Ralph, M. A., Graham, K. S., Patterson, K., Wilkin, H., Rowland, J., et al. (2003). A duck with four legs: investigating the structure of conceptual knowledge using picture drawing in semantic dementia. *Cognitive Neuropsychology, 20,* 27–47.

Butter, C. M., Mark, V., & Heilman, K. M. (1989). An experimental analysis of factors underlying neglect in line bisection. *Journal of Neurology, Neurosurgery and Psychiatry, 51,* 1581–1583.

Chatterjee, A. (1995). Cross-over, completion and confabulation in unilateral spatial neglect. *Brain, 118,* 455–465.

Chatterjee, A., Mennemeier, M., & Heilman, K. M. (1994). The psychophysical power law and unilateral spatial neglect. *Brain and Cognition, 25,* 92–107.

Chatterjee, A., Ricci, R., & Calhoun, J. (2000). Weighing the evidence for cross over in neglect. *Neuropsychologia, 38,* 1390–1397.

Desgranges, B., Matuszewski, V., Piolino, P., Chétat, G., Mézenge, F., Langeau, B., et al. (2007). Anatomical and functional alterations in semantic dementia: a voxel-based MRI and PET study. *Neurobiology of Aging, 28,* 1904–1913.

Devlin, J. T., Gonnerman, L. M., Andersen, E. S., & Seidenberg, M. S. (1998). Category-specific semantic deficits in focal and widespread brain damage: a computational account. *Journal of Cognitive Neuroscience, 10,* 77–94.

Diehl, J., Grimmer, T., Drzezga, A., Riemenschneider, M., Förstl, H., & Kurz, A. (2004). Cerebral metabolic patterns at early stages of frontotemporal dementia and semantic dementia. A PET study. *Neurobiology of Aging, 25,* 1051–1056.

Geschwind, N. (1965). Disconnexion syndromes in animals and man. *Brain, 88,* 237–294, 585–644.

Gleick, J. (1987). Chaos: Making a New Science. New York: Viking.

Grossman, M., & Ash, S. (2004). Primary progressive aphasia: a review. *Neurocase, 10,* 3–18.

Harm, M. W., & Seidenberg, M. S. (2004). Computing the meanings of words in reading: cooperative division of labor between visual and phonological processes. *Psychological Review, 111,* 662–720.

Heilman, K. M., Watson, R. T., & Valenstein, E. (2003). Neglect and related disorders. In K. M. Heilman & E. Valenstein (Eds.), *Clinical Neuropsychology* (4th ed., pp. 296–346). Oxford: Oxford University Press.

Hinton, G. E., & Shallice, T. (1991). Lesioning an attractor network: investigations of acquired dyslexia. *Psychological Review, 98*, 74–95.

Hodges, J. R., Graham, N., & Patterson, K. (1995). Charting the progression in semantic dementia: implications for the organization of semantic memory. *Memory, 3*, 463–495.

Hodges, J. R., Patterson, K., Oxbury, S., & Funnell, E. (1992). Semantic dementia. Progressive fluent aphasia with temporal-lobe atrophy. *Brain, 115*, 1783–1806.

Hollingworth, H. L. (1909). The indiference point. In H. L. Hollingworth (Ed.), *The Inaccuracy of Movement.* New York: Science Press.

Hovius, M., Kellenbach, M. L., Graham, K. S., Hodges, J. R., & Patterson, K. (2003). what does the object decision task measure? Reflections on the basis of evidence from semantic dementia. *Neuropsychology, 17*, 100–107.

Jewell, G., & McCourt, M. E. (1999). Pseudoneglect: a review and meta-analysis of performance factors in line bisection tasks. *Neuropsychologia, 38*, 93–110.

Kilgard, M. P., & Merzenich, M. M. (1998). Cortical map reorganization enabled by nucleus basalis activity. *Science, 279*, 1714–1718.

Kiran, S. (2007). Complexity in the treatment of naming disorders. *American Journal of Speech-Language Pathology, 16*, 18–29.

Lambon Ralph, M. A., & Ehsan, S. (2006). Age of acquisiton effects depend on the mapping between representations and the frequency of occurrence: empirical and computational evidence. *Visual Cognition, 13*, 928–948.

Lambon Ralph, M. A., Graham, K. S., & Patterson, K. (1999). Is a picture worth a thousand words? Evidence from concept definitions by patients with semantic dementia. *Brain and Language, 70*, 309–335.

Marshall, R. S., Lazar, R. M., Krakauer, J., & Sharma, R. (1998). Stimulus context in hemineglect. *Brain, 121*, 2003–2010.

McClelland, J. L., McNaughton, B. L., & O'Reilly, R. C. (1995). Why there are complementary learning systems in the hippocampus and neocortex: insights from the successes and failures of connectionist models of learning and memory. *Psychological Review, 102*, 419–457.

McClelland, J. L., & Rumelhart, D. E. (1985). Distributed memory and the representation of general and specific information. *Journal of Experimental Psychology: General, 114*, 159–188.

McClelland, J. L., Rumelhart, D. E., & PDP Research Group. (1986). *Parallel Distributed Processing.* Cambridge, MA: MIT Press.

McCourt, M. E., & Jewell, G. (1999). Visuospatial attention in line besection: stimulus modulation of pseudoneglect. *Neuropsychologia, 37*, 843–855.

McRae, K., De Sa, V. R., & Seidenberg, M. S. (1997). On the nature and scope of featural representations of word meaning. *Journal of Experimental Psychology: General, 126*, 99–130.

Mennemeier, M., Pierce, C. A., Chatterjee, A., Anderson, B., Jewell, G., Dowler, R., et al. (2005). Biases in attentional orientation and magnitude estimation explain crossover: neglect is a disorder of both. *Journal of Cognitive Neuroscience, 17*, 1194–1211.

Mennemeier, M., Rapcsak, S. Z., Dillon, M., & Vezey, E. (1998). A search for the optimal stimulus. *Brain and Cognition, 37*, 439–459.

Mennemeier, M., Rapcsak, S. Z., Pierce, C., & Vezey, E. (2001). Crossover by line length and spatial location. *Brain and Cognition, 47*, 412–422.

Mennemeier, M., Vezey, E., Lamar, M., & Jewell, G. (2002). Crossover is not a consequence of neglect: a test of the orientation/estimation hypothesis. *Journal of the International Neuropsychological Society, 8*, 107–114.

Milner, A. D., Brechman, M., & Pagliarini, L. (1992). To have and halve not: an analysis of line bisection judgments in normal subjects. *Neuropsychologia, 30*, 515–526.

Na, D. L., Adair, J. C., Williamson, D. J., Schwartz, R. L., Haws, B., & Heilman, K. M. (1998). Dissociation of sensory-attentional from motor-intentional neglect. *Journal of Neurology, Neurosurgery and Psychiatry, 64*, 331–338.

Nadeau, S. E. (2001). Phonology: A review and proposals from a connectionist perspective. *Brain and Language, 79*, 511–579.

Neumann, O., & Niepel, M. (2004). Timing of "perception" and perception of "time." In C. Kaernbach, E. Schröger & H. Müller (Eds.), *Psychophysics beyond Sensation. Laws and Invarients of Human Cognition* (pp. 245–269). Mahwah, NJ: Lawrence Erlbaum Associates.

Patterson, K. (2007). The reign of typicality in semantic memory. *Philosophical Transactions of the Royal Society, B, 362,* 813–821.

Patterson, K., Lambon Ralph, M. A., Jefferies, E., Woollams, A. M., Jones, R., Hodges, J. R., et al. (2006). "Presemantic" cognition in semantic dementia: six deficits in search of an explanation. *Journal of Cognitive Neuroscience, 18,* 169–183.

Plaut, D. C., McClelland, J. L., Seidenberg, M. S., & Patterson, K. (1996). Understanding normal and impaired word reading: computational principles in quasi-regular domains. *Psychological Review, 103,* 56–115.

Randall, B., Moss, H. E., Rodd, J. M., Greer, M., & Tyler, L. K. (2004). Distinctiveness and correlation in conceptual structure: behavioral and computational studies. *Journal of Experimental Psychology: Learning, Memory, and Cognition, 30,* 393–406.

Rapcsak, S. Z., & Beeson, P. M. (2000). Agraphia. In S. E. Nadeau, L. J. Gonzalez Rothi & B. Crosson (Eds.), *Aphasia and Language. Theory to Practice* (pp. 184–220). New York: Guilford Press.

Ricci, R., & Chatterjee, A. (2001). Context and crossover in unilateral neglect. *Neuropsychologia, 39,* 1138–1143.

Rogers, T. T., Ivanoiu, A., Patterson, K., & Hodges, J. R. (2006). Semantic memory in Alzheimer's disease and the frontotemporal dementias: a longitudinal study of 236 patients. *Neuropsychology, 20,* 319–335.

Rogers, T. T., Lambon Ralph, M. A., Garrard, P., Bozeat, S., McClelland, J. L., Hodges, J. R., et al. (2004). Structure and deterioration of semantic memory: a neuropsychological and computational investigation. *Psychological Review, 111,* 205–235.

Rogers, T. T., Lambon Ralph, M. A., Hodges, J. R., & Patterson, K. (2004). Natural selection: the impact of semantic impairment on lexical and object decision. *Cognitive Neuropsychology, 21,* 331–352.

Rogers, T. T., & McClelland, J. L. (2004). *Semantic Cognition. A Parallel Distributed Processing Approach.* Cambridge: MIT Press.

Rolls, E. T., & Treves, A. (1998). *Neural networks and brain function.* New York: Oxford University Press.

Rumelhart, D. E., Smolensky, P., McClelland, J. L., & Hinton, G. E. (1986). Schemata and sequential thought processes in PDP models. In J. L. McClelland, D. E. Rumelhart & the PDP Research Group (Eds.), *Parallel distributed processing* (Vol. 2, pp. 7–57). Cambridge, MA: MIT Press.

Sarris, V. (2004). Frame of reference models in psychophysics: a perceptual-cognitive approach. In C. Kaernbach, E. Schröger & H. Müller (Eds.), *Psychophysics behond Sensation. Laws and Invariants of Human Cognition* (pp. 69–88). Mahwah, NJ: Lawrence Erlbaum Associates.

Sarter, M., & Bruno, J. P. (1997). Cognitive functions of cortical acetylcholine: Toward a unifying hypothesis. *Brain Research Reviews, 23,* 28–46.

Sartori, G., & Job, R. (1988). The oyster with four legs: a neuropsychological study on the interaction of visual and semantic information. *Cognitive Neuropsychology, 5,* 105–132.

Seidenberg, M. S., & McClelland, J. L. (1989). A distributed, developmental model of word recognition and naming. *Psychological Review, 96,* 523–568.

Shallice, T. (1988). *From Neuropsychology to Mental Structure.* Cambridge: Cambridge University Press.

Squire, L. R., & Zola-Morgan, S. (1991). The medial temporal lobe memory system. *Science, 253,* 1380–1386.

Stevens, S. S. (1957). On the psychophysical law. *Psychological Review, 64,* 153–181.

Stevens, S. S. (1970). Neural events and the psychophysical law. *Science, 170,* 1043–1050.

Tegnér, R., & Levander, M. (1991). The influence of stimulus properties on visual neglect. *Journal of Neurology, Neurosurgery and Psychiatry, 54,* 882–887.

Warrington, E. K. (1975). The selective impairment of semantic memory. *Quarterly Journal of Experimental Psychology, 27*, 635–657.

Warrington, E. K., & Shallice, T. (1984). Category specific semantic impairments. *Brain, 107*, 829–854.

Werth, R., & Pöppel, E. (1988). Compression and lateral shift of mental coordinate systems in a line bisection task. *Neuropsychologia, 26*, 741–745.

Woollams, A. M., Cooper-Pye, E., Hodges, J. R., & Patterson, K. (2008). Anomia: a doubly typical signature of semantic dementia. *Neuropsychologia, 46*, 2503–2514.

Woollams, A. M., Lambon Ralph, M. A., Plaut, D. C., & Patterson, K. (2007). SD-squared: on the association between semantic dementia and surfact dyslexia. *Psychological Review, 114*, 316–339.

Worth, R., & Poppel, E. (1988). Compression and lateral shift of mental coordinate system in a line bisection task. *Neuropsychologia, 26*, 741–745.

CHAPTER 16

Plasticity

Victor W. Mark

Introduction

In recent years clinical studies that have stop imputed neurologic plasticity, or neuroplasticity, have become rampant. The topic has cachet in both the scientific literature and the popular press,[1] in reaction to the long held but now diminishing perception that the adult central nervous system (CNS) is either incapable or at best minimally capable of intrinsic modification and repair. The original reasons for such an inflexible and pessimistic view of the nervous system were never clear. After all, adults routinely learn new names, games, faces of colleagues, routes to work, and motor skills such as using chopsticks. Indeed, it has long been recognized that with advancing age adults significantly improve their vocabulary.[2] Given that an adult''s skills can improve with practice in so many ways, how could such phenomena possibly occur except from substantial modification of the nervous system? Furthermore, in view of the considerable learning that can occur in healthy adults—albeit with less efficiency than in juveniles and children—it is surprising that such a faculty was long considered beyond the reach of individuals who had become disabled by acute brain injury, despite their often showing gradually relearned neurologic functions such as speech or walking during inpatient rehabilitation. Indeed, this author has found that some of his physical and occupational therapy co-workers would routinely reject the pleas of stroke patients to be hospitalized to train their motor deficits if they had been more than a month post-injury, even if they had never had a rehabilitation trial in the first place. The explanation given was that they would likely be too set in their often maladaptive ways to benefit. (No credible citations were provided upon request to support these denials of care.)

However, considerable experimental work in the past several decades demonstrates that the adult human is indeed capable of substantial neuroplasticity and moreover that this can be harnessed for functional benefit following disabling neurologic illness. This chapter will review the historical background that, first, undermined confidence in adult neuroplastic reorganization and, second, supported its occurrence. However, before reviewing the foundations and extent of our modern understanding, first a clarification for how the term ""plasticity"" will be used.

The term plasticity is widely used imprecisely and inconsistently.[3, 4] It has been applied to diverse phenomena that included behavioral changes without specifying their neurobiological substrates, alterations in synaptic conductivity, differences in regional brain activation either between clinical populations or longitudinally within individuals following specific interventions, or use-dependent CNS morphological changes identified from either microscopic or *in vivo* neuroimaging investigations. Because this chapter describes neurobiological changes that are impressive and contrary to the standard wisdom concerning the inflexibility of the nervous system, particularly in adult humans, the emphasis will be on anatomically large-scale changes in CNS activity or structure. Furthermore, we will specify such changes in the adult and particularly following a considerable change in the individual''s experiences, either as a result of training or reduction in activity.This is termed *use-dependent plasticity.* Such anatomically described physiologic or structural changes, moreover, should *persist* (if not permanently) after the termination of the change in activity.[5] These neuroplastic changes thus are enduring rather than elastic.

The case for neurological stasis in the adult

In the neurological literature one seldom finds an overt declaration that the adult CNS cannot or does not change with experience. And yet, over and over, literature reviews have indicated that this was the common understanding for much of the 20th century.[4, 6–10] In retrospect the situation resembles an unverified rumor, one that ""everybody knew"" but which nonetheless was seldom put into writing and supported by credible citations. Here and there, though, one may find such intimations. For example, in the first edition of the venerable Adams and Victor text *Principles of Neurology,* one reads without attribution that after the onset of disabling stroke, ""whatever motor paralysis remains after 5 to 6 months will probably be permanent.""[11] A similarly bleak forecast appears in Church and Peterson''s text.[12] Such statements were probably correct with regard to standard care in the 20th century. They also implied an inalterable hopelessness that, coming from major textbooks, likely discouraged serious academic challenge. Such was the case despite numerous reports across the first part of the century that indicated the substantial malleability of hemiparesis in humans that could follow various interventions.[13–17] Apparently, such studies escaped common notice or their methods and outcomes were so unorthodox as not to merit consideration. Ruch and Fulton''s physiology text at least acknowledged that hemiplegia could improve with training, but only as a result of compensatory actions by ""unaffected"" muscles and not through any neurological repair.[18] Again, no citations were provided. Other general neurological texts from the 20th century simply avoided discussing altogether the patterns or prospects for neurologic recovery after CNS injury. This practice was in keeping with the emphasis of much of medicine at the time, which was devoted to the manifestations, pathobiological bases, and management of acute illness, but had little or nothing to say about the long-term consequences of disease. So dismal was the situation that neurologists were mocked with the slogan ""diagnose and *adios*","" to indicate that their practical skills were of little value.

The 20th century Zeitgeist that discredited neurologic remodeling, repair and recovery in the adult probably arose not from one particular influence but instead from the cumulative contributions of a variety of investigations that appeared to cohere to and thus reinforce this view. The following sources most likely contributed:

1) *The functional mapping of the cerebral cortex* was largely inaugurated by the studies of Paul Broca, French neuroanatomist and anthropologist who in the 1860s posited that the left third frontal convolution is the ""seat"" of articulate language, following his seminal post-mortem investigation of the chronically aphasic inpatient ""Tan.""[19] Broca did not comment on the capacity for aphasia to recover, and therefore in the assault on neuroplasticity he is blameless. (Indeed, it has been noted that Broca had ascribed the differences in head circumferences between medical students and nurses to their different amounts of training![20]) However, Broca''s publications inspired a new viewpoint, which held that from localizing sharply demarcated and solitary cerebral injuries in adults in regard to their subsequent effects on specific neurologic functions, one could establish a cartography of normal cognitive function in the nervous system. Following similarly meticulous clinicopathological investigations of subsequent European investigators, a veritable patchwork quilt of neurologic functions became stitched onto the cerebral cortex (notable examples are reviewed by Heidi Roth in this volume). Thus, one inferred that the functions that were mapped from the lesion technique represented a fixed and predictable arrangement for all humans,[21] regardless of potentially modifying factors (e.g., level of education, handedness, cultural background, or history of prior neurologic injury).

This mapping of functions to structure was reinforced in the early 20th century by the *in vivo* cortical stimulation research of the American neurosurgeon Harvey Cushing, who determined in humans that a narrow vertical motor strip lies immediately anterior to the Rolandic fissure and a similarly narrow somatosensory strip just behind it. In artistry that presaged the conservative vs. liberal contrasts of latter-day American politics, Cushing colored the motor area red and the somatosensory area blue, and the twain did not overlap. This convention thereafter became the norm in neurosurgery textbooks. The simplification withstood the contemporary challenges by other investigators that indicated a substantial anatomical overlap between motor and somatosensory areas in the human cerebral cortex.[22] Finally, yet another milestone in the history of human brain mapping came with the surgical investigations of Wilder Penfield. While at Montreal, Penfield determined that Cushing''s sensory and motor cortices could be subdivided into respective "homunculi," miniature inverted mannequins draped along the brain''s lateral convexity that elongated parts of the body as if seen in a funhouse mirror, in proportion to their contribution to either tactile resolution or precision movements.[23] Penfield himself was blameless in the popular promulgation of a fixed correspondence between structure and function, aware as he was not only of the considerable inter-individual variation in the somatotopical charts that were derived from cortical stimulation studies, but also that such mapping could change *within* the individual from pre- to post-surgery.[24] (Later research showed that the homunculus could change simply by inducing transient ischemia to the arm.[25]) Nonetheless, so persuasive were the graphic depictions of the mapmakers that by the mid-20th century the conventional teaching held that cerebral real estate comprised a motley arrangement of multiple, non-overlapping functional districts segregated by inflexible boundaries, corresponding to specific cognitive and perceptual abilities or somatosensory and motor somatotopical maps, despite contemporary reports indicating that such inflexibility and non-overlap were not the rule.

2) *Doubt for the existence or functional value of cerebral regeneration.* The Spanish Nobel Prize laureate and histologist Santiago Ramón y Cajal initially held that the adult CNS does not undergo plastic reorganization. Cajal, whose microscopic investigations established that the neuron is the fundamental cellular unit of the nervous system,[26] determined that sectioned peripheral nerves could regenerate. He agreed with the orthodox view at the time among histologists that regeneration within the adult CNS was not possible. However, his later research suggested to him that post-injury axonal sprouting could occur within the adult CNS but had no adaptive value.[27] However, Cajal also speculated that use-dependent axonal and dendritic sprouting could be fundamental to normal cognitive maturation, although such changes would diminish during the lifespan of the individual.[28] In retrospect, Cajal''s bivalent views on structural neuroplasticity are confusing,[27] and later investigators either did not appreciate or disregarded his diverse opinions on the existence and value of post-natal CNS structural plasticity.[29]

3) The concept of a *critical period for plastic reorganization* became established in the 20th century. Among its prominent contributors was the Yale experimental neuroscientist Margaret Kennard. Her research in the 1930s-1940s on monkeys found that recovery of motor function after focal cortical ablation was greater in infants than in adults,[30] which became known as the ""Kennard principle."" Subsequent research by other investigators doubted the general consistency or validity of this principle.[31-33] Nonetheless, the basic theory, while not excluding use-dependent relearning in brain-injured adults, has considerably influenced experimental and clinical opinion to the present day concerning the relative abilities of adults vs. children to recover from acute brain injury[34] and thus may have dampened optimism for functional recovery after CNS injury in adults. In contrast, however, as a kind of anti-Kennard principle, the Nobel Prize-winning work of the Harvard visual system neurobiologists David Hubel and Torsten Wiesel in the 1960s-1970s found that the temporary deprivation of light input to one eye of kittens at a certain age would more likely cause permanent degeneration along the associated visual pathway and depressed physiologic responsiveness of associated visual cortical areas, compared to older cats treated the same way.[35] This finding considerably discouraged later investigators from any hope for use-dependent functional recovery following permanent CNS injury.[10]
4) *Disbelief in post-natal neurogenesis.* Early in the 20th century Cajal had declared that neurogenesis does not occur in the adult mammalian brain.[4] This pessimism was reinforced decades later by the failure of Pasko Rakic at Yale University in the 1980s to find evidence for cerebral neurogenesis in adult monkeys, despite numerous attempts.[36, 37] So persuasive were these negative findings, and Rakic''s influence, that earlier positive findings of other neuroscientists were widely disregarded.[38-40]

The turning of the tide: investigations in support of adult neuroplasticity

Although a surge in research interest in neurologic plasticity occurred in the final third of the 20th century (summarized below) and continues to the present, numerous historical reviews indicate that speculation on CNS plasticity in the adult extended as far back as late in the 19th century, including discussions by William James, Eugenio Tanzi, and Ernest Lugaro, among others.[5, 41, 42] However, the pivotal 20th century figure in inspiring wide acceptance for plastic reorganization in the brain was the Canadian experimental psychologist Donald Hebb of Dalhousie University. Hebb was impressed by anatomical reports of fiber tract loops in the brain, which led him to suggest that neuronal signals could be amplified in physiological feedback loops and thus could maintain a percept after removal of the original stimulus.[43] This foundation inspired Hebb''s landmark 1949 text *The Organization of Behavior,*[44] which postulated that ""cell assemblies"" exist in the brain that are fundamental for learning specific associations between stimuli. Neuronal assemblies that initially were tapped to process a particular stimulus were subsequently reinforced to strengthen their activations. Such neural enhancement occurred either morphologically by synaptic growth or physiologically by changing the efficacy of synaptic conduction. In turn, such enhanced neural activity could allow the generalization of percepts following exposure to a restricted set of stimuli (e.g., recognizing that geometric shapes differing only in size are essentially the same shape) without requiring the burdensome recruitment of additional neurons for every different stimulus encountered.

For much of the mid-20th century, learning was widely considered to occur through such postulated excitatory synaptic activation. Later modifications in the theory for a synaptic basis for learning invoked inhibitory synapses in neural circuitry as well. Subsequent empirical findings on longterm potentiation were consistent with Hebb''s hypotheses.[45]

At Berkeley in the 1960s, Mark Rosenzweig, Edward Bennett, and colleagues showed that immersion of rats in spatially challenging environments could increase brain mass, even with exposure confined to adulthood.[9] The increased brain mass that followed training coincided with increased cholinesterase but reduced acetylcholinesterase activity per unit volume of cortex. This observation suggested to these investigators that the histological changes were from elements low in acetylcholine, including non-cholinergic neurons, glia, and blood vessels.[20] Structural changes from exposure to such enriched environments were later shown to include thickened occipital cortex, gliosis, synaptogenesis, dendritic arborization,[46] and even new neurons in the hippocampus.[47]

A major impetus to the study of experience-dependent adult neuroplasticity was the plethora of somatotopic cortical mapping studies in the late 20th century performed in rats and primates following various forms of experimental neurologic injury or tactile training. In 1971 Patrick Wall and M. David Egger at University College, London, reported that they had unexpectedly found that the thalamic somatotopic map in rats had remarkably changed several days to weeks after unilateral nucleus gracilis ablation, such that the forelimb representation had expanded and invaded the territory formerly inhabited by the now deafferented hindlimb.[48] Subsequently, Michael Merzenich and colleagues at the University of California at San Francisco and John Donoghue and Jerome Sanes and colleagues at the National Institutes of Health (NIH) and Brown University commenced a large series of studies in monkeys and rats on the changes in somatotopical sensory maps within the brain following manipulations such as peripheral denervation, digit amputation, surgical fusion of digits, and practice at tactile discrimination (summarized in Mark and Taub[49]).

These basic neuroscience studies set the stage for non-invasive investigations of use-dependent neuroplasticity in humans. Alon Mogilner and colleagues at New York University in 1993 demonstrated with magnetoencephalography the individuation of the receptive fields of the fingers on one hand following the surgical relief of congenital syndactyly (fusion of the fingers).[50] At the same time, Alvaro Pascual-Leone and Fernando Torres at the NIH found significantly enlarged digital maps overlying somatosensory cortex based on evoked potential recordings when stimulating the scanning fingers of blind individuals who were proficient with reading Braille, compared to the fingers of the opposite hand and the hands of control subjects.[51] These and numerous other clinical studies that followed established that use-dependent changes in somatosensory function in humans could be identified by using various forms of non-invasive cortical mapping.

Further advances soon followed that indicated that efficacious physical therapy for chronic post-stroke hemiparesis was associated with significantly changed cortical motor representations of the paretic hand. These studies, based on the work of Edward Taub of the University of Alabama at Birmingham (UAB) and affiliated laboratories, utilized Constraint-Induced Movement therapy (CI therapy), a treatment developed by Taub that promotes sustained improved use of a chronically hemiparetic extremity.[52] In the late 1990s several studies from this group showed that CI therapy significantly alters hand representations based on neuroelectric source localization and transcranial magnetic stimulation mapping.[53–55]

While the foregoing studies used various physiologic imaging methods, advances in quantitative *structural in vivo* neuroimaging on MRI have further supported the idea of use-dependent neuroplasticity. Early in the present century studies that used voxel-based morphometry from quantitative structural MRI suggested that the brain''s grey matter can increase in healthy individuals with activities such as proficient taxi driving, juggling, and studying for examinations.[56-58] Work by our laboratory at UAB extended these structural discoveries for the first time to stroke patients, finding that grey matter can significantly increase in bilateral sensorimotor cortices and the hippocampi after only 2 weeks of CI therapy.[59] The histologic basis for such use-dependent changes in humans has not yet been established. Candidates include angiogenesis, gliosis, dendritic arborization, and possibly even neuronal mitosis (i.e., neurogenesis).[60]

After considerable debate, late in the 20th century the scientific consensus finally accepted that neural progenitor cells (sometimes termed stem cells) can undergo mitosis in the cerebrum of human adults. This consensus was based on a post-mortem study of terminally ill cancer patients who had undergone the antemortem infusion of bromodeoxyuridine, a thymidine analog that labels dividing cells with an immunofluorescent marker.[61]Thus far, neuronal generation in the adult mammalian CNS has been found only in the hippocampus, the olfactory bulb,[62] and the spinal cord.[63] Although use-dependent neurogenesis has not so far been confirmed in humans *in vivo*,[64] recent MRI research indicates that exercise in humans can augment regional cerebral blood flow in the adult human dentate gyrus, which would be expected to occur following the induction of focal neurogenesis and angiogenesis.[65] Therefore, we may not be far from having the *in vivo* confirmation of use-dependent focal neurogenesis in adult humans.

Implications of neuroplasticity for understanding the neurologically-impaired individual

The foregoing findings imply that the human CNS is constantly modified in response to persisting environmental or internal challenges, changes, or pressures. In this way it behaves like other ""systems"" of the natural world, such as ecosystems (e.g., populations" gene pools changing following environmental upheavals) or the solar system (e.g., the orbit of a body becoming thrown off course by the close approach of another, massive body). Furthermore, spontaneous modifications in the adult CNS can be functionally adaptive. For example, the brain"s plasticity can mitigate the damaging effects of a large cerebral infarction. Thus, Marcel Kinsbourne showed in 1971 that the speech of adults with aphasia following left cerebral infarction became much worse by transient inactivation of the right hemisphere with intracarotid sodium amobarbital. This suggested that the right hemisphere had compensated for acute language impairment prior to the barbiturate infusion.[66] In another example, functional imaging research by Maurizio Corbetta and colleagues showed that left unilateral spatial neglect in humans after right cerebral infarction was initially associated with relative left hemispheric overactivity during spatial tasks.[67] However, after several months this interhemispheric functional asymmetry was significantly reduced during the same tasks, coinciding with reduced spatial neglect. Thus, the findings suggested that the spontaneous anatomical shift over time in the activation of surviving brain regions that mediated directional spatial attention could ameliorate acute spatial neglect. In still another example, recent findings from our laboratory at UAB have demonstrated that *chronic* cerebral infarction size does not predict the severity of motor deficits in patients, in contrast to the majority of studies that report that *acute* infarction size *does* predict concurrent clinical status.[68] We postulate that long-term reorganization in the surviving CNS permits at least partial recovery from the initially damaging volumetric effects of acute cerebrovascular injury.

The ameliorating effects of neuroplastic reorganization following CNS disease may be maximal when the spatial extent of a focal illness progresses slowly over an extended period. Neurologists commonly recognize that slowly growing brain tumors are either clinically silent or at least subdued compared to acute infarctions at the same location and size.[21,69] A recent study of a right-handed man with a progressive left frontotemporal glioma demonstrated a gradual shift of metabolic activity over several years toward the right hemisphere with only minimal effects on language.[70] This suggests that intact parts of the brain when given enough time can functionally compensate for the effects of focal chronic injury, perhaps through unmasking previously suppressed functions. The spinal cord in humans similarly adapts to slowly compressive lesions.[71]

However, not all neuroplastic responses are adaptive. For example, acute spinal cord injury can gradually induce severe, enduring, and spontaneous electric shock-like sensations in the dermatomes affected by the level of injury. The mechanism of such ""neuropathic pain"" is not well understood but is currently believed to reflect the disinhibition or over-excitation of pain-associated pathways from the site of injury.[72] The delayed appearance and progression of limb hypertonia, or spasticity, can involve severe and very disabling flexor spasms triggered by mild tactile stimulation and often follows paralyzing acute, congenital, or degenerative CNS injury (e.g., stroke, traumatic brain injury, spinal cord injury, cerebral palsy, multiple sclerosis[73]). Spasticity, at least following acute CNS injury, is believed to reflect neuroplastic reorganization of reflex pathways.[74] Within the same individual, spasticity can even be both adaptive and maladaptive. Thus, spasticity following hemiparetic stroke can help to stabilize the paretic leg during walking and transfers, while at the same time its involvement in the ipsilateral upper extremity can hinder functional activities.[75] Another disorder that suggests maladaptive plasticity is chronic tinnitus (the noxious experience of a constant high-pitched auditory tone, or ""ringing in the ears""), which is associated with tonotopic remapping of the auditory cortex in humans.[76] The mechanism that incites tinnitus and such reorganization is not understood. Recent research suggests that repetitive transcranial magnetic stimulation to the temporal cortex can ameliorate the symptom.[77] Finally, numerous reports have indicated that in professional musicians, focal hand dystonia (the inability of the main performing hand to play a specialty instrument) is associated on magnetoencephalography with significantly altered somatosensory maps of the digits of the affected hand compared to the opposite hand.[78] This is believed to result from overuse of the performing hand. Such maps in turn can be normalized by a controlled therapeutic program of individuated finger exercises over an extended period, with simultaneous improvement of the dystonia.[78]

Thus, neuroplastic responses to CNS injury or illness can either be ameliorative or detrimental. It is unclear why biological processes that repair neurological injury may in many instances (particularly after spinal cord injury) extend suffering and thus inhibit functional activities. It seems that such responses lack sufficient feedback to adjust the strength or quality of their reparative processes. In this way, neuroplastic responses are like autoimmune responses, which can control somatic infections but can also have punishing effects when they fail to distinguish between intruders and one''s own tissues, as for example when

Guillain-Barré syndrome follows bacterial or viral exposure.[79] Another example is scar formation in the skin, which for minor penetrating injuries conveniently excludes infection or toxins, but after more severe injuries such as extensive burns can lead to disabling contractures.[80]

As the above examples from tinnitus and performance dystonia suggest, however, therapists can directly harness neuroplastic mechanisms to improve function in the neurologically impaired individual. As a result, illnesses or conditions that formerly were thought to have little prospect for clinical improvement at the hands of therapists have instead been shown to respond favorably to specific practice regimens. As noted above, post-stroke hemiparesis, at least if it is mild or moderate, can significantly improve with one such approach, CI therapy. Similarly, an adaptation of CI therapy (Constraint-Induced Aphasia Therapy) has been repeatedly shown to improve speech output in individuals with chronic, primarily expressive aphasia.[81] Unexpectedly, such treatment can also benefit *receptive* language skills, through a process that has yet to be understood. Studies that used a variety of functional brain imaging techniques have preliminarily identified significantly altered regional brain activation following this treatment.[82-84] Another therapy for aphasia, Melodic Intonation Therapy, has been associated with increased fiber bundle counts in the arcuate fasciculus as evaluated by diffusion tensor imaging,[85] thus suggesting that efficacious aphasia rehabilitation can promote structural neuroplastic changes.

Another promising intervention is prism adaptation training for left spatial neglect, which involves practicing reaching while wearing goggles that shift the subject"s view 10-15° to the right. Such training over approximately 10-15 sessions over a few weeks can be followed by significantly reduced spatial neglect on laboratory measures for as long as 1 year,[86] although functional carryover to real-world activities has thus far been little evaluated, and results have not been consistent.[87] Nonetheless, functional brain imaging studies indicate significant alterations in regional brain activity following this training in neurologically impaired as well as healthy subjects.[88, 89]

Further innovations in cognitive rehabilitation have recently been shown in community-living, generally healthy elders who have undergone visual speed of processing training. Normal aging includes a constriction of the ""useful field of view"" (UFOV),[90] which is the region of the visual field from which salient information is efficiently extracted against cluttered backgrounds. Extracting this information is particularly difficult when rapidly judging simultaneous central and peripheral transient events.[91] The UFOV is measured with a tachistoscopic test on a touchscreen on which subjects must touch the location of a briefly presented peripheral target and verbally identify a simultaneous briefly shown central silhouette. ""Not surprising, a reduced UFOV predicts traffic accidents by drivers.[92]

However, training to improve the UFOV through repetitive practice on the test can significantly reduce dangerous driving maneuvers, with benefits lasting as long as 18 months following the few weeks of training.[93, 94] Although as of this writing no studies have evaluated neuroplastic responses to UFOV training, recent findings in traumatic brain injury indicate that other forms of visual attention training are accompanied by elevated metabolic activity in the anterior cingulate and precuneus areas.[95] UFOV training may induce similar changes. The UFOV treatment results represent another instance where cognitive remediation has lasting improvements that can transfer to the real life situation, as a result of neuroplastic reorganization. The old dog can learn new tricks.

However, despite the enthusiastic reception for demonstrations of neuroplastic responses to disease or treatment, one must cautiously interpret the evidence. It has become very common to evaluate neuroplastic changes in the brain with functional neuroimaging techniques, particularly fMRI or PET scanning. These methods generally require the participant to perform a specific task (such as moving the paretic hand repetitively to a metronome) while being scanned. The associated regional cerebral metabolic profile is then compared either to different clinical populations or longitudinally within individuals from pre- to post-intervention.

The approach is problematic for a few reasons. First, it requires the cooperation of an individual who may be markedly impaired in the specific function of interest. Consequently, the procedure risks considerable difficulty with subject compliance or the reliable and repeated elicitation of the precise activity that is required, and thus may engender highly variable responses.[96] Second, the technique does not exclude the functional imaging effects from possible changes in the ways subjects actually undertake the task following an intervention.[97] Thus, if over the course of time a research subject adopts a different approach to the particular task for any reason, the regional pattern of metabolic activation could change without strictly requiring an associated physiologic or histologic structural change. To no surprise functional imaging studies of CI therapy after stroke show enormous inconsistency among subjects, complicating the understanding of training-associated neuroplasticity.[98] For these reasons, imaging methods that do not require the subject to perform a specific task, such as transcranial magnetic stimulation mapping, structural MRI, or resting network analyses are more reliable for assessing use-dependent neuroplasticity.

Concluding remarks

The studies of neuroplasticity teach us that the adult CNS is considerably reactive and adaptive, not stagnant. The anatomical distributions of specific brain functions are much more fluid than were formerly thought. Although there are probable limits to the beneficial outcomes of therapies that harness use-dependent plasticity, our understanding that spontaneous plastic reorganization and remodeling of the CNS is normal, not exceptional, and occurs even (or especially) after illness, inspires optimism for continuing to develop practice-based interventions to overcome the functional limitations of chronic CNS disease.

In short, it is a good time to be a neurologist.

Literature Cited

1. Buchtel HA. On defining neural plasticity. *Arch Ital Biol* 1978;116:241–247.
2. Verhaegen P. Aging and vocabulary scores: a meta-analysis. *Psychol Aging* 2003;18:332–339.
3. Jones EG. NEUROwords 8. Plasticity and neuroplasticity [review]. *J Hist Neurosci* 2000;9:37–39.
4. Stahnisch FW. Making the brain plastic: early neuroanatomical staining techniques and the pursuit of structural plasticity, 1910-1970 [review]. *J Hist Neurosci* 2003;12:413–435.
5. Berlucchi G, Buchtel HA. Neuronal plasticity: historical roots and evolution of meaning. *Exp Brain Res* 2009;192:307–319.
6. Illis LS. Central nervous stimulation in neurological disease [review]. *J R Soc Med* 1983;76:905–909.
7. Raineteau O. Plastic responses to spinal cord injury [review]. *Behav Brain Res* 2008;192:114–123.
8. Kaas JH. The reorganization of sensory and motor maps in adult mammals [review]. In: Gazzaniga M, ed. *The Cognitive Neurosciences*. Cambridge, Massachusetts: MIT Press, 1995: 51–71.
9. Bennett EL, Diamond MC, Krech D, Rosenzweig MR. Chemical and anatomical plasticity of brain [review]. *Science* 1964;146:610–619.
10. Schwartz JM, Begley S, eds. *The Mind & The Brain*. New York: Harper Collins, 2002.
11. Adams RD, Victor M. *Principles of Neurology*. New York: McGraw-Hill, 1977.
12. Church A, Peterson F. *Nervous and Mental Diseases*, 9th ed. Philadephia: W.B. Saunders, 1919.
13. Meige H. Les amnésies motrices fonctionnelles et le traitement des hémiplégiques. *Rev Neurol (Paris)* 1905;13:183–184.
14. Franz S, Scheetz M, Wilson A. The possibility of recovery of motor function in long-standing hemiplegia. *JAMA* 1915;65:2150–2154.
15. Jelliffe SE, White WA. *Diseases of the Nervous System*. 6th ed. Philadelphia: Lea & Febiger, 1935.
16. Ince LP. Escape and avoidance conditioning of response in the plegic arm of stroke patients: a preliminary study. *Psychon Sci* 1969;16:49–50.
17. Halberstam JL, Zaretsky HH, Brucker BS, Guttman AR. Avoidance conditioning of motor responses in elderly brain-damaged patients. *Arch Phys Med Rehabil* 1971;52:318–327, 336.
18. Ruch TC. The cerebral cortex: its structure and motor functions. In: Ruch TC, Fulton JF, eds. *Medical Physiology and Biophysics*. Philadelphia: W.B. Saunders Company, 1960: 249–276.
19. Broca P. Remarques sur le siège de la faculté du langage articulé, suivies d''une observation d''aphémie (perte de la parole). *Bulletin de la Société Anatomique de Paris* 1861;6:332–333, 343–357.
20. Rosenzweig M, Bennett E, Diamond M. Brain changes in response to experience [review]. *Sci Am* 1972;226(2):22–29.
21. Desmurget M, Bonnetblanc F, Duffau H. Contrasting acute and slow-growing lesions: a new door to brain plasticity [review]. *Brain* 2007;130:898–914.
22. Uematsu S, Lesser RP, Gordon B. Localization of sensorimotor cortex: the influence of Sherrington and Cushing on the modern concept. *Neurosurgery* 1992;30:904–913.
23. Penfield W, Boldrey E. Somatic motor and sensory representation in the cerebral cortex of man as studied by electrical stimulation. *Brain* 1937;60:389–443.

24. Schott GD. Penfield''s homunculus: a note on cerebral cartography [editorial]. *J Neurol Neurosurg Psychiatry* 1993;56:329–333.
25. Amassian V, Cracco R, Maccabee P, Cracco J. Is the classical motor homunculus representation correct? [Abstract.]. *Neurology* 1992;42:216.
26. DeFelipe J. Sesquicentennary of the birthday of Santiago Ramón y Cajal, the father of modern neuroscience. *Trends Neurosci* 2002;25:481–484.
27. Stahnisch FW, Nitsch R. Santiago Ramón y Cajal''s concept of neuronal plasticity: the ambiguity lives on. *Trends Neurosci* 2002;25:589–591.
28. Jones EG. Santiago Ramón y Cajal and the Croonian lecture, March 1894. *Trends Neurosci* 1994;17:190–192.
29. DeFelipe J. Brain plasticity and mental processes: Cajal again [review]. *Nat Rev Neurosci* 2006;7:811–817.
30. Kennard M. Reorganization of motor function in the cerebral cortex of monkeys deprived of motor and premotor areas in infancy. *J Neurophysiol* 1938;1:477–486.
31. Schneider G. Is it really better to have your brain lesion early? A revision of the ""Kennard Principle."". *Neuropsychologia* 1979;17:557–583.
32. Passingham R, Perry V, Wilkinson F. The long-term effects of removal of sensorimotor cortex in infant and adult rhesus monkeys. *Brain* 1983;106:675–705.
33. Duval J, Braun CM, Montour-Proulx I, Daigneault S, Rouleau I, Bégin J. Brain lesions and IQ: recovery versus decline depends on age of onset. *J Child Neurol* 2008;23:663–668.
34. Johnson DA, Rose FD, Brooks BM, Eyers S. Age and recovery from brain injury: legal opinions, clinical beliefs and experimental evidence. *Pediatr Rehabil* 2003;6:103–109.
35. Hubel D, Wiesel T. The period of susceptibility to the physiological effects of unilateral eye closure in kittens. *J Physiol* 1970;206:419–436.
36. Rakic P. DNA synthesis and cell division in the adult primate brain. *Ann NY Acad Sci* 1985;457:193–211.
37. Rakic P. Limits of neurogenesis in primates. *Science* 1985;227:1054–1056.
38. Gross C. Neurogenesis in the adult brain: death of a dogma. *Nat Rev Neurosci* 2000;1:67–73.
39. Kaplan M. Environment complexity stimulates visual cortex neurogenesis: death of a dogma and a research career. *Trends Neurosci* 2001;24:617–620.
40. Gross CG. Three before their time: neuroscientists whose ideas were ignored by their contemporaries. *Exp Brain Res* 2009;192:321–334.
41. Jones EG. Plasticity and neuroplasticity [letter]. *J Hist Neurosci* 2004;13:293.
42. Johansson B. Regeneration and plasticity in the brain and spinal cord [review]. *J Cereb Blood Flow Metab* 2007;27:1417–1430.
43. Milner P. The mind and Donald O. *Hebb. Sci Am* 1993;268(1):124–129.
44. Hebb DO. *The Organization of Behavior*. New York: John Wiley & Sons, 1949.
45. Brown RE, Milner PM. The legacy of Donald O.Hebb: more than the Hebb Synapse. *Nat Rev Neurosci* 2003;4:1013–1019.
46. Markham JA, Greenough WT. Experience-driven brain plasticity: beyond the synapse. *Neuron Glia Biol* 2004;1:351–363.
47. Kempermann G, Kuhn HG, Gage FH. More hippocampal neurons in adult mice living in an enriched environment. *Nature* 1997;386:493–495.
48. Wall PD, Egger MD. Formation of new connexions in adult rat brains following partial deafferentation. *Nature* 1971;232:542–545.
49. Mark VW, Taub E. Cortical reorganization and the rehabilitation of movement by CI therapy after neurologic injury. In: Pessoa L, de Weerd P, eds. *Filling-in: From Perceptual Completion to Skill Learning*. Oxford: Oxford University Press, 2003.
50. Mogilner A, Grossman J, Ribary U, et al. Somatosensory cortical plasticity in adult humans revealed by magnetoencephalography. *Proc Natl Acad Sci USA* 1993;90:3593–3597.
51. Pascual-Leone A, Torres F. Plasticity of the sensorimotor cortex representation of the reading finger in Braille readers. *Brain* 1993;116:39–52.

52. Taub E, Miller NE, Novack TA, et al. Technique to improve chronic motor deficit after stroke. *Arch Phys Med Rehabil* 1993;74:347–354.
53. Kopp B, Kunkel A, Mühlnickel W, Villringer K, Taub E, Flor H. Plasticity in the motor system correlated with therapy-induced improvement of movement after stroke. *NeuroReport* 1999;10:807–810.
54. Liepert J, Miltner WHR, Bauder H, et al. Motor cortex plasticity during constraint-induced movement therapy in stroke patients. *Neurosci Lett* 1998;250:5–8.
55. Liepert J, Bauder H, Miltner WHR, Taub E, Weiller C. Treatment-induced cortical reorganization after stroke in humans. *Stroke* 2000;31:1210–1216.
56. Maguire EA, Gadian DG, Johnsrude IS, et al. Navigation-related structural change in the hippocampi of taxi drivers. *Proc Natl Acad Sci USA* 2000;97:4398–4403.
57. Draganski B, Gaser C, Busch V, Schuierer G, Bogdahn U, May A. Neuroplasticity: changes in grey matter induced by training. *Nature* 2004;427:311–312.
58. Draganski B, Gaser C, Kempermann G, et al. Temporal and spatial dynamics of brain structure changes during extensive learning. *J Neuroscience* 2006;26:6314–6317.
59. Gauthier LV, Taub E, Perkins CE, Ortmann M, Mark VW, Uswatte G. Remodeling the brain: plastic structural brain changes produced by different motor therapies after stroke. *Stroke* 2008;39:1520–1525.
60. Colcombe SJ, Erickson KI, Scalf PE, et al. Aerobic exercise training increases brain volume in aging humans. *J Gerontol A Biol Sci Med Sci* 2006;61:1166–1170.
61. Eriksson P, Perfilieva E, Björk-Eriksson T, et al. Neurogenesis in the adult human hippocampus. *Nat Med* 1998:1313–1317.
62. Rakic P. Neurogenesis in adult primates. *Progr Brain Res* 2002;138:3–14.
63. Mothe AJ, Tator CH. Proliferation, migration, and differentiation of endogenous ependymal region stem/progenitor cells following minimal spinal cord injury in the adult rat. *Neuroscience* 2005;131:177–187.
64. Couillard-Despres S, Aigner L. *In vivo* imaging of adult neurogenesis. *Eur J Neurosci* 2011;33:1037–1044.
65. Pereira AC, Huddleston DE, Brickman AM, et al. An *in vivo* correlate of exercise-induced neurogenesis in the adult dentate gyrus. *Proc Natl Acad Sci USA* 2007;104:5638–5643.
66. Kinsbourne M. The minor cerebral hemisphere as a source of aphasic speech. *Arch Neurol* 1971;25:302–306.
67. Corbetta M, Kincade MJ, Lewis C, Snyder AZ, Sapir A. Neural basis and recovery of spatial attention deficits in spatial neglect. *Nat Neurosci* 2005;8:1603–1610.
68. Mark VW, Taub E, Perkins C, Gauthier L, Uswatte G. MRI infarction load and CI therapy outcomes for chronic post-stroke hemiparesis. *Restor Neurol Neurosci* 2008;26:13–33.
69. Anderson SW, Damasio H, Tranel D. Neuropsychological impairments associated with lesions caused by tumor or stroke. *Arch Neurol* 1990;47:397–405.
70. Rosenberg K, Liebling R, Avidan G, et al. Language related reorganization in adult brain with slow growing glioma: fMRI prospective case-study. *Neurocase* 2008;14:465–473.
71. van Nuenen B, Grotenhuis A, Vliet T, Gijtenbeek A. Spinal cord compression by an arachnoid cyst: a case report and review of the literature. *Zentralbl Neurochirurg* 2008;69:155–157.
72. Kalous A, Osborne P, Keast J. Spinal cord compression injury in adult rats initiates changes in dorsal horn remodeling that may correlate with development of neuropathic pain. *J Comp Neurol* 2009;513:668–684.
73. Thompson AJ, Jarrett L, Lockley L, Marsden J, Stevenson V. Clinical management of spasticity [editorial]. *J Neurol Neurosurg Psychiatry* 2005;76:459–463.
74. Frigon A, Rossignol S. Functional plasticity following spinal cord lesions. *Prog Brain Res* 2006;157:231–260.
75. Rosales RL, Kanovsky P, Fernandez HH. What''s the ""catch"" in upper-limb post-stroke spasticity: expanding the role of botulinum toxin applications [review]. *Parkinsonism Relat Disord* 2011;17:S3–S10.

76. Mühlnickel W, Elbert T, Taub E, Flor H. Reorganization of auditory cortex in tinnitus. *Proc Natl Acad Sci USA* 1998;95:10340–10343.
77. Mennemeier M, Chelette KC, Myhill J, et al. Maintenance repetitive transcranial magnetic stimulation can inhibit the return of tinnitus. *Laryngoscope* 2008;118:1228–1232.
78. Candia V, Wienbruch C, Elbert T, Rockstroh B, Ray W. Effective behavioral treatment of focal hand dystonia in musicians alters somatosensory cortical organization. *Proc Natl Acad Sci USA* 2003;100:7942–7946.
79. Hardy TA, Blum S, McCombe PA, Reddel SW. Guillain-barré syndrome: modern theories of etiology [review]. *Curr Allergy Asthma Rep* 2011;11:197–204.
80. Parry I, Walker K, Niszczak J, Palmieri T, Greenhalgh D. Methods and tools used for the measurement of burn scar contracture [review]. *J Burn Care Res* 2010;31:888–903.
81. Cherney LR, Patterson JP, Raymer A, Frymark T, Schooling T. Evidence-based systematic review: effects of intensity of treatment and constraint-induced language therapy for individuals with stroke-induced aphasia. *J Speech Lang Hear Res* 2008;51:1282–1299.
82. Breier JI, Maher LM, Novak B, Papanicolaou AC. Functional imaging before and after constraint-induced language therapy for aphasia using magnetoencephalography. *Neurocase* 2006;12:322–331.
83. Meinzer M, Elbert T, Wienbruch C, Djundja D, Barthel G, Rockstroh B. Intensive language training enhances brain plasticity in chronic aphasia. *BMC Biol* 2004;2:20.
84. Richter M, Miltner W, Straube T. Association between therapy outcome and right-hemispheric activation in chronic aphasia. *Brain* 2008;131:1391–1401.
85. Schlaug G, Marchina S, Norton A. Evidence for plasticity in white-matter tracts of patients with chronic Broca"s aphasia undergoing intense intonation-based speech therapy. *Ann NY Acad Sci* 2009;1169:385–394.
86. Humphreys G, Watelet A, Riddoch M. Long-term effects of prism adaptation in chronic visual neglect: a single case study. *Cogn Neuropsychol* 2006;23:463–478.
87. Nys GMS, de Haan EHF, Kunneman A, de Kort PLM, Dijkerman HC. Acute neglect rehabilitation using repetitive prism adaptation: a randomized placebo-controlled trial. *Restor Neurol Neurosci* 2008;26:1–12.
88. Luauté J, Michel C, Rode G, et al. Functional anatomy of the therapeutic effects of prism adaptation on left neglect. *Neurology* 2006;66:1859–1867.
89. Luauté J, Schwartz S, Rossetti Y, et al. Dynamic changes in brain activity during prism adaptation. *J Neurosci* 2009;29:169–178.
90. Edwards J, Ross L, Wadley V, et al. The Useful Field of View test: normative data. *Arch Clin Neuropsychol* 2006;21:275–286.
91. Sekuler A, Bennett P, Mamelak M. Effects of aging on the useful field of view. *Experimental Aging Research* 2000;26:103–120.
92. Owsley C, Ball K, McGwin G, et al. Visual processing impairment and risk of motor vehicle crash among older adults. *JAMA* 1998;279:1083–1088.
93. Ball K, Owsley C. Increasing mobility and reducing accidents of older drivers. In: Schaie KW, Pietrucha M, eds. *Mobility and Transportation in the Elderly*. New York: Springer, 2000: 213–251.
94. Roenker D, Cissell G, Ball K, Wadley V, Edwards J. Speed-of-processing and driving simulator training result in improved driving performance. *Hum Factors* 2003;45:218–233.
95. Kim YH, Yoo WK, Ko MH, Park CH, Kim ST, Na DL. Plasticity of the attentional network after brain injury and cognitive rehabilitation. *Neurorehabil Neural Repair* 2009;23:468–477.
96. Nelles G. Cortical reorganization—effects of intensive therapy [review]. *Restor Neurol Neurosci* 2004;22:239–244.
97. Rosenberger PB, Rottenberg DA. Does training change the brain? [Editorial.]. *Neurology* 2002;58:1139–1140.
98. Mark VW, Taub E, Morris DM. Neuroplasticity and Constraint-Induced Movement therapy. *Eura Medicophys* 2006;42:269–284.

CHAPTER 17

Visual Art

Anjan Chatterjee

Introduction

Katherine Sherwood was 44 years old when she had a massive left hemisphere stroke. This catastrophic event left her with an aphasia and right-sided weakness. She was (and is, as of this writing) an artist and a professor. After recovering from the psychological impact and some of the neurological deficits from her stroke, she began to paint again using her left hand. She laid canvasses horizontally, and moved around them in a mobile chair. She also noticed a curious thing. The style and content of her painting changed (Waldman, 2000). She previously regarded herself as a particularly cerebral painter, approaching her work in an over-intellectualized manner. After her stroke, she felt that images flowed from her more easily and expressively (Sherwood, 2012) (Figure 17.1). Something changed about her process of making art (Chatterjee, 2008). What changed?

More generally, cases like Professor Sherwood raise questions about what we can learn from the neuropsychology of art. Neuropsychology has been critical to advancing our knowledge of various cognitive systems, including perception, memory and language, as evidenced by other chapters in this book. But its impact on the study of aesthetics has been limited. Why is that? Certainly, an important factor is that as a domain of inquiry, neuroaesthetics is relatively immature (Chatterjee, 2004b; Chatterjee, 2011). The data from which one might draw inferences are sparse. Beyond the constraints of limited data, fundamental questions about proper methods remain. It is easy to be seduced by the striking phenomenology and to construct interesting "just so" stories to account for these observations. Cognitive neurology and neuropsychology has had a long tradition of starting with careful clinical observations before applying rigorous quantitative methods to the phenomena under consideration. The neuropsychology of art is at this threshold and seems poised to make the quantitative shift (Chatterjee, 2009).

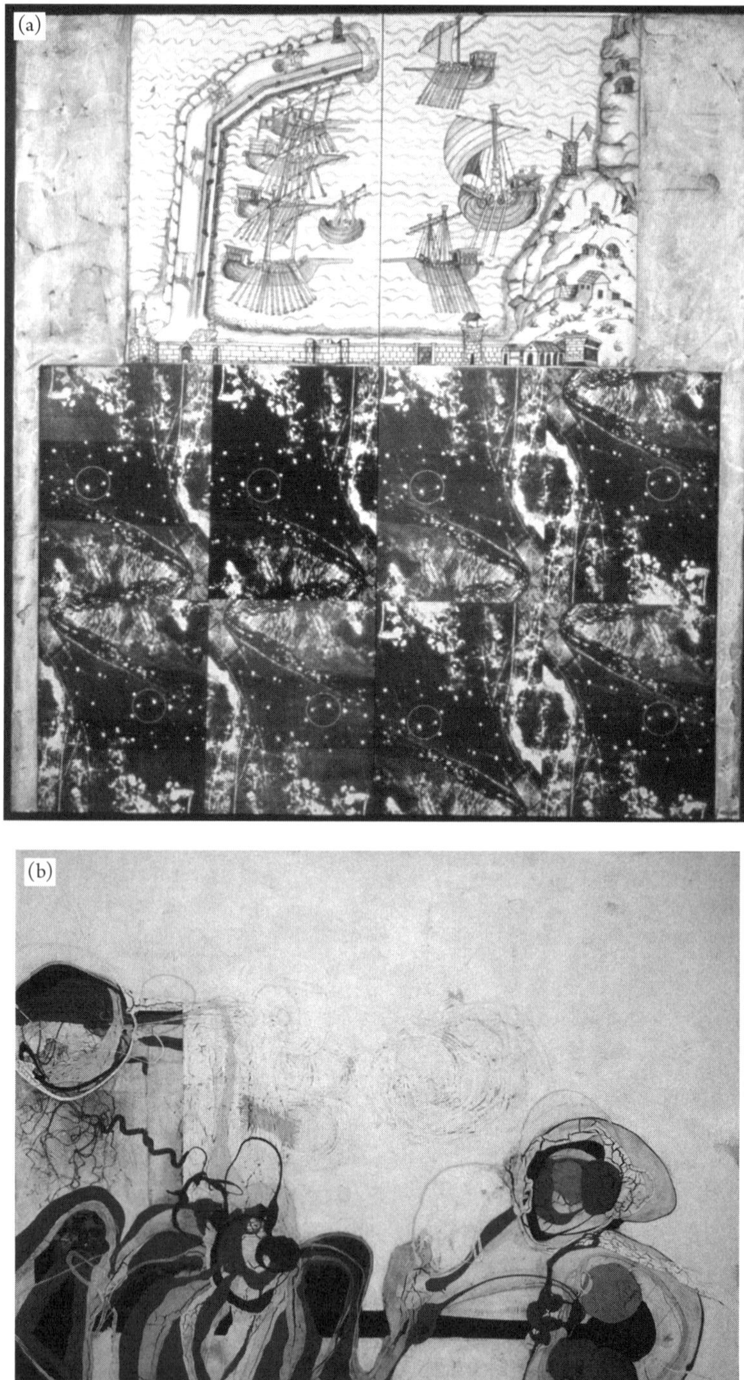

Figure 17.1 Examples of Katherine Sherwood's paintings. Permission obtained from Katherine Sherwood. a) Test Sites, painted before her stroke b) The Cart Before the Horse, painted after her stroke (see color insert).

One could speculate that artists, by virtue of their developed visuomotor skills, might be relatively protected from the visuomotor deficits associated commonly with brain damage. Such speculation appears not to be true when we consider the effects of brain damage on artistic production (Bogousslavsky & Boller, 2005; Chatterjee, 2004a, 2004b; Rose, 2006; Zaidel, 2005). Unilateral spatial neglect is a disorder in which patients are unaware of one side of space (Chatterjee, 2003; Heilman, Watson, & Valenstein, 1993). Artists with unilateral spatial neglect demonstrate neglect in their artwork (Jung, 1974). Visual agnosia is the inability to perceive or recognize objects visually. Artists with visual agnosias have difficulty depicting objects in their art (Wapner, Judd, & Gardner, 1978). Achromatopsia is the inability to apprehend color. Artists with achromatopsia may be unable to use color properly in their images (Sacks, 1995a). In these cases, the artwork illustrates the nature of neuropsychological deficits. While the depictions may be beautiful and captivating, they do not offer insight into the nature of artistic production itself.

In this chapter, I focus on two aspects of the neuropsychology of art. First, I will examine situations in which brain damage produces a paradoxical facilitation (Kapur, 1996) of artistic output. The effects of brain damage on the ability to produce visual art stand in sharp contrast to virtually all other complex human abilities. Diseases of the brain can impair our ability to communicate, coordinate movements, recognize objects, apprehend emotions and make rational decisions. By contrast, while diseases of the brain often alter the ability to produce art, the alterations are sometimes interesting and occasionally even regarded as improvements (Chatterjee, 2006). Second, I will discuss the issue of measurement in art. One might approach the idea of measuring aesthetic experiences with some trepidation. The fear is that quantifying these experience robs them of that which is fundamental. However, if neuropsychology of art is to advance as a science, it must incorporate some form of quantification in its methods (Chatterjee, Thomas, Smith, & Aguirre, 2009). I will describe our attempts to do so.

The Paradoxical Facilitation of Visual Art

Implicit in a discussion of the paradoxical facilitation of art is the view that there is no single art center in the brain. Nor does one hemisphere play a privileged role in art production per se. Rather, the production of art is highly complex with different components mediated by different parts of the brain. The final artistic output emerges from a coordination of these different components. Brain damage alters the available parts of the brain dedicated to the overall artistic output that becomes the product of a different coordination of components. By analogy, we might think of these neural systems like a suspended mobile. The mobile rests in some equilibrium of its weights. If a particular weight is removed, the entire configuration might collapse. However, the configuration might also find itself in a new resting state that is different from the original, but is also appealing. Similarly, brain damage may render an artist incapable of continuing to work analogous to the collapse of the mobile. Or it may create a new equilibrium in which the art proceeds in new and interesting configurations.

There are four ways in which neurological disorders might improve art production (Chatterjee, 2006). These are the 1) disposition to produce visual art; 2) provision of a unique visual vocabulary; 3) aids to descriptive accuracy; and 4) changes in expressive powers.

DISPOSITION TO PRODUCE ART

Fronto-temporal dementias (FTD) are a group of degenerative neurological diseases in which people undergo profound changes in their social interactions. They can be disinhibited and disorganized. They can have problems with language, attention, and the ability to make decisions. In addition to these alterations in personality and cognition, a few people with FTD develop a propensity to produce art for the first time. Miller and colleagues (Miller et al., 1998) note that their art is realistic, not abstract or symbolic. It is highly detailed and has an obsessive quality. The patients themselves seem intensely preoccupied with their art. The artistic output of people with FTD appears to be a consequence of changes in their personalities. The acquired obsessive-compulsive traits find a graphic expression and they produce striking visual images as a part of their repetition and attention to detail.

Several other examples show that obsessive-compulsive traits rendered by neurological diseases can predispose people to produce art. Sacks (Sacks, 1995b) described the Italian painter, Franco Magnani, living in San Francisco. Magnani painted hundreds of realistic scenes of an Italian town, Pontito, where he grew up. At the age of 31, Magnani probably had an encephalitic illness. Following that illness, he painted compulsively. Pontito preoccupied his thoughts and conversations. Sacks speculated that he had partial complex seizures and was in part demonstrating an obsessive "sticky" personality sometimes associated with temporal lobe epilepsy (Waxman & Geschwind, 1975). Such patients are also sometimes hypergraphic, meaning they write incessantly. Magnani's hypergraphia was being expressed visually rather than verbally.

Lythgoe and colleagues (Lythgoe, Polak, Kalmus, de Haan, & Khean Chong, 2005) reported the case of a builder with a sub-arachnoid hemorrhage. He also had no interest in art premorbidly but became an obsessive artist after recovery from the initial injury. After the hemorrhage, he had a normal verbal and performance IQ and normal behavior except for some degree of verbal disinhibition. He did well on most neuropsychological tasks except for those that involved mental flexibility. He also began to draw hundreds of sketches, mostly faces. He then moved to large-scale drawings sometimes covering entire rooms, while confining his art to a few themes.

Finally, about 10 percent of children with autism develop savant-like abilities (Rimland & Fein, 1988). A subset of these children produce striking visual images (Sacks, 1995c). The most detailed description of such a case was Nadia, reported by Selfe (Selfe, 1977). As a baby, Nadia did not respond to her mother, and as she got older she lacked social empathy. As a child, she was obsessively concerned with the presence of other children without forming any substantial bonds with them. Her acquisition of language was delayed. Despite these developmental abnormalities, she was remarkably skilled at drawing. By the age of three she was drawing life-like horses. She drew intensively for a few moments at a time, always copying images. She also focused on specific kinds of images like horses, of which she drew hundreds of examples. While Nadia's abilities were striking, she was not unique. Autistic children with these striking drawing skills seem to focus on specific subjects and draw them repeatedly.

Thus neurological disorders that produce obsessive-compulsive traits can also dispose people to produce art. These artists produce realistic images and focus on a narrow range of themes. While the neural basis for obsessive-compulsive disorders is not completely understood, dopamine and alterations of reward circuits are probably involved. We reported a patient with Parkinson's disease who produced art obsessively after being placed on dopamine agonists (Chatterjee, Hamilton, & Amorapanth, 2006). Interestingly, despite profound impairments in his motor control, which were evident when he wrote, he could make graceful sinuous movements when drawing. Obsessive-compulsive traits are also associated with dysfunction of the orbito-frontal and medial temporal cortices and fronto-striatal circuits (Kwon et al., 2003; Saxena et al., 1999; Ursu, Stenger, Shear, Jones, & CS, 2003). Notably, in cases such as those described in this section, these regions may have been damaged, leaving posterior occipito-temporal cortices intact. The preservation of posterior cortices ensures that the neural substrate that represents faces, places, and objects are preserved and are available as the focus of these patients' obsessions.

VISUAL VOCABULARY

Neurological disorders such as migraine and epilepsy are associated with productive visual phenomena. Of over 200 entries submitted to the first National Art Competition sponsored by the British Migraine Association and WB Pharmaceuticals, 70 percent showed spectral appearances, 48 percent showed fortifications, 16 percent showed areas of visual loss and 2.5 percent showed mosaic visions (Wilkinson & Robinson, 1985).

The artist, Ignatius Brennan, (Podoll & Robinson, 2000) eloquently expressed how migrainous auras inspired his art. His migraines, beginning at the age of 11, were experienced frightening episodes of visual loss, often with a zigzag cloud obscuring much of his visual fields. As he got older, he saw triangles and rounded forms as well as mosaics. He also experienced visual distortions of things getting larger or smaller. He recounts the effects of migraines on his art as follows: "I started with pictures of my migraine experiences unconsciously rather than deliberately, when I was in art school. I used to do a lot of drawings of landscapes at that time and often found that I would be drawing clouds not just in the sky, but everywhere, which I think was a reference to the visual voids experienced during visual loss. I also used serrated zigzag shapes in my drawings, symbolizing the experience of a whole being broken up... Clouds, zigzags, and other imagery are part of my own personal visual vocabulary, but which certainly has come out of migraine experiences. I'm absolutely sure. I don't tend to do that deliberately, but when it suits a particular subject, e.g., to represent a feeling or an emotion, I make use of these images in different ways...."

Such patients offer insights into how artists generally have a visual vocabulary at their disposal. Greater analyses of these cases may inform us about how artists develop this visual vocabulary and how they develop a visual grammar in concatenating this visual vocabulary.

DESCRIPTIVE ACCURACY

For centuries, visual artists have been preoccupied with rendering objects and their surroundings accurately. Underlying the problem of descriptive accuracy in drawing and painting is the role of knowledge. Visual agnosias are a class of disorders in which patients have difficulty recognizing objects (Farah, 1990). Since Lissauer's classic descriptions of visual agnosias, object recognition deficits are known to lie on a continuum between perceptual and conceptual deficits (Lissauer, 1890). Perceptually based agnosias, called apperceptive agnosias, impair the ability to process the visual information into a coherent object. Conceptually based agnosias, called associative agnosias, involve impairments of semantic knowledge of the object (Farah, 1990).

Wapner, Judd and Gardner (Wapner et al., 1978) described an artist with an apperceptive agnosia who had difficulty copying images despite being able to convey depth and shading in drawings that were otherwise fragmented. His preserved semantic system did not help guide his artistic production. Thus, when asked to draw a telephone, he constructed images by reasoning "It needs a base for it to stand on, a place to speak into, something to hear with a wire to plug in for communication and a place to dial." This verbal strategy was not effective in rendering accurate images. Semantic knowledge by itself does not help render objects accurately.

This patient contrasts with two people with associative agnosias (Franklin, van Sommers, & Howard, 1992; Schwartz & Chawluck, 1990). In both cases, when asked to draw objects from verbal labels, these people drew crude, simplified images similar to those drawn by a young child. However, when drawing from complex visual images, the results were strikingly different. For example, one of these people could copy a portrait originally painted by Botticelli or draw a portrait of a staff worker beautifully (Franklin et al., 1992). People can render objects accurately and beautifully without semantic knowledge.

The case of a Polish aphasic artist is also informative about the relationships between semantics and art (Kaczmarek, 1991). Profoundly influenced by the events of the World War II, his premorbid paintings were antiwar statements. They often included numbers, letters, and ideograms. Following his stroke, he was non-fluent and only produced a few words. At its core, our semantic system functions to abstract and generalize. The use of abstracted symbols could be considered a marker for a preserved semantic system. Although testing of his semantic system was not reported, from the descriptions of his aphasia one might infer that it was impoverished. His inability to make use of verbal symbols extended to his artwork. He was no longer able to produce paintings in his previous style of using symbols to communicate his antiwar sentiments. However, he was still able to draw realistic landscapes and portraits well, despite having lost his ability to manipulate symbols!

Does semantic knowledge of an object hinder artistic production? The art historian Gombrich (Gombrich, 1960) observed that even trained artists impose knowledge of what they are looking at in their depictions in a way that can compromise their accuracy. Thus impaired knowledge, provided visual-motor systems are intact, might aid in the ability to depict objects and scenes accurately. Perhaps such impaired knowledge accounts for cases of autistic children with savant–like artistic abilities.

Autistic artists need only to look at an object for a few minutes before drawing them rapidly and accurately (Sacks, 1995c; Selfe, 1977). Nadia's abilities were not an accelerated version of other children's drawing development. She did not first pass through a phase of drawing simple schematic images before learning to draw realistically. Rather her skills developed very early and did not change much over time. Nadia initially drew horses deftly and without hesitation. Two observations suggest that she treated horses as visual patterns rather than as objects. Firstly, she would start drawing anywhere on the page. Rather than trying to squeeze the whole horse into a page, she would stop drawing when she came to the paper's edge even if it meant only drawing part of the horse. Secondly, most people draw horses by starting at the head. Nadia could start her drawing at the neck and seemed unaffected by critical features associated with a specific object, such as the head of a horse. Her remarkable skill at drawing horses, and later, pelicans were not hindered by semantic associations that interfere with the ability to "see" the visual object. As Nadia eventually acquired language her drawings became more prosaic. Presumably, the acquisition of language indicated development of a richer semantic system and detracted from her artistic skills.

CHANGED EXPRESSIVITY

Visual art is, of course, not restricted to rendering objects and scenes accurately. Perhaps driven by the advent of photography, visual art diverged into many forms of expression. Among the most intriguing effects of brain damage on artists are a class of phenomena in which the inability to make accurate depictions results in surprisingly appealing stylistic changes. These changes can occur in the use of color and form and in the content of images.

Sacks (Sacks, 1995a) described an artist with an acquired achromatopsia following a traumatic brain injury. His earlier paintings were colorful and abstract. After the accident everything appeared "dirt gray" to him. His initial attempts to use color did not work and he resigned himself to painting in black and white. Eventually, he incorporated a limited set of colors to his paintings. After an initial sense of helplessness, he considered his new way of seeing as a strange gift. He thought he saw the world as pure form, uncluttered by color and endowed with a new range of expressions.

Right hemisphere damage can produce left spatial neglect and artists with neglect omit the left side of images that they draw or paint (Blanke, Ortigue, & Landis, 2003; Cantagallo & Sala, 1998; Halligan & Marshall, 1997; Jung, 1974; Marsh & Philwin, 1987; Schnider, Regard, Benson, & Landis, 1993). As they recover from their neglect, their use of line may still be altered. Two examples show how this change in the use of line can produce art that comes to be regarded highly. Lovis Corinth, an important German artist, had a right hemisphere stroke in 1911. As he recovered, he resumed painting. His self portraits and portraits of his wife showed clear changes in style, with details on the left sometimes left out and textures on the left blended with the background. Alfred Kuhn characterized this work as follows (quoted in Gardner (Gardner, 1975)) "He [Corinth] had become prescient for the hidden facets of appearance… The contours disappear, the bodies are often as ript asunder, deformed, disappeared into textures…. also the faithfulness of portraits had ceased almost entirely…With wide stripes the person is captured in essence. Characterization is now exaggerated, indeed, often to caricature… Corinth always seems to be painting a picture behind the picture, one which he alone sees… at this point Corinth shifted from the ranks of the great painters into the circle of the great artists."

Heller (Heller, 1994) reported the experience of the artist Loring Hughes, who after a right hemisphere stroke had difficulty coordinating the spatial relationship between lines. This forced her to abandon her premorbid style of depictive accuracy. Instead she turned to her own imagination and emotions. Initially, she was too ashamed to display her paintings. Once she became comfortable with her new style, she began to show her work. The artistic community responded well to these distorted images. The critic Eileen Watkins described her work as now delivering "an emotional wallop," that was not present previously.

The stylistic changes, when they occur with left brain damage, might be different from those observed with right brain damage. The specific changes reported are the introduction of more vivid colors and a change in content. These changes are exemplified in the Bulgarian painter, Zlatio Boiyadjiev, the Californian artist Katherine Sherwood who was mentioned in the introduction, and a Swiss painter reported by Annoni and colleagues.

Boiyadjiev's premorbid artistic style was natural and pictorial and he tended to use earth tones in his paintings. Following the onset of his aphasia, Boiyadjiev's paintings have been described as richer, more colorful and containing more fluid and energetic lines (Brown, 1977; Zaimov, Kitov, & Kolev, 1969). The imagery in his work became more inventive and at times even bizarre and fantastical. Similarly, as already mentioned, Katherine Sherwood suffered a left hemisphere hemorrhagic stroke that left her with an aphasia and right-sided weakness (Waldman, 2000). She trained herself to paint with her left hand, and since then her career has flourished. Premorbidly, her images were described as "highly cerebral," incorporating a range of esoteric images such as cross-dressers, medieval seals, and spy photos. After her stroke she felt that she could not produce such images if she wanted. Her new style is described as "raw" and "intuitive," with large irregular circular movements. She says her left hand enjoys an ease and a grace with the brush that her right hand never had, and describes it as "unburdened" (Sherwood, 2012). Finally, Annoni and colleagues (Annoni, Devuyst, Carota, Bruggimann, & Bogoousslavsky, 2004) recently described a Swiss landscape painter whose art was described as being "figurative-impressionist." He had a small stroke in the left thalamus. His wife thought he had mild emotional dyscontrol after his stroke. He felt that he was more sensitive to the hidden beauty of images and used bolder colors. He switched from realistic to more impressionistic images. He thought that he was less likely to use lines, contours and perspective clearly, and was more creative.

A final stylistic change rendered by brain damage is a move towards simplicity. Annoni and colleagues (Annoni et al., 2004) described a person with a left occipital lesion. A month after his stroke he resumed drawing and painting. His new artwork was simplified, stylized, increasingly abstract and confined to a limited use of colors. It is not known if damage to visual association cortices would consistently result in simplification and abstraction. A few artists with Alzheimer's disease have continued to paint (Crutch, Isaacs, & Rossor, 2001; Maurer & Prvulovic, 2004; Miller & Hou, 2004) and demonstrate a similar pattern.[1] William Utermohlen painted a series of self-portraits several years into the course of his illness. As these portraits became increasingly simplified and distorted, they appear as haunting psychological self-expressions.

Willem DeKooning is probably the best-known artist who continued to paint after the onset of Alzheimer's disease (Storr, 1995). After the onset of his neurological disease, DeKooning's ex-wife and students provided the structure for him to continue to work. They stretched his canvases and mixed his colors. Experts think this late period represents a new and coherent style. His paintings were simpler and he confined his palette to primary colors. Traces of shapes from earlier works are evident, but were pared down. Garrels (Garrels, 1995), the senior curator at the San Francisco Museum of Modern Art, thought "the vocabulary of forms was retained, but clarified... the results are paintings of an openness and freedom not seen before, paintings that are extraordinarily lyrical, immediately sensual, and exhilarating."

Quantification in the Neuropsychology of Art

Despite the fascinating observations recounted above, much needs to be done if neuropsychology is to make substantive contributions to empirical aesthetics. For the field to mature, it needs to go beyond describing fascinating anecdotes. Methodologically, it is critical to quantify features of artwork in order to assess change. Most of the cases reported are devoid of measurement. Claims about changes in art after brain damage are usually post-hoc comments supported by a few illustrative examples of artwork.

We need an instrument to assess art quantitatively. Such an instrument should have at least two characteristics. First, it should assess artwork along a comprehensive set of attributes, which would include formal properties (use of line, color, composition, etc.) and content properties (abstract, realism, etc.) Second, it should distinguish between descriptive and evaluative judgments. With such an instrument one could begin to impose quantitative structure on otherwise casual observations about works of art.

With these considerations in mind, we developed the Assessment of Art Attributes (AAA) (Chatterjee, Widick, Sternschein, Smith II, & Bromberger, 2010). The AAA assesses 12 descriptive attributes that would apply to any piece of visual art. Six attributes refer to formal/perceptual properties and six to content/conceptual properties. The six formal/perceptual attributes are: *Balance, Color Saturation, Color Temperature, Depth, Complexity,* and *Stroke Style*. The six content/conceptual attributes are: *Abstractness, Animacy, Emotionality, Realism, Representational Accuracy,* and *Symbolism*. The stimuli in the AAA consist of 24 paintings from the Western canon. These are paintings by well-known artists, but not their most famous works and encompass a range in the six formal/perceptual and six content/conceptual attributes of interest. The paintings are also evaluated for preference or liking and their interestingness.

Art Production

We have used the AAA to examine changes in art production as well as art perception following brain damage. For art production, we examined the work of three artists that have already been mentioned (Chatterjee, Bromberger, Smith, Sternshein, & Widick, 2011). These are Sherwood and Boiyadjiev, both with left brain damage, and Corinth with right brain damage. In each case we sampled several paintings completed before and after their stroke. Average ratings on each attribute were obtained for each painting. Then the average ratings for all the pre- and post-morbid paintings were obtained for each participant for each artist.

We examined Sherwood and Boiyadjiev's work to determine if left brain damage produces consistent changes in art. Sherwood describes her approach to her work pre-morbidly as over-intellectualized (Chatterjee, 2008). Post-morbidly, her work has been described as raw and more expressive, and less forced (Sherwood, 2012). In concordance with these descriptions, raters found her work following brain injury to be more abstract, more symbolic, more distorted, more vibrant, less realistic, and depicted with looser strokes. Raters also found her work to be flatter and to contain warmer colors, changes not mentioned previously by critics describing her work. Boiyadjiev's work has been described as becoming fantastic and sometimes bizarre with richer, more colorful forms and having fluid, energetic lines (Brown, 1977). Consistent with these descriptions, raters found his work to be more abstract, more symbolic, less realistic, more distorted as well as having a looser stroke style. They also found his work to be flatter and less animate, changes also not mentioned by critics before.

Could motor deficits for Sherwood and Boiyadjiev have caused these changes? Both were right-handed artists who began to paint with their left hands after their strokes, From these data, it is not clear if some pictorial aspects of the artwork, such as the coarser brushstroke, changed because of hemispheric brain damage or because they began to use their left hand. However, a shift to the left hand is unlikely to explain the use of increasingly vibrant colors or changes in conceptual attributes of their artwork, such as greater symbolism or abstraction.

A priori, one could be pessimistic about the prospects of identifying systematic effects of brain damage on art production. After all, artistic styles and content vary so much across different artists that one might be comparing changes in qualitatively different kinds of objects. Our observations of Sherwood and Boiyadjiev's art suggest that this pessimism might not be warranted. Sherwood and Boiyadjiev's artistic styles are quite different from each other. For example, Sherwood's paintings started out being substantially flatter than Boiyadjiev's paintings. Critically, both artists' paintings were judged as becoming flatter following their strokes, despite the fact that Sherwood's paintings *before* her stroke were more similar to Boiyadjiev's paintings *after* his stroke in depicting depth. Thus, it would be a mistake to think that people with left brain damage produce a *prototypic style* of painting. Rather, it appears that left brain damage produces a *prototypic shift* in style of painting.

Sherwood and Boiyadjiev's paintings became more abstract, symbolic, and distorted as well as less realistic, and were painted with looser strokes, more vibrant colors, and less depth (Chatterjee et al., 2011). Examining Corinth's work would test the specificity of these changes. Corinth's paintings after his stroke were described as "deformed" and attempts at producing faithful portraits "ceased almost entirely." Blanke (Blanke, 2006) describes a broadening of brush strokes, a lack of depth, less spatial detail, and several deformities on the left side of his self-portrait paintings. Raters found Corinth's paintings to be more abstract, more distorted, less realistic, and also to exhibit looser strokes and a flatter perspective.

When Sherwood, Boiyadjiev and Corinth's paintings are considered together, the following changes were found in all three artists. Their paintings became more abstract and distorted, and less realistic and accurate. They were also rendered with looser strokes, less depth, and with more vibrant colors. Thus, none of these changes can be ascribed to laterality of brain functions. Also, their paintings did not change in complexity or emotionality. It remains to be seen whether these attributes would be susceptible to change with other kinds of neurological illness. For example, we might expect the art of people with Alzheimer's disease to become less complex over time.

All the changes observed in Corinth's paintings were also observed in Sherwood and Boiyadjiev (Chatterjee et al., 2011). Thus, chronic right hemisphere damage does not appear to produce specific patterns of change in artistic production. By contrast, both Sherwood and Boiyadjiev's paintings became more symbolic. This could mean that artists with left brain damage, because of an unfettered right hemisphere, engage meaning more loosely, specifically in the use of symbolism. These data show that the popular idea that right hemisphere is the artistic hemisphere is wrong. Clearly, both hemispheres participate in artistic production as evidenced by the fact that the art of these artists changed regardless of which hemisphere was damaged. If anything, damage to the left hemisphere produced more significant alterations in artistic production than did damage to the right hemisphere.

We have also used the AAA to assess gradual changes in artistic styles in two patients with Alzheimer's disease. Investigating artists with AD allows us to look for gradual changes in art production rather than sudden changes brought about by a stroke.

William Utermohlen was diagnosed with AD after a long, successful painting career (Crutch et al., 2001). He was born in Philadelphia and studied at the Pennsylvania Academy of Fine Arts from 1951 to 1957. He moved to England in 1957 where he enrolled at the Ruskin School of Art in Oxford before settling in London. His early work was characterized by linear expressionism, with frequent inclusion of Pop imagery and styles, including a use of strong colors. His earliest symptoms began four years before diagnosis, and involved difficulties with tying a necktie, calculating household finances, and memory for day-to-day events. Formal neuropsychological examination revealed a moderate degree of global cognitive deterioration, while MRI indicated generalized cerebral atrophy. Following the initial diagnosis at the age of 61, regular clinical assessments documented the expected gradual decline in cognitive function (Crutch & Rossor, 2006). We used five self-portraits executed by William Utermohlen in the four-year period following his diagnosis.

The second artist, Lester Potts, was diagnosed with Alzheimer's disease around age 70. He had worked in a rural Alabama sawmill during the Great Depression. He served in the Korean War and was regarded as a dependable civic leader. He had not painted before his enrollment at an adult day care center. At the center, he learned to use watercolors with a retired artist, as part of a community outreach program. By the time he died at age 78 Lester Potts had painted over a 100 original watercolors.

Using the AAA, we found that both artists' paintings became more abstract and more symbolic. They also became less depictively accurate and less realistic. Potts' paintings also showed more color saturation, shifts in hues, less complexity, and less emotion as his disease progressed. Notably, changes were not seen with balance, depth, or stroke quality in either person's art.

Our observations were in general accord with other observations of the relationship between AD and artistic production and offered greater detail in the nature of change observed. For example, Fornazzari (Fornazzari, 2005) describe changes in the portraiture of a woman who suffered from AD. These changes include trends toward "unusual figure fond, loss of proportion in the facial features, and loss of proportionality...." The changes that they mention might parallel those observed in Utermohlen and Potts. "Unusual figure fond" and "loss of proportionality" might correspond to a decline in depictive accuracy. However, it is not clear if loss of proportionality could refer to loss of balance, which we did not see in either person. This uncertainty highlights one of our points, which is that clear operational definitions of art attributes are needed if we are to compare results across studies.

Our findings also validate anecdotal observations of changes in abstraction and increased symbolism among artists with AD (Crutch, 2001 #2984; Cummings, 1987 #3873; Rankin, 2007 #3401; Chatterjee, 2004 #2545). For example, art historians describe a heightened trend towards abstraction in paintings executed by Willem de Kooning during the progression of his AD (Garrels, 1995). Maurer & Prvulovic (Maurer & Prvulovic, 2004) thought that in the later works of the painter Carolus Horn, "ornamental symbols and mythical creatures appeared, which were derived from a conjunction of different species." Cummings and Zarit (Cummings & Zarit, 1987) reported that an artist with AD over a period of two and a half years moved towards simplicity and distortion. Miller and Hou (Miller & Hou, 2004) observed AD artists to produce works with less precision and attention to spatial relationships.

Art Perception

We know virtually nothing about the neuropsychology of the perception of art. One might expect that sensitivity to different attributes within a work of art would be affected by different kinds of brain damage. Recently, we used the AAA to examine the effects of brain damage on art perception (Bromberger, Sternschein, Widick, Smith, & Chatterjee, 2011). We focus our investigation on the role of the right hemisphere. The right hemisphere participates prominently in visuospatial attention and representation (Chatterjee, 2003; Heilman et al., 1993). As a first step, we wished to avoid confounding language comprehension with perceptual judgments in our study. For example, if a participant does not understand what the word *symbolic* means, it would not be difficult to assess their perception of symbolism in any painting. We also use contemporary lesion analysis methods in our study. Voxel-lesion-symptom mapping (VLSM) techniques allow us to formally assess the way in which damage to a brain area correlates with behavioral scores (Bates et al., 2003; Kimberg, Coslett, & Schwartz, 2007; Wu, Waller, & Chatterjee, 2007) with the advantage that one does not have to establish a deficit cut-off. Rather, behavior in VLSM considered a continuous variable.

In this study, the judgments of 20 people with right brain damage were compared to 30 healthy age-matched control participants. Of the content/conceptual qualities, damage to the right frontal lobe was associated with differences in judgments of abstractness, realism, animacy, and symbolism in visual art. In addition, damage to the right parietal lobe was related to deviations in judgments of animacy and symbolism. There were no brain behavior relationships for differences in evaluative judgments, those of preference or interestingness.

Any aesthetic experience is built upon at least three components (Chatterjee, 2004b; Chatterjee, 2011). These components are the experience of sensory qualities, the associated sets of meanings, and the emotional responses evoked by the aesthetic object. Broadly, one might regard the formal-perceptual attributes of the AAA as probing the sensory experience, the content-conceptual attributes as probing the meaning, and the evaluative questions as probing the emotional response to these paintings. The data from this study suggests that these three components of visual aesthetic experiences might segregate broadly in the organization of the brain. Most of our participants had damage in the distribution of the right middle cerebral artery. This distribution of brain damage involving lateral frontal-parietal and temporal cortices was more likely to affect judgments of conceptual attributes. We would predict that damage in the posterior cerebral artery distribution affecting ventral occipital and temporal cortices might be more likely to affect the perceptual attributes. Furthermore, given the extensive data implicating the ventral striatum and orbitofrotal cortex in subjective rewards (Kable & Glimcher, 2009), damage to ventro-medial prefrontal cortices is plausibly more likely to affect people's evaluation of paintings.

These recent results demonstrate the feasibility of conducting systematic quantitative studies in the neuropsychology of art. This point by no means implies that theoretical analyses or qualitative approaches to art are not useful. It does mean that if the neuropsychology of art is to mature *as a science*, it needs to incorporate quantitative approaches, and formal tests of hypotheses as part of its research program.

Conclusions

In reviewing the literature of the neuropsychology of art production, I emphasized the possible enhancing effects of brain damage on artistic production. Of course, these observations are based on selected artists. It is likely that many more artists are devastated by their brain injury and these cases are not reported. We simply do not know the base rate of facilitation effects. Yet, the examples of changed and possibly improved art following brain damage point to the multifaceted nature of art. In my view, exploring the mechanisms underlying the alterations and gaining insights into these facets is one way that neuropsychology can advance neuroaesthetics. Looking forward, unless the neuropsychology of art can incorporate the basic rigors of any experimental science, we will not get past the description of seductive artistic phenomenology under consideration. We are in a position to augment qualitative insights with quantitative approaches. The observations from patients can also serve to generate hypotheses to be tested using functional imaging techniques. For example, the hypothesis that the perception of art dissociates from the evaluation of art is amenable to functional imaging methods. We can be guardedly optimistic that the neuropsychology of art may mature and serve as a fundamental anchor in the new field of neuroaesthetics.

Note

1. My clinical experience is that such patients become too disorganized to bring art projects to completion. I have cared for several artist-patients who spend hours in their studio puttering around without producing much art.

References

Annoni, J., Devuyst, G., Carota, A., Bruggimann, L., & Bogoousslavsky. (2004). Changes in artistic style after minor posterior stroke. *Journal of Neurology, Neurosurgery, and Psychiatry, 76*, 797–803.

Bates, E., Wilson, S., Saygin, A., Dick, F., Sereno, M., Knight, R., & Dronkers, N. (2003). Voxel-based lesion symptom mapping. *Nature Neuroscience, 6*, 448–450.

Blanke, O. (2006). Visuo spatial neglect in Lovis Corinth's self portraits. *International Review of Neurobiology, 74*, 193–214.
Blanke, O., Ortigue, S., & Landis, T. (2003). Color neglect in an artist. *Lancet, 361*, 264.
Bogousslavsky, J., & Boller, F. (2005). *Neurological Disorders in Famous Artists*. Basel: Karger.
Bromberger, B., Sternschein, R., Widick, P., Smith, W., & Chatterjee, A. (2011). The Right Hemisphere in Aesthetic Perception. [Original Research]. *Frontiers in Human Neuroscience, 5*. doi:10.3389/fnhum.2011.00109
Brown, J. (1977). *Mind, Brain, and Consciousness. The Neuropsychology of Cognition*. New York: Academic Press.
Cantagallo, A., & Sala, S. D. (1998). Preserved insight in an artist with extrapersonal spatial neglect. *Cortex, 34*, 163–189.
Chatterjee, A. (2003). Neglect. A disorder of spatial attention. In M. D'Esposito (Ed.), *Neurological Foundations of Cognitive Neuroscience* (pp. 1–26). Cambridge, MA: The MIT Press.
Chatterjee, A. (2004a). The neuropsychology of visual artists. *Neuropsychologia, 42*, 1568–1583. doi:http://dx.doi.org/10.1016/j.neuropsychologia.2004.03.011
Chatterjee, A. (2004b). Prospects for a cognitive neuroscience of visual aesthetics. *Bulletin of Psychology and the Arts, 4*, 55–59.
Chatterjee, A. (2006). The neuropsychology of visual art: conferring capacity. *International Review of Neurobiology, 74*, 39–49. doi:http://dx.doi.org/10.1016/S0074-7742(06)74003-X
Chatterjee, A. (2008). Apoplexy and personhood in Katherine Sherwood's Paintings. In K. Sherwood (Ed.), *Golgi's Door* (pp. 44–52). Washington, DC: National Academy of Sciences Exhibition Catalogue.
Chatterjee, A. (2009). Prospects for a neuropsychology of art. In M. Skov & O. Vartanian (Eds.), *Neuroaesthetics* (pp. 131–143). Amityville, New York: Baywood Publishing Company.
Chatterjee, A. (2011). Neuroaesthetics: a coming of age story. *The Journal of Cognitive Neuroscience, 23*(1), 53–62. doi:10.1162/jocn.2010.21457
Chatterjee, A., Bromberger, B., Smith, W. B., Sternshein, R., & Widick, P. (2011). Artistic Production Following Brain Damage: A Study of Three Artists. *Leonardo, 44*(5), 405–410. doi:10.1162/LEON_a_00240
Chatterjee, A., Hamilton, R. H., & Amorapanth, P. X. (2006). Art produced by a patient with Parkinson's disease. *Behavioural Neurology, 17*, 105–108.
Chatterjee, A., Thomas, A., Smith, S. E., & Aguirre, G. K. (2009). The neural response to facial attractiveness. *Neuropsychology, 23*(2), 135–143.
Chatterjee, A., Widick, P., Sternschein, R., Smith II, W. B., & Bromberger, B. (2010). The assessment of art attributes. *Empirical Studies of the Arts, 28*(2), 207–222. doi:10.2190/EM.28.2.f
Crutch, S., Isaacs, R., & Rossor, M. (2001). Some workmen can blame their tools: artistic change in an individual with Alzheimer's disease. *Lancet, 347*, 1096–1098. doi:10.1016/S0140-6736(00)05187-4
Crutch, S. J., & Rossor, M. N. (2006). Artistic Changes in Alzheimer's Disease. [10.1016/S0074-7742(06)74012-0]. *International Review of Neurobiology00747742, 74*, 147–161. doi:10.1016/S0074-7742(06)74012-0
Cummings, J. L., & Zarit, J. M. (1987). Probable Alzheimer's disease in an artist. *The Journal of the American Medical Association, 258*(19), 2731–2734. doi:10.1001/jama.1987.03400190113039
Farah, M. J. (1990). *Visual Agnosia*. Cambridge, MA: The MIT Press.
Fornazzari, L. R. (2005). Preserved painting creativity in an artist with Alzheimer's disease. *European Journal of Neurology, 12*(6), 419–424. doi:10.1111/j.1468-1331.2005.01128.x
Franklin, S., van Sommers, P., & Howard, D. (1992). Drawing without meaning?: dissociations in graphic performance of an agnosic artist. In R. Campbell (Ed.), *Mental Lives. Case Studies in Cognition* (pp. 179–198). Cambridge, USA: Blackwell.
Gardner, H. (1975). *The Shattered Mind. The Person After Brain Damage*. New York: Alfred A. Knopf.
Garrels, G. (1995). Three toads in the garden: line, color, and form. In J. Jenkins & S. Engberg (Eds.), *Willem de Kooning. The Late Paintings, The 1980s* (pp. 9–37). Minneapolis: San Francisco Museum of Modern Art and Walker Arts Center.

Gombrich, E. (1960). *Art and Illusion*. Princeton: Princeton University Press.

Halligan, P. W., & Marshall, J. C. (1997). The art of visual neglect. *Lancet, 350*, 139–140.

Heilman, K. M., Watson, R. T., & Valenstein, E. (1993). Neglect and related disorders. In K. M. Heilman & E. Valenstein (Eds.), *Clinical Neuropsychology* (3rd ed., pp. 279–336). New York: Oxford University Press.

Heller, W. (1994). Cognitive and emotional organization of the brain: Influences on the creation and perception of art. In D. Zaidel (Ed.), *Neuropsychology* (pp. 271–292). New York: Academic Press.

Jung, R. (1974). Neuropsychologie und neurophysiologie des kontur und formsehens in zeichnerei und malerei. In H. Weick (Ed.), *Pyschopathologie Mususcher Gestaltungen* (pp. 27–88). Stuttgart: FK Shattauer.

Kable, J. W., & Glimcher, P. W. (2009). The Neurobiology of Decision: Consensus and Controversy. *Neuron, 63*(6), 733–745.

Kaczmarek, B. (1991). Aphasia in an artist: A disorder of symbolic processing. *Aphasiology, 5*, 361–371.

Kapur, N. (1996). Paradoxical functional facilitation in brain-behavior research. *Brain, 119*, 1775–1790.

Kimberg, D. Y., Coslett, H. B., & Schwartz, M. F. (2007). Power in Voxel-based Lesion-Symptom Mapping. *Journal of Cognitive Neuroscience, 19*(7), 1067–1080.

Kwon, J., Kinm, J., Lee, D., Lee, J., Lee, D., Kim, M., . . . , Lee, M. (2003). Neural correlates of clinical symptoms and cognitive dysfunctions in obsessive-compulsive disorder. *Psychiatry Research, 122*, 37–47.

Lissauer, H. (1890). Ein Fall von Seelenblindheit Nebst Einem Beiträge zur Theori derselben. *Archiv fur Psychiatrie und Nervenkrankheiten, 21*, 222–270.

Lythgoe, M., Polak, T., Kalmus, M., de Haan, M., & Khean Chong, W. (2005). Obsessive, prolific artistic output following subarachnoid hemorrhage. *Neurology, 64*, 397398.

Marsh, G. G., & Philwin, B. (1987). Unilateral neglect and constructional apraxia in a right-handed artist with a left posterior lesion. *Cortex., 23*(1), 149–155.

Maurer, K., & Prvulovic, D. (2004). Paintings of an artist with Alzheimer's disease: visuoconstructive deficits during dementia. *Journal of Neural Transmission, 111*, 235–245. doi:10.1007/s00702-003-0046-2

Miller, B., & Hou, C. (2004). Portraits of artists: Emergence of visual creativity in dementia. *Archives of Neurology, 61*, 842–844.

Miller, B. L., Cummings, J., Mishkin, F., Boone, K., Prince, F., Ponton, M., & Cotman, C. (1998). Emergence of artistic talent in frontotemporal dementia. *Neurology, 51*, 978–982.

Podoll, K., & Robinson, D. (2000). Migraine experiences as artistic inspiration in a contemporary artist. *Journal of the Royal Society of Medicine, 93*(5), 263–265.

Rimland, B., & Fein, D. (1988). Special talents of autistic savants. In L. Obler & D. Fein (Eds.), *The Exceptional Brain* (pp. 474–492). New York: Guilford.

Rose, F. E. (2006). *The Neurobiology of Painting*. London: Academic Press.

Sacks, O. (1995a). The case of the color blind painter. *An Anthroplogist on Mars* (pp. 3–41). New York: Alfred A. Knopf, Inc.

Sacks, O. (1995b). The landscape of his dreams. *An Anthropologist on Mars* (pp. 153–187). New York: Alfred A. Knopf.

Sacks, O. (1995c). Prodigies. *An Anthropologist on Mars* (pp. 188–243). New York: Alfred A. Knopf.

Saxena, S., Brody, A., Maidment, K., Dunkin, J., Colgan, M., Alborzian, S., . . . , Baxter, L. J. (1999). Localized orbitofrontal and subcortical metabolic changes and predictors of response to paroxetine treatment in obsessive-compulsive disorder. *Neuropsychopharmacology, 21*, 683–693.

Schnider, A., Regard, M., Benson, D. F., & Landis, T. (1993). Effect of a right-hemisphere stroke on an artist's performance. *Neuropsychiatry, Neuropsychology, & Behavioral Neurology, 6*(4), 249–255.

Schwartz, M., & Chawluck, J. (1990). Deterioration of language in progressive aphasia: a case study. In M. Schwartz (Ed.), *Modular Deficits in Alzheimer-Type Dementia* (pp. 245–296). Cambridge, MA: The MIT Press.

Selfe, L. (1977). *Nadia. A case of extraordinary drawing ability in an autistic child.* New York: Academic Press.

Sherwood, K. (2012). How a cerebral hemorrhage altered my art. [10.3389/fnhum.2012.00055/abstract]. *Frontiers in Human Neuroscience, 6.* doi:papers2://publication/doi/10.3389/fnhum.2012.00055/abstract

Storr, R. (1995). At last light. *Willem de Kooning. The Late Paintings, The 1980s* (pp. 37–79). In J. Jenkins & S. Engberg (Eds.), Minneapolis: San Franscisco Museum of Modern Art and Walker Arts Center.

Ursu, S., Stenger, V., Shear, M., Jones, M., & CS, C. (2003). Overactive action monitoring in obsessive-compulsive disorder. *Psychological Science, 14,* 347–353.

Waldman, P. (2000, Friday May 12). Master stroke: A tragedy transforms a right-handed artist into a lefty—and a star. *Wall Street Journal, CXLII,* 94.

Wapner, W., Judd, T., & Gardner, H. (1978). Visual agnosia in an artist. *Cortex, 14,* 343–364.

Waxman, S., & Geschwind, N. (1975). The interictal behavior syndrome associated with temporal lobe epilepsy. *Archives of General Psychiatry, 32,* 1580–1586.

Wilkinson, M., & Robinson, D. (1985). Migraine art. *Cephalalgia, 5*(3), 151–157.

Wu, D. H., Waller, S., & Chatterjee, A. (2007). The functional neuroanatomy of thematic role and locative relational knowledge. *The Journal of Cognitive Neuroscience, 19,* 1542–1555.

Zaidel, D. (2005). *Neuropsychology of Art.* New York: Psychology Press.

Zaimov, K., Kitov, D., & Kolev, N. (1969). Aphasie chez un peintre. *Encephale, 58,* 377–417.

CHAPTER 18

Creativity

Valeria Drago and Glen R. Finney

Introduction

Creativity is a multifaceted concept. It underlies the arts, such as painting, sculpting, dance, song, poetry, music, photography, as well as the sciences, such as mathematics, physics, cosmology, chemistry, geology, biology, and psychology. Creativity crops up in small acts of personal novelty to grand works of genius that transform the way we live, think, and believe. Hard to define, hard to capture, yet creativity is an essential part of human culture.

In this chapter, we review the construct of creativity, and demonstrate how neurological diseases influence creativity and delineate the brain mechanisms that underlie these effects, including a discussion of case reports of artists with neurological diseases and how the disease interfered with their abilities.

The construct of creativity is of great interest in psychology and neuroscience, but the findings of investigations are not always consistent. The reason for inconsistent findings may partially be because creativity is a very difficult domain to study. Different researchers define creativity differently, use different paradigms, and provide different explanations for the mechanisms that might underlie creative thinking.

Definitions of Creativity

COMMON DEFINITION

What is creativity? Webster's II University Dictionary (1988) provides a common definition of creativity as: "having the power or ability to create," "productive," "marked by originality," "new." Emphasized in this common defining of creativity is the idea of production and that of novelty.

PRODUCTION

The importance of production to creativity makes sense in that a workable idea in the abstract may fail in the execution. By this definition of creativity, a concept must move beyond the mind of the imaginer to the actual production of a creative work. However, even with production, and skillful production at that, an act or work still may not be creative. There is a difference between being creative and being skillful. Skill is often a necessary prerequisite for creativity, in that skilled musicians, artists, writers, and scientists replicating or providing minor flourishes on the works of others can be very productive without being creative.

NOVELTY

Novelty can be considered from two different perspectives; novelty for a person versus novelty for the world. Researchers often find that what they initially believed were original or new ideas for future studies have already been conducted once they conduct a literature review. This represents a reinventing of the wheel. Are these instances of creativity, even though the idea was not new? They seemed to be so initially to those who conceived them, until they discovered another had done so before. This certainly represents an act of creativity at the level of the individual. The creative process or creative thinking encompasses activities that engender novel products to an individual, so long as they had no prior knowledge of the concept.

THE PROBLEM OF RANDOMNESS

Production and novelty, as defined here, are both necessary, but not sufficient to define creativity. For instance, a list of words or colors randomly applied to a canvas are produced, and most likely novel, but lack creativity. It is highly unlikely that a room full of monkeys typing on typewriters (or should we say computers) would produce the equivalent of Shakespeare, or anything of value whatsoever. One way to get around this problem of randomness is to require that the act of creative production have an intentional component or goal. Another way is to summon the criterion of value.

VALUE

Several researchers add that, in addition to being novel, a work should also have value in order to be considered creative (Shavinina, 2003, Sternberg, 1999). Csikszentmihalyi (1988, 1996, 1999) provided a detailed analysis of the relevance of both novelty and value to creativity. A novel product becomes creative only when it is accepted as "part of the domain" or valued by "the field"(which can refer to any external audience or consumers). In this view, if a product is rejected by "the field," that work is not creative regardless of its novelty.

There are problems with the addition of value as a defining feature of creativity. Sometimes a work is not valued at the time it is produced, but only later. For example, the impressionist painters were criticized when they first developed their style. There is also the problem of who deems the work of value. In many daily cases of creativity, the creative work may be of value only to its creator. This is similar to the problem of the individual versus general novelty of a work. Thus, it may be more useful to separate creativity from the value of a work, and to consider a work as creative if it is produced (intentionally) and novel to its creator.

UNITY IN DIVERSITY

A somewhat different approach to the definition of creativity used in some research is that of Bronowski (1972): *"Creativity is finding unity in what appears to be diversity."* The concept of unity in diversity is an old one, known to St. Augustine in the 5th century. Frances Hutcheson in 1725 was one of the first to write about unity in diversity as applied to an artistic endeavor such as music. Many great visual artworks use a wide palette of colors and forms, and similarly, we can hear in several great musical pieces a variety of melodies and rhythms. For both paintings and symphonies, the creators develop a thread that unifies these diverse elements, bringing order to seeming (or potential) chaos. This definition highlights the concept of a "global approach" as a common feature in creativity. Unfortunately, this definition lacks the previously mentioned features of novelty and productivity. Heilman and colleagues provided a related definition of creativity that expanded on this, defining creativity as the ability to understand, develop, and express in a systematic fashion novel orderly relationships (Heilman, 2004).

ASSOCIATED CONCEPTS: CONVERGENT AND DIVERGENT THINKING

J.P. Guilford first defined (1950), then elaborated (1967), two modes of thinking that play a role in both intelligence and creativity to varying degrees: convergent and divergent thinking. Convergent thinking can be defined as the ability to come up with the "correct" answer to a question or problem, when there is one known specific solution to a problem. Convergent thinking is most heavily involved in activities that normally are classified as intelligence tasks, but convergent thinking can be part of the creative process depending on the task and the stage of creativity in question, especially in scientific and technological endeavors. In contrast to convergent thinking, divergent thinking can be defined as the generation of novel ideas or solutions to a question or problem. This process requires the thinker to go beyond known answers and processes and generate new ones, and thus is a key component of the creative process.

Prerequisites of Creativity

Guilford and Christensen (1973) thought creativity was a subset of intelligence. Guilford developed psychometric tests to "measure" creativity. His findings indicate that students with low IQ consistently performed poorly on these tests, but for those students with high IQ, performance on creativity tests did not highly correlate with their performance on IQ tests. After reviewing the relationship between intelligence and creativity, Torrance (1974) suggested that IQ and creativity are only moderately related (Heilman, 2005).

Intelligence and Creativity

A significant change in the direction of creativity research started around 1950. J.P. Guilford, an expert on intelligence testing, proposed that psychology had not done enough to examine thinking that went beyond the kind measured by traditional I.Q. tests, specifically creative thinking. Similar to creativity itself, there are many definitions of intelligence, such as the ability to do well in school, but for most, intelligence is the measure of a person's ability to acquire and apply knowledge.

Sternberg & O'Hara (1999) suggest several possible relationships between intelligence and creativity: 1) they are the same; 2) one is a subset of another, such as creativity is a subset of intelligence; 3) they are unrelated; 4) they are overlapping but independent constructs. Another way to look at the difference between intelligence and creativity, at least as is often assessed on psychological testing, is in defining intelligence as the ability to come to a correct answer, whereas creativity is the ability to generate a new answer.

The founder of intelligence testing, Alfred Binet, may have initially thought that creativity and intelligence were the same or closely overlapping constructs because the first intelligence test he devised in 1896 used inkblots to explore the imagination of children. Later, according to Sternberg & O'Hara (1999), he discontinued this inkblot test because he was unable to develop a reliable means of scoring it, a problem that still plagues creativity assessment to this day. Guilford & Christensen (1973) thought creativity was a subset of intelligence. Terman (1954) found that the later day success (or lack thereof) of children in the gifted range of the intelligence quotient (IQ) did not demonstrate increased creativity, at least by their self-report of their careers and achievements. Guilford and Christensen in 1973 used a divergent product battery to compare creativity to

IQ and found that divergence ability was closely correlated at IQs of lower levels, but became less so as IQ approached 130. Barron & Harrington (1981) focused on the relationship between intelligence and creativity, studying creative peoples' intelligence. Their article on creativity, intelligence, and personality suggested a curvilinear relationship between intelligence and creativity, with intelligence presumably becoming less and less relevant at the higher levels of intelligence.

These observations suggest that there might be an IQ threshold, such that a person needs to be above this threshold for her or him to be successfully creative.

Simonton (1994) and Herr (1965) in their studies also found that the correlation between intelligence and creativity is weak. This weak correlation, however, might be related to the tests that were used to measure intelligence.

Cattell (1963) posited that there are two types of intelligence, which he termed, "crystallized" and "fluid." Crystallized intelligence refers to specific knowledge and skills that accumulate over a lifetime, including but not limited to such areas as declarative memories, knowing that Rome is the capital of Italy, or lexical-semantic knowledge such as knowing the meaning of the word *impale*. Fluid intelligence has been defined as the ability to reason and think abstractly. Most intelligence tests, such as the Wechsler Adult Intelligence Scale (WAIS), assess both crystallized (e.g., vocabulary-definitions) and fluid intelligence (e.g., How are a fly and a tree similar?). Cattell posited that while crystallized knowledge is important as a prerequisite for creativity, it is fluid intelligence that more directly relates to creative ability. Although fluid intelligence may be the best predictor of creativity, there are no formal studies that have studied this relationship, and little has been little written about the brain mechanisms of fluid intelligence and cognitive flexibility (Heilman, 2004, 2012).

Stages of Creativity

Socrates thought "inspired thinking" was bestowed by the gods, specifically the nine daughters of Zeus, the Muses, who were each responsible for a specific form of the arts. Thus, geniuses were thought to be the inspired instruments of the gods through which Nature revealed knowledge to humanity. Unlike antiquity, the modern era has focused on identifying the brain mechanisms that underlie creativity (Weisberg, 2006).

Helmholtz (1826) with elaboration by Wallas (1926) parsed the creative act into four stages:

- Preparation
- Incubation
- Illumination
- Verification

PREPARATION

The model begins with a "pre-creative" stage, preparation. It posits that in order to be creative an individual must learn to some degree the basic background knowledge and skills necessary to engage in the specific creative endeavor. The most creative acts may require training or preparation in disparate, previously unconnected areas of knowledge or skill, whose synthesis results in a truly novel innovation. For some activities preparation may take years or even decades.

Kuhn (1996) and others have noted that many important discoveries are initiated by the observation of an anomaly and recognition of its potential significance, as in the example of the "ruined" petri dishes that led to Alexander Fleming's discovery of penicillin. Louis Pasteur's famous quote, "Chance favors the prepared mind," perhaps has multiple meanings; that it takes knowledge and skill to identify and move forward when an anomalous observation or idea appears, but also that it takes a curious mind to even look for such anomalies.

INCUBATION

As previously intimated, the more rich and varied the experiences and training of a person, the more the imagination will have to work with (the proverbial "grist for the mill"). Imagination takes advantage of the ability of our brain to displace different life events in a new and original way. The creative person may engage in an active search for a creative answer to an unknown question, but in many cases at least part of this work is performed preconsciously, which may take advantage of the massively parallel processing ability of the subconscious brain, as opposed to conscious thought which seems more serial in nature. The final phase of incubation seems to be best performed in a relaxed or low arousal state. Heilman has hypothesized that such a relaxed state might allow for weaker semantic connections to be made, whereas in an excited state only the strongest semantic connections tend to come to consciousness. Ramòn y Cajal in his book entitled *"Advice for a young investigator"* suggests: *"If a solution fails to appear . . . and yet you feel success is just around the corner, try resting for a while."*

ILLUMINATION

The third stage is typically the briefest, but it often marks the moment of recognition of a creative concept. This is illumination, sometimes referred to as the "Aha!" or "Ha!" or "Ah!" moment. Henri Poincare' (1854–1912), the mathematician and scientist (Miller, 1996), reported several instances of illuminations when describing his creative achievements. It should be noted that scientists and artists can develop this illumination without necessarily observing an anomaly. The occurrence of illuminations in the absence of a consciously deliberative process is suggestive of unconscious processing, replacing the gift of the gods of Socrates with the products of the subconscious brain.

Other famous examples from Incubation to Illumination.

- The Bath—Greek inventor Archimedes, third century B.C.E.; the original "Eureka!" experience while relaxing in a bath, discovery of using water displacement to discern volume of irregularly shaped objects, such as the crown he was charged to check if pure gold or not without melting it.
- Newton and the Apple—English mathematician and physicist Sir Isaac Newton, 1666; inspired in his mother's garden by idea of an apple's fall, led to the surmise of gravity.
- Kekulé and the Dream of Ouroborus—German chemist Friedrich August Kekulé, 1865; discovery of the ring-shaped structure of benzene that came to him as a daydream of snake seizing its tail, an Ouroborus.
- Einstein and Light—Austrian physicist Albert Einstein worked in the patent office, engaged in thought experiments that led to theory of relativity.
- Mullis and the Endless Highway—American chemist Kary Mullis had a breakthrough on polymerase chain reaction in 1983 driving late at night down the highway with his girlfriend.

Often the "Aha!" moment of illumination changes the state of arousal of the creating individual from one of relaxation to excitement or exhilaration. Of course, it is possible to have the sensation of illumination incorrectly, a false positive. Metcalfe and Wiebe (1987) demonstrated that the subjective feeling of knowing (the "Aha!") did not predict performance on insight problems. The constructs of incubation and illumination have received criticism for this and other reasons. Weisberg (1986) suggested that creativity does not always require great leaps (illumination) and the processes that led to many great discoveries might not involve subconscious incubation, but rather a series of conscious steps. Helmholtz and later, Wallas, saw illumination as the culmination of the incubation process rather than being an independent factor.

John Kounios and Marc Beeman have written and set up experimental paradigms to test the neural correlates of the illumination stage, using EEG and functional magnetic resonance imaging (fMRI) to examine the neural correlates of the "Aha! moment" and its antecedents. Their results suggest that this illumination or "insight" phenomenon is the "culmination of a series of brain states and processes operating at different time scales" (Kounios & Beeman, 2009). In their study, they used a type of test called the compound remote association test. This test consists in three words (e.g., crab, pine, sauce). Participants need to provide a single word that can form a compound or a familiar two word phrase with each of the three problem words (e.g., apple for pineapple, crabapple, applesauce). The EEG results indicated that insight solutions were associated with a burst of high frequency activity starting about 300 milliseconds before the solution was reached by the subjects over the right anterior temporal lobe. The insight effect was also evaluated with fMRI, with findings localizing to the right anterior superior temporal gyrus, underneath where the electrodes found the corresponding EEG signal (Kounios & Beeman, 2009).

VERIFICATION

In this last stage, creative people validate their creative insight, such as when scientists perform experiments to test their hypotheses. The verification stage can be further divided into a production and a confirmation stage. For successful production, there must be appropriate initiation, persistence, and disengagement. Whether the work can be produced successfully is the first form of verification. Confirmation is a more controversial part of the verification stage, where the work created is reviewed for its novelty, and in many instances, its value. This confirmation step is unnecessary for those models of creativity that only require personal novelty and do not place any value stipulation. For those that require more general novelty and/or value, however, it is a vital part of the process.

Neurobiology of Creativity

The following section will provide examples on the potential influence of neurological diseases on various cognitive mechanisms that may be important in serving as a foundation for creative thinking. The specific brain mechanisms that potentially explain the effects of neurological diseases on creativity will also be reviewed.

THE ROLE OF NONDOMINANT (RIGHT) HEMISPHERE IN CREATIVITY

Bruce Miller and colleagues (Miller et al., 1998; Miller, Boone, Cummings, Read & Mishkin, 2000) have a series of reports on the emergence of artistic talents in patients affected by frontotemporal lobar degeneration. As the name implies, the most devastated part of the brain in the course of frontotemporal lobar degeneration are the frontal and temporal lobes. There are three main syndromic types to frontotemporal lobar degeneration; progressive nonfluent aphasia (impacting dominant hemisphere frontotemporal regions), behavioral variant frontotemporal dementia (impacting nondominant hemisphere frontotemporal regions), and semantic dementia (impacting the bilateral anterior temporal lobes predominantly). Additionally, the logopenic variant of primary progressive aphasia [also referred to as logopenic progressive aphasia (LPA)] is the most recently identified variant of primary progressive aphasia. This disorder, characterized by a unique speech and language profile, occurs due to damage to the left temporo-parietal junction (Gorno-Tempini et al., 2004).

Several of the patients described by Miller (1998–2000) started drawing or painting around the time they had the symptoms and signs of dementia or at the time when the disease was just beginning. It is remarkable that these patients in spite of their progressive dementia continued to paint and some even improved their artistic skill. While it can be debated whether these types of dementias actually enhance creativity and abstraction as opposed to releasing productivity with increasing distortion of works as the dementia progresses, that they could create works of art at all is amazing.

It is important to note that the left hemisphere in right-handed individuals is almost always dominant for language and primarily mediates verbal activities, whereas the right hemisphere ("nondominant") appears to be more important for affective, spatial, and musical skills. Miller noted that brain atrophy in these patients who developed artistic activities had a predominance in the left frontal and temporal lobes, relatively sparing the right side of the brain, possibly sparing their creative skills in nonverbal activities.

An important question is what effect does frontotemporal lobar degeneration have on people who have already acquired the skills of an artist? The first case report to address this question was by Mell (2003). who reported a woman who had been trained as an artist long before the onset of her disease. There was continued art production through the course of her disease, and an increasing trend towards more "abstract" works, though in the late stage of her disease her art began to show severe degradation and signs of hemispatial neglect. Finney & Heilman (2007) conducted a study in another patient with progressive nonfluent aphasia and used an artistic quality rating tool to quantify the differences in her artwork before and after the onset of dementia, having independent judges rate the art works. The qualities assessed included novelty, aesthetics, representation, technique, and closure. Interestingly, during the period for which art was available, in this already trained artist, no changes in skill were noted, and even though the raters did not know the order of the paintings, they rated those done latest in the course of the disease as the least novel. It should be noted that the patient did show lightening of her color palette, simplification of her details, and distortion of angles in her artwork.

Drago et al. (2006) conducted a similar investigation by studying 40 paintings of an artist affected by semantic dementia. Their findings were consistent with previous studies, showing an increase of some visual artistic skills over time. To help explain why brain dysfunction can result in the emergence of a new or improved skill, Kapur (1996) suggested that facilitation of a function might be induced by a lesion that destroys an inhibitory circuit (i.e., a "paradoxical functional facilitation"). Miller and his coworkers (1998 and 2000) suggested that perhaps a similar phenomenon was occurring in their patients and the left anterior temporal lobe degeneration "contributed to the unexpected emergence of talent in our patients."

The aforementioned studies are interesting and provide important insights concerning visuospatial ability and visual artistic skills in patients affected by FTD, and some would suggest they also illuminate the systems subsuming creativity. It is important to mention all those studies indicating the effects of brain damage on the capacity to produce visual art.

The effects of brain damage on the capacity to produce visual art contrast sharply with many other human capacities. Disease of the brain commonly impairs our ability to speak or comprehend language, to coordinate movements, and to recognize objects. By contrast, while diseases of the brain can certainly alter the ability to produce art, in many cases, it is not so clear that the results are "impaired." Paradoxically, on some cases, patients' creativity is enhanced and their art seems to improve (Chatterjee, 2006).In a paper about "conferring capacity," Chatterjee (2006) argues that in these cases and in those of autism (Selfe, 1977) and subarachnoid hemorrhage (Lythgoe, 2005), the issue is a change in personality that produces obsessive compulsive disease characteristics, predisposing individuals to produce art. Caution is needed to discuss the "enhancing" effects of brain damage on artistic production; it not at all clear if it is "creative" in the true sense.

Support for the hypothesis that the nondominant (typically right) hemisphere is important in creativity comes from several sources. One prominent view of creativity is that it is based on the processing of remote or loose associations between ideas (Mednick, 1962). Recent research implicates the brain's right hemisphere in the processing of remote associates and the left hemisphere in the processing of close association (for a review, Jung-Beeman, 2005). Asari (2008) examined unique perception using functional MRI by having 68 healthy participants view 10 ambiguous figures from the Rorschach inkblot test (Rorschach, 1921) and state what they thought the figures looked like. There was greater activity in the right temporopolar region at times when participants gave a unique response when compared to times of frequent responses. Carlsson (2000) found that cerebral blood perfusion differed between high and low creativity individuals during the alternate use of object task, with bilateral frontal activation response seen in the high creativity individuals, but only left (presumably dominant) frontal activation response in low creativity individuals. This may be due to more efficient but less extensive processing in the less creative individuals. It may also reflect that there is a specific role for the non-dominant hemisphere.

Drago et al. (2009) studied an artist with Parkinson's disease who subsequently had a left deep brain stimulator (DBS) implanted. DBS can induce activation in one or both hemispheres. Based on the hypothesis of a "paradoxical functional facilitation," the study sought to learn if DBS of the left hemisphere, presumably inducing left hemisphere activation, would impact the creativity of a professional artist and her ability to judge art. The patient completed a test of creativity with the stimulator on and then with it off. The patient was also asked to judge the artwork of others in both the on and off stimulation states. The results suggested the possibility that left ventral STN/SNr (subthalamic nuclei/substantia nigra reticular) DBS reduced creativity as well as appreciation of art. The reason for this might be related to enhanced activation of the left hemisphere and reciprocal deactivation of the right hemisphere which mediates both visuospatial skills and global attention, both of which might be important in artistic creativity and appreciation of art.

The hemispheric lateralization model grew in the 1970s. Researchers espousing this model postulated that the nondominant hemisphere was specialized for creative activities such as holistic pattern recognition, art, and music. At the beginning of the chapter when creativity was defined, we discussed the concept of "finding the thread that unites" and "finding unity in what appears to be diversity" (Bronowski, 1972). The nondominant right hemisphere is thought to be more important in global than local processing (Robertson et al., 1988) and if a key component to creativity is the ability to unify disparate elements, then a global approach may be important in "finding the thread that unites." The nondominant right hemisphere is also thought to be important in mediating visual-spatial functions (Benton & Tranel, 1993), which may be important for a number of creative endeavors. The hemispheric lateralization model suggests nondominant right hemisphere mediates functions that are important for creative processing. An EEG study conducted by Jausovec (2000) recorded the EEGs of 115 healthy individuals during resting, "eyes open" and "eyes closed" condition and found that when they were stratified by measures of creativity and intelligence, EEG coherence (obtained during "rest" with eyes open) was significantly related to creativity scores, particularly in the right hemisphere.

Coherence provides information about the cooperation of different areas of the brain and functional relations between brain regions. Coherence measures may be sensitive to differences in intelligence and creativity Haier's (1992) cortical efficiency theory suggests that differences between individuals with good and poor achievements are indicated by the amount of neural activity required to sustain a given level of cognitive activity (Reiterer, 2002). The concept originally introduced by Ertl (1969), was reintroduced by the group of Richard Haier by investigating the relationship between intelligence and brain glucose metabolism with the help of positron emission tomography (PET) (1992). Haier and his co-authors (Haier et al., 1988, 1995, 1992) found a negative correlation between intelligence measures and glucose consumption. Their results have been interpreted as an expression of higher cortical efficiency in performance groups with higher intellect ("smarter brains burn less glucose") and vice versa.

THE ROLE OF THE FRONTO-TEMPORAL LOBES

Thomas Edison is commonly quoted as saying that being a creative genius required "ninety-nine percent perspiration and one percent inspiration" (Beals, 1996). To be successful, creative people often need to have perseverance and persistence. Goal-oriented behaviors and volition rely predominantly on the frontal lobes. Patients with degeneration of the frontal lobes often present with a loss of initiative and drive (abulia). The ability to generate and maintain long-term goals and to suppress biological drives when they interfere with those goals, as well as the ability to persist and not be distracted, is what Heilman calls "frontal intelligence" (Heilman, 2004). Frontal intelligence as conceptualized by Heilman is probably one of the major factors underlying success in any profession, including those that require creativity. Additionally, the frontal lobe networks have another function that appears to be important for creativity, divergent thinking.

Divergent thinking as alluded to previously is the ability to take a different direction from prevailing modes of thought or expression (Williams James, 1890). Zangwell (1966) and Milner (1984) suggested frontal lobe dysfunction would disrupt divergent thinking. As previously mentioned, highly creative individuals possess higher baseline frontal lobe activity and greater increases in frontal lobe activity measured by regional cerebral blood flow while performing creative tasks (Carlsson, 2000). There is also evidence that transcranial magnetic stimulation applied to the frontal lobes can increase creativity in healthy participants during drawing and writing tasks (Snyder, 2004). Case reports of patients whose creativity increased after receiving subcortical deep brain stimulation with the electrodes placed near the nucleus accumbens, which has strong connections to the frontal and temporal lobes, have also been reported (Flaherty, 2005; Gabriëls, 2003). The dorsolateral prefrontal cortex supports the planning and organization, while the cingulate cortex has been implicated in the modulation of drive and emotion. In addition, there is evidence suggesting that creative drive may be controlled through interactions among the frontal lobes, temporal lobes, and the limbic system (Flaherty, 2005), with creative drive increasing with temporal lobe dysfunction and increasing dopaminergic activity. Creative block occurs with deficits in frontal lobe activity or decreasing dopaminergic activity.

OTHER GRAY MATTER SYSTEMS IMPLICATED IN CREATIVITY

The neurobiology of creativity has also been addressed using single photon emission computerized tomography (SPECT), positron emission tomography (PET), and functional magnetic resonance imaging (fMRI). Chavez et al. (2004) used SPECT to study 12 highly creative subjects while performing figural and verbal creative tasks. These authors found a positive relationship between the creativity index and cerebral blood flow in the right postcentral gyrus, bilateral rectus gyrus, right inferior parietal lobule, and right parahippocampal gyrus. These findings were interpreted as supporting a "highly distributed brain system" underlying creativity (Chavez et al., 2004). PET was used to study normal subjects as they performed verbal creativity tasks, with significant brain activation being observed in the left parieto-temporal brain regions (Brodmann's areas 39 and 40), which are considered to be "crucial" to the creative process (Bechtereva et al., 2004). An fMRI study attempted to localize creative story generation within the brains of a cohort of 8 normal subjects (Howard-Jones, 2005). The results indicated that when creative story generation was contrasted to uncreative story generation, significant activations were observed within bilateral medial frontal gyri (Brodmann's areas 9 and 10) and the left anterior cingulate gyrus (BA 32). Across all studies, no clear consensus has emerged as to whether frontal or more posterior brain regions are more central to creative processes.

THE ROLE OF WHITE MATTER IN CREATIVITY

Given that creativity often draws on novel connections, it may require intra and interhemispheric communication between several brain systems. Works of scientific or artistic creativity often require skills and knowledge known to be subserved by both cerebral hemispheres. For example, the sculptor must imagine the rotation of spatial images mediated by the nondominant right hemisphere, while at the same time he uses motor skills mediated by the dominant left hemisphere. Thus, intra- and interhemispheric communication could be crucial for integrating, especially in novel ways, knowledge and skills that depend on both hemispheres. The largest white matter structure connecting the "independent" modular systems represented by the two hemispheres is the corpus callosum. Lewis (1979) administered the Rorschach test to eight patients with drug resistant epilepsy before and after cerebral commissurotomy. Disconnection of the two cerebral hemispheres tended to destroy "creativity" as measured by this test. Frederic Bremer suggested that the corpus callosum subserves the highest and most elaborate activities of the brain, including, conceivably, creativity. The corpus callosum is primarily comprised of myelinated axons whose cells bodies are in the pyramidal layers of the cerebral cortex. The cerebral connections important for creativity, however, might not only be inter-hemispheric, but also intra-hemispheric.

In addition to the myelinated axons that carry information between the hemispheres, from the thalamus and basal ganglia to the cortex, and from the cortex to the basal ganglia, thalamus, brain stem, and spinal cord, these myelinated axons also carry information between cortical regions in the same hemisphere. These intra-hemispheric connections facilitate intra-hemispheric communication, which also might be important for creative innovation because widespread connectivity allows creative people to combine the representations of ideas that have been previously isolated (Heilman, 2003). In addition, these intra-hemispheric white matter connections that include connections between the frontal lobes and the posterior association area in the temporal and parietal lobes might allow the selective activation or inhibition of cognitive modules.

Connectionist and parallel distributed processing (PDP) models are based on using processing units or nodes that are thought to be similar to the neurons found in the brain. PDP models strongly simulate the fundamental properties of neural networks. Information in PDP networks is stored in the strengths of connections between units (as in the brain) and concepts are represented as patterns of activity involving many units (as distributed representations) (Rumelhart, 1986). A large number of units linked by a set of connections define a domain of knowledge from which any one of a large number of concepts can be generated. Psychological studies of priming effects on lexical decision latency tasks are a good demonstration of the ability of this model to account for empirical results. Mednick (1962) suggested that in generating associative responses to a stimulus, creative individuals are characterized by a broader associative hierarchy or network than less creative individuals. Hence, creative people might be able to activate broader, more highly distributed networks.

RELAXATION, SEMANTIC NETWORK ACTIVATION, AND CREATIVITY

As previously noted, several scientists have reported solving difficult scientific problems during sleep or during transitions from sleep to wake and vice versa. These moments of insight appear to occur at times when people are relaxed or at rest. Eysenck (1995) suggested that during conscious problem solving, cortical arousal is high and this high level of cortical arousal narrows the associative field or semantic network and thus suppresses the ability to make remote associations, but that lowered arousal might allow these remote associations to emerge. Support for the theory that the level of arousal might determine the size of neural networks comes from some recent research by Contreras and Llinas (2001). Using high-speed optical imaging, they electrically stimulated subcortical white matter in the slices of brain from a guinea pig to record the portion of the neocortex activated by subcortical stimulation. Low-frequency stimulation cortical activation was limited at the beginning, and then, after a few milliseconds, the activation spread into nearby areas. High frequency stimulation, on the other hand, saw the excitation remain fixed to a small column of neurons directly above the stimulating electrode. Intracellular recording from the neurons around the excited column during rapid stimulation actually revealed increased inhibitory synaptic activity that probably helped account for the inhibition of the spread of activation.

Several researchers have investigated reports of depression and bipolar disorder in creative individuals (Kraepelin, 1921, Post, 1996). Through the study of biographies of composers, scientists, artists, and writers, a high incidence of affective disorders was identified in this population and even their families. It would be reasonable to think that depression might facilitate creative innovation. However, the verification and productivity portions of the creative process require a high level of arousal and focus, and thus, it might be that depressed individuals have very creative ideas but it would be very difficult for them to produce creative products.

THE ROLE OF DOPAMINE IN CREATIVITY

Creative people have higher baseline arousal and heightened responses to sensory stimulation (Martindale, 1999). Dopamine raises baseline arousal and decreases latent inhibition, a behavioral index of the ability to habituate to sensation (Ellenbroek et al., 1996; Swerdlow et al., 2003). The focused aspect of creative drive may be driven by mesolimbic dopaminergic activity, though this drive system is known to be involved in other drive activities and is not specific to creativity. Dopamine also mediates reward-seeking activity, ranging from gambling and cocaine addiction to the appreciation of beautiful faces and music (Aharon et al., 2001; Breiter et al., 2001). However, as in many brain systems, too much dopamine may cause excessively focused, highly complex motor stereotypes, such as repeatedly disassembling and reassembling one's motorcycle engine or performing obsessive painting (Fernandez & Friedman, 1999; Chatterjee et al., 2006). Dopamine may also play a role in creative discovery through its effect on novelty seeking, possibly an element in curiosity. An allele of the D4 receptors has been postulated somewhat controversially to increase novelty-seeking (Keltikangas-Jarvinen et al., 2003; Savitz & Ramesar, 2004). Drago (2009) examined the performance on a test of creativity in a group of Parkinson's disease patients. Patients were divided by side of onset, with the a priori hypothesis that patients with a right hemibody, and thus left hemisphere, onset Parkinson's disease would be more impaired in verbal creativity whereas patients with left hemibody (right hemisphere) onset would have more problems with a test of visuospatial creativity, as compared to healthy controls. The results indicated a decline in verbal creativity in the group of patients with right hemibody onset Parkinson's disease compared to controls. Foster (2008) also performed a study looking at dopamine levels and sematic networks in a population of Parkinson's patients. They sought to investigate the effects of Parkinson's disease (PD), which is associated with dopamine depletion, on spreading activation in the lexical networks, looking at the average word frequency of the controlled oral word association test in Parkinson's patients and controls. This measure was treated as an index of spreading activation. The PD patients exhibited a lower average word frequency, suggesting increased spreading activation, and a significant relationship between the strength of the initial activation and subsequent extent of spreading activation.

Catecholamines are believed to modulate the size of neuronal networks as demonstrated in the priming study of Kischka (1996) that used a lexical priming task with either real words or pseudowords flashed on screen; participants were instructed to press a computer key as quickly as possible when the word on the screen was real, but not to press the key if it was a pseudoword. Sometimes these real words and pseudowords were preceded by another word that served as a prime. The more the prime and the target word were associated (direct priming), the more rapid the recognition of the real target word. The less the two real words were related (indirect priming), the less the influence of the prime on word recognition and response time. When healthy participants were administered L-Dopa, the indirect priming effect decreased, suggesting that dopamine reduced the spread of semantic activation, which was the conclusion reached by Kischka et al. However, L-Dopa is a precursor not solely of dopamine, but also of norepinephrine, and the administration of L-Dopa to these individuals may have also increased the level of norepinephrine, which could be constricting the spread of semantic activation seen in this experiment.

It has been suggested that all these different states (such as relaxation, depression, resting, etc.) share an alteration of the brain's neurotransmitter systems, specifically a reduction of catecholamines including norepinephrine (McCarley, 1982) that might increase creative thinking.

INHIBITORY EFFECTS OF NOREPINEPHRINE ON CREATIVITY

To test the influence of norepinephrine on cognitive flexibility, Beversdorf (1999) tested participants with anagrams when taking either placebo, the pro-adrenergic drug ephedrine, or the beta-adrenergic blocker propanolol. Performance on the anagram task improved after participants took propanolol. Further support for the idea that high levels of adrenergic activity might reduce cognitive performances comes from a study where students with test anxiety improved their score on the scholastic aptitude test when given the beta adrenergic blocker propanolol (Faigel, 1991). Martindale (1973) found that during stressful conditions, when it would be expected that sympathetic tone would be elevated, performance on the remote association test declined.

Farah et al. (2008) did a study looking at Adderall (mixed amphetamine salts) and creativity, to find out whether Adderall impairs creativity in healthy young adults. Their preliminary evidence was consistent with the hypothesis that Adderall has an overall negative effect on creativity. Its effects on divergent creative thought cannot be inferred with confidence from this study because of the ambiguity of null results. Its effects on convergent creative thought appear to be dependent on the baseline creativity of the individual. Those in the higher range of the normal distribution may be unaffected or impaired, whereas those in the lower range of the normal distribution experience enhancement (Farah et al., 2008).

Ghacibeh (2006) studied people with vagus nerve stimulators for medically intractable partial epilepsy, assessing its impact on creativity and cognitive flexibility. He found that creativity and cognitive flexibility were both reduced during stimulation, in keeping with the hypothesis that since vagus nerve stimulation could activate the neurons in the locus coeruleus (LC), resulting in increased release of norepinephrine, vagus nerve stimulation should reduce creativity and cognitive flexibility.

Closure on Creativity

This chapter serves to introduce the concept, theories, investigation, and understanding of creativity. We are just beginning to understand the neuroanatomical and neurochemical correlates of creativity, and are still at an early stage in our understanding. How much of the observed differences in the brains of highly creative people is the source of their creativity or the result of that creativity remains to be seen. Creativity is a necessary and important part of living successfully in a world where we do not know all the answers, a world that we are still exploring. Understanding the neurological underpinnings of creativity will allow us to identify and develop treatment and rehabilitation strategies for those who have difficulty engaging in creative activity.

Many of the greatest acts of creativity, or genius, were presaged by the simple act of relaxation. At the beginning of the 21st century, as information technology blurs the lines between work and recreation and relaxation, truly relaxed periods of time are in danger of disappearing. If we value creativity and set as a goal to increase creativity and innovation, we need to build into our lives and society protected time simply to be, and allow our brains to find their own way to new heights of achievement that we otherwise may miss in our hectic day-to-day lives.

References

Aharon, I., Etcoff, N., Ariely, D., Chabris, C. F., O'Connor, E., & Breiter, H. C. (2001). Beautiful faces have variable reward value: fMRI and behavioral evidence. *Neuron, 32*(3), 537–551.

Asari, T., Konishi, S., Jimura, K., Chikazoe, J., Nakamura, N., & Miyashita, Y. (2008). Right temporal activation associated with unique perception. *Neuroimage, 41*, 142–152.

Barron, F., & Harrington, D. M. (1981). Creativity, intelligence and personality. *Annual Review of Psychology, 32*, 439–476.

Beals, G. (1996). Thomas Edison's home page. Retrieved from www.thomasedison.com

Bechtereva, N. P., Korotkov, A. D., Pakhomov, S. V., Roudas, M. S., Starchenko, M. G., & Medvedev, S. V. (2004). PET study of brain maintenance of verbal creative activity. *International Journal of Psychophysiology, 53*(1), 11–20.

Benton, A., & Tranel, D. (1993). Visuoperceptual, visuospatial, and visuoconstructive disorders. In K. M. Heilman, & E. Valenstein (Eds.), *Clinical Neuropsychology*: New York: Oxford University Press.

Beversdorf, D. Q., Hughes, J. D., Steinberg, B. A., Lewis, L. D., Heilman, K. M. Noradrenergic modulation of cognitive flexibility in problem solving. (1999). *Neuroreport, 10*(13), 2763–2767.

Binet, A. (1886). La psychologie du raisonnement. Paris, Alcan. (Published in English as The psychology of reasoning. Chicago, IL: Open Court, 1896).

Breiter, H. C., Aharon, I., Kahneman, D., Dale, A., & Shizgal, P. (2001). Functional imaging of neural responses to expectancy and experience of monetary gains and losses. *Neuron, 30*(2), 619–639.

Bronowski, J. (1972). *Science and Human Values*. New York: Harper & Row.

Carlsson, I., Wendt, P. E., & Risberg, J. (2000). On the neurobiology of creativity. Differences in frontal activity between high and low creative subjects. *Neuropsychologia, 38*, 873–885.

Cattell, R. B. (1963). The theory of fluid and crystallized intelligence: A critical experiment. *Journal of Educational Psychology*, 54, 1–22.

Chatterjee, A. (2006). The neuropsychology of visual art: conferring capacity. *International Review of Neurobiology, 74*, 39–49.

Chavez, R. A., Graff-Guerrero, A., Garcia-Reyna, J. C., Vaugier, V., & Cruz-Fuentes, C. (2004). Neurobiology of creativity: preliminary results from a brain activation study. *Salud Mental, 27*(3), 38–46.

Contreras, D., & Llinas, R. (2001). Voltage-sensitive dye imaging of neocortical spatiotemporal dynamics to afferent activation frequency. *Journal of Neuroscience, 21*(23), 9403–9413.

Csikszentmihalyi, M. (1988) Motivation and creativity: Toward a synthesis of structural and energistic approaches to cognition. *New Ideas in Psychology, 6*(2), 159–76.

Csikszentmihalyi, M. (1999) Implications of a Systems Perspective for the study of creativity. In R. J. Sternberg (Ed.), *Handbook of Creativity* (pp. 313–335). New York: Cambridge University Press.

Csikszentmihalyi, M. (1996). *Creativity: Flow and the psychology of discovery and invention.* New York: Harper Collins.

Drago, V., Foster, P. S., Trifiletti, D., FitzGerald, D. B., Kluger, B. M., Crucian, G. P., & Heilman, K. M. (2006). What's inside the art? The influence of frontotemporal dementia in art production. *Neurology, 67*(7), 1285–1287.

Drago, V., Foster, P. S., Okun, M. S., Haq, I., Sudhyadhom, A., Skidmore, F. M., & Heilman, K. M. (2009). Artistic creativity and DBS: A case report. *Journal of the Neurological Sciences, 276*, 138–142.

Drago, V., Foster, P. S., Skidmore, F. M., & Heilman, K. M. (2009). Creativity in Parkinson's disease as a function of right versus left hemibody onset. *Journal of the Neurological Sciences, 276*(1–2), 179–183.

Ellenbroek, B. A., Budde, S., & Cools, A. R. (1996). Prepulse inhibition and latent inhibition: The role of dopamine in the medial prefrontal cortex. *Neuroscience, 75*(2), 535–542.

Ertl, J. & Schafer, E. (1969). Brain Response correlates of psychometric intelligence. *Nature*, 223, 421–422.

Eysenck, H. L. (1995). *Genius*. New York and Cambridge: Cambridge University Press.

Faigel, H. C. (1991). The effect of beta blockade on stress-induced cognitive dysfunction in adolescents. *Clinical Pediatrics, 30*, 441–445.

Flaherty, A. W. (2005). Frontotemporal and dopaminergic control of idea generation and creative drive. *Journal of Comparative Neurology, 493*, 147–153.

Fernandez, H. H., & Friedman, J. H. (1999). Punding on L-dopa. *Movement Disorders, 14*, 836–838.

Finney, G. R., & Heilman, K. M. (2007). Artwork before and after onset of progressive nonfluent aphasia. *Cognitive and Behavioral Neurology, 20*, 7–10.

Foster, P. S., Drago, V., FitzGerald, D. B., Skoblar, B. M., Crucian, G. P., Heilman, K. M. (2008). Spreading activation of lexical–semantic networks in Parkinson's disease. *Neuropsychologia, 46*(7), 1908–1914.

Gabriëls, L., Cosyns, P., Nuttin, B., Demeulemeester, H., & Gybels, J. (2003). Deep brain stimulation for treatment-refractory obsessive-compulsive disorder: Psychopathological and neuropsychological outcome in three cases. Preview. *Acta Psychiatrica Scandinavica, 107*(4), 275–282.

Ghacibeh, G. A., Shenker, J. I., Shenal, B., Uthman, B. M., & Heilman, K. M. (2006). Effect of vagus nerve stimulation on creativity and cognitive flexibility. *Epilepsy and Behavior*, 8(4), 720–725.

Goff, K., & Torrance, E. P. (2002). *Abbreviated Torrance test for Adults Manual*. Bensenville, IL: Scholastic Testing Service.

Gorno-Tempini, M. L., Dronkers NF, Rankin KP, Ogar JM, Phengrasamy L, Rosen HJ, Johnson JK, Weiner MW, Miller BL (2004) Cognition and anatomy in three variants of primary progressive aphasia. *Annals of Neurology, 55*, 335–346.

Guilford, J. P. (1950). Creativity research: Past, present, and future. *American Psychologist, 5*, 444–454.

Guilford, J. P., & Christensen, P. W. (1973). The one way relationship between creative potential and IQ. *Journal of Creative Behavior, 7*, 247–252.

Haier, R. J., Siegel, B. V., Nuechterlein, K. H., Hazlett, E., Wu, J. C., Peak, J., Browning, H. L., & Buchsbaum, M. S. (1988). Cortical glucose metabolic rate correlates of abstract reasoning and attention studied with Positron Emission Tomography. *Intelligence*, 11, 199–218.

Haier, R. J., Siegel, B. V., Maclachlan, A., Soderling, E., Lottenberg, S., Buchsbaum, M. S. (1992). Regional glucose metabolic changes after learning a complex visuospatial/motor task: A positron emission tomographic study. *Brain Research*, 570, 134–143.

Haier, R., Siegel, B., Tang, Ch., Abel, L., Buchsbaum, M. (1992). Intelligence and changes in regional cerebral glucose metabolic rate following learning. *Intelligence*, 16, 415–426.

Haier, R., Larson, G., LaCasse, L., Hazen, K. (1995). Evaluation of a Mental Effort Hypothesis for Correlations between Cortical Metabolism and Intelligence. *Intelligence*, 21, 267–278.

Heilman, K. M. (2004). *Creativity and the Brain*. New York: Oxford.

Heilman, K. M., Nadeau, S. E., Beversdorf, D. O. (2003), Creative Innovation: Possible Brain Mechanisms, *Neurocase, 9*, 369–379.

Heilman, K. M. & Valenstein E. (2012). *Clinical Neuropsychology* (5th ed., pp. 637–654). New York: Oxford University press.

Helmholtz, H. (1826/1995). Vortrage und reden. In H. Eysenck (Ed.), *Genius. The natural history of creativity*. Cambridge, UK: Cambridge University Press.

Herr, Edwin L., et al. (1965). Creativity, intelligence, and values: A study of relationships. *Exceptional Children, 32*(2), 114–115.

Howard-Jones, P. A., Blakemore, S. J., Samuel, E. A., Summers, I. R., & Claxton, G. (2005). Semantic divergence and creative story generation: An fMRI investigation. *Cognitive Brain Research, 25*(1), 240–250.

Hutcheson, F., An Inquiry into the Original of our Ideas of Beauty and Virtue…, London: J. Darby, 1725, 4/1738, Treatise I, section 2, in le Huray/Day, p. 24.

James, W. (1890). *The Principles of Psychology*. New York: Dover.

Jausovec, N., & Jausovec, K. (2000). Differences in resting EEG related to ability. *Brain Topography, 12*, 229–240.

Kapur, N. (1996). Paradoxical functional facilitation in brain-behavior research. *Brain, 119*, 1775–1790.

Keltikangas-Järvinen, L., Elovainio, M., Kivimäki, M., Lichtermann, D., Ekelund, J., & Peltonen, L. (2003). Association between the type 4 dopamine receptor gene polymorphism and novelty seeking. *Psychosomatic Medicine, 65*, 471–476.

Kischka, U., Kammer, T., Maier, S., Weisbrod, M., Thimm, M., & Spitzer, M. (1996). Dopaminergic modulation of semantic network activation. *Neuropsychologia, 34*, 1107–1113.

Kraepelin, E. (1921). *Manic-depressive insanity and paranoia* (R. M. Barclay, trans.). Edinburgh: E. & S. Livingstone.

Kuhn, T. S. (1996). *The Structure of Scientific Revolutions* (3rd ed.). Chicago: University of Chicago Press.

Lewis, R. T. (1979). Organic sign, creativity, and personality characteristic of patients following cerebral commissurotomy. *Clinical Neuropsychologist, 1*, 29–33.

Lythgoe, M., Polak, T., Kalmus, M., de Haan, M., & Khean Chong, W. (2005). Obsessive, prolofic artistic output following subarachnoid hemorrhage. *Neurology, 64*, 397–398.

Martindale, C. (1999). Biological bases of creativity. In R. J. Sternberg (Ed.), Handbook of creativity (pp. 137–152). New York, NY: Cambridge University Press.

Martindale C., & Greenough, J. (1973). The differential effect of increased arousal on creative and intellectual performance. *Journal of Genetic Psychology, 123*, 392–335.

McCarley, R. W. (1982). REM sleep and depression: Common neurobiological control mechanisms. *American Journal of Psychiatry, 139*, 565–570.

Mednick, S. A. (1962). The associative basis of the creative process. *Psychological Review, 9*, 220–232.

Mell, J. C., Howard, S. M., Miller, B. L. (2003, May 27). Art and the brain: the influence of frontotemporal dementia on an accomplished artist. *Neurology, 60*(10), 1707–1710.

Metcalfe, J., & Wiebe, D. (1987). Intuition in insight and noninsight problem solving, *Memory & Cognition, 15*, 238–246.

Miller, B. L., Boone, K., Cummings, J. L., Read, S. L., & Mishkin, F. (2000). Functional correlates of musical and visual ability in frontotemporal dementia. *British Journal of Psychiatry, 176*, 458–463.

Miller B. L., Cummings J., Mishkin, F., Boone K., Prince F., Poton, M., & Cotman, C. (1998). Emergence of artistic talent in frontotemporal dementia. *Neurology, 51*, 978–982.

Milner, B. (1984). Behavioural effects of frontal-lobe lesions in man. *Trends in Neurosciences, 7*, 403–407.

Post, F. (1996). Verbal creativity, depression, and alcoholism. An investigation of one hundred American and British writers. *British Journal of Psychiatry, 168*, 545–555.

Reiterer, S. M. (2002). EEG coherence analysis and foreign language processing. Differences Between Language Students (English) and Students of Other Disciplines During the Processing of Natural Language Stimuli (TV texts) in British English, American English and German. Dissertation zum Erlangen des Doktorgrades der Naturwissenschaften an der Human und Sozialwissenschaftlichen Fakultät der Universität Wien in dem Studienfach Psychologie.

Robertson, L. C., Lamb, M. R., & Knight, R. T. (1988). Effects of lesions of temporal parietal junction on perceptual and attentional processing in humans. *Journal of Neurosciences, 8*, 3757–3769.

Rorschach, H. (1921). Psychodiagnostik: Methodik und ergebnisse eines wahrnehmungsdiagnostischen experiments. Bern: Ernst Bircher.

Rumelhart, D. E., & McClelland, J. L. (1986). *Parallel Distributed Processing: Explorations in the Microstructure of Cognition*, Vols. 1 and 2. Cambridge, MA: MIT Press.

Savitz, J. B., & Ramesar, R. S. (2004). Genetic variants implicated in personality: A review of the more promising candidates. *American Journal of Medical Genetics B Neuropsychiatric Genetics, 131B*(1), 20–32.

Shavinina, L. V. (Ed) (2003), *The International Handbook on Innovation*. New York, NY, US: Elsevier Science.

Simonton, D. K. (1994). *Greatness: Who Makes History and Why?* New York: Guilford Press.

Simonton, D. K. (1999). *Origins of Genius: Darwinian Prospective on Creativity*. New York: Oxford.

Snyder, A., Bossomaier, T., & Mitchell, D. J. (2004). Concept formation: "Object" attributes dynamically inhibited from conscious awareness. *Journal of Integrated Neurosciences*, 3, 31–46.

Sternberg, R. J., & O'Hara, L. A. (1999). Creativity and intelligence. In R. J. Sternberg (Ed.), *Handbook of Creativity* (pp. 251–272). New York: Cambridge University Press.

Sternberg, R. J. (Ed.). (1999a). *Handbook of Creativity*. New York: Cambridge University Press.

Swerdlow, N. R., Stephany, N., Wasserman, L. C., Talledo, J., Sharp, R., & Auerbach, P. P. (2003). Dopamine agonists disrupt visual latent inhibition in normal males using a within-subject paradigm. *Psychopharmacology (Berl)*, *169*, 314–320.

Torrance, E. P. (1974). The Torrance test of creative thinking. Bensenville: Scholastic Testing Service.

Wallas, G. (1926). *The Art of Thought*. New York: Harcourt Brace.

Weisberg, R. W. (1986). *Creativity: Genius and Other Myths*. New York: W. H. Freeman.

Weisberg, R. W. (2006). Creativity: Understanding Innovation in Problem Solving, Science, Invention, and The Arts. Hoboken, NJ: John Wiley.

Zangwell, O. L. (1966). Psychological deficits associated with frontal lobe lesions. *International Journal of Neurology*, *5*, 395–402.

Afterword

Kenneth M. Heilman, Edward Valenstein, and Robert T. Watson

Note: The authors each knew Ken Heilman early in his neurology career. Ken was a year ahead of E.V. in the Neurology residency program at Boston City Hospital, and Ken later recruited him to join the faculty at the University of Florida (UF). R.T.W. began his neurology residency at UF on the same day that Ken joined the faculty.

Ken Heilman likes to tell of the customs officer who, after questioning passengers on the line before him in detail to verify their citizenship, told Ken to pass right through. "Aren't you going to even ask where I'm from?" Ken said. "You're from Brooklyn! Now move on." After eight years at the University of Virginia, two years in Turkey, three years in Boston, and forty years in north central Florida, Ken still talks and acts as if he never left Brooklyn. There may have been something about the Borough Park/Bensonhurst neighborhood that fostered individuality and academic success. Ken learned many years after he left Brooklyn that Norman Geschwind, Mel Greer, and Arthur Benton had grown up in the same neighborhood. Each of them had a profound influence on Ken's career.

A Little Early History

Ken's early education in Brooklyn did not always presage his success. He failed to complete an early achievement test, and was labeled as a non-honors student, a label that his difficulty mastering the niceties of English tended to support. But he was resilient and persistent, an avid reader with talent in the sciences, so he eventually overcame the label, and gained admittance to the University of Virginia, where he spent his undergraduate and medical student years, and where he met Patricia Phillips, who later became his wife.

Ken graduated from the University of Virginia School of Medicine, and did his internship and a year of residency on the Cornell Medical service at Bellevue

Hospital in New York. After serving two years in the Army based in Turkey, he chose to do his neurology residency at the Neurological Unit of the Boston City Hospital under Derek Denny-Brown. During Ken's first year of residency, in 1967, Denny-Brown suffered a heart attack, and retired from teaching and clinical responsibilities to continue his research at the New England Primate Center. During the search for a new Chief of Neurology, Simeon Locke and then Flaviu Romanul served as Interim Directors. In 1969, in the middle of Ken's second year of neurology residency, Norman Geschwind was appointed as the James Jackson Professor of Neurology to direct the neurological unit.

Neurology at the Boston City Hospital

The Harvard-associated neurological unit had been the premier training program in neurology in the middle of the 20th century (see Vilensky, Gilman and Sinish, 2004). The unit was founded in 1930, with Stanley Cobb as its first director. In 1934, Cobb was succeeded by Tracy Putnam, who with H. Houston Merritt had developed an experimental model for epilepsy in cats and discovered that diphenylhydantoin (phosphenytoin, Dilantin®) was effective in preventing experimentally induced seizures. Putnam resigned in 1939 to become chair of neurology and neurosurgery at the College of Physicians and Surgeons at Columbia University. Harvard President James Conant appointed Cobb to direct a search committee, and selected Derek Denny-Brown, who had established a reputation as a clinical researcher in England, initially in Sherrington's lab. Denny-Brown's research accomplishments spanned the field of neurology, with important discoveries in muscle histology, electromyography, the neurological control of micturition, and the cortical control of movement based on studies in humans and primates. Denny-Brown used the 10th floor of the Medical Building at Boston City Hospital to house his primates. The administrative offices, library, EEG lab, and conference room were on the ninth floor, and the neurology wards were on floors seven and eight. Denny-Brown's rigorous clinical training program and active research interests attracted some of the best physicians, many of whom became chairs of neurology at other institutions. His residents responded to his expectation that all residents would have a thorough command of their patients, including compulsive neurological assessments. To present a patient with sensory loss to Denny-Brown without a detailed sensory map was risking public humiliation.

Denny-Brown was a hard act to follow, and EV recalls that several of Denny-Brown's last residents did not think that Norman Geschwind would be up to the task of maintaining the stature of the neurological unit. Indeed, Geschwind had a very different pedagogical approach. Whereas Denny-Brown was dictatorial and aloof, Geschwind was affable and accessible. Every morning between work rounds and attending rounds, Geschwind would join residents and students in a small room opposite the conference room on the ninth floor of the Medical Building, and shoot the breeze over coffee, Cokes, and peanut butter crackers. These conversations were wide-ranging and always interesting, even more so when Ken was there.

While Geschwind's easy manner and enthusiasm signaled a change in leadership style, it became clear that his dedication to academics and to research was not less than Denny-Brown's. Geschwind retained Denny-Brown's primate facility (on the 10th floor of the Medical Building), and brought in Dee Pandya to continue his important anatomic investigations of cortical connectivity in primates. Geschwind had landed the job largely on the basis of his brilliant two-part treatise, "Disconnection Syndromes in Animals and Man" published in Brain in 1965. In this remarkable paper, Geschwind had reasserted the significance of anatomical connections in the brain in the analysis of the most complex behaviors. He demonstrated the relevance of animal studies to the understanding of human behavior, and had shown how hypotheses about cognitive activity could be tested scientifically. He was deeply schooled in the work of the classical neurologists, and resurrected syndromes that had been neglected for decades. For the young clinician attracted to neurology by the power of clinical analysis to localize pathology in the nervous system, expanding this to include the full range of cortical function was tremendously exciting. Geschwind's achievements, his unbounded enthusiasm, and his interest in and support of any resident or student who expressed an interest, inspired residents to consider academic careers. Ken was fascinated by the phenomenon of hemispatial neglect, and with Geschwind's encouragement, proposed to see if he could devise a primate model of this syndrome. With Dee Pandya's generous support and assistance, Ken operated on rhesus monkeys, and demonstrated that monkeys with parietal and frontal lesions evidenced features similar to patients with unilateral neglect (Heilman, Pandya, & Geschwind, 1970).

Ken realized that a host of questions about the neglect syndrome begged for additional studies both in animals and humans. But his experience working with monkeys, however productive, left him with an abiding dislike of the primate lab. Although he later supported primate work, and was actively engaged in designing experiments, he was careful to encourage others to perform the experiments. There was, after all, plenty of research that needed to be done with humans.

Moving to the University of Florida

At the conclusion of his residency, Ken was offered an instructorship at Harvard, but, with Geschwind's encouragement, he decided to look at other opportunities. Geschwind knew Mel Greer, then chief of the division of eurology at UF, and recommended him to Ken. Ken's visit to Gainesville was productive: he realized that Mel was a leader who would fully support his junior faculty. For his part, Mel immediately liked the young Dr. Heilman, and liked him even more when he heard Ken's requirements for research start-up: "Time, paper, and a pencil." What a deal!

Ken thrived at UF. Dr. Greer, known to all in the division of neurology as "the Chief," provided an ideal environment for junior faculty. The Chief treated his faculty and residents as well as students and staff as one big family; he created a safe environment in which everyone could focus on doing well. Not only did he shoulder the entire burden of administration; but he also took on himself the lion's share of clinical work, enough to support not only his own salary, but also a significant portion of his faculty's salaries. Ken could therefore concentrate on his research without the threat of losing his protected research time. For Mel, this turned out to be a very good investment. In a few years, Ken had secured research grants from the National Institutes of Health (NIH) and from the Veteran's Administration (VA), and his program has enjoyed almost continual grant support ever since. Even more important, Gainesville soon became recognized as a center for behavioral neurology research and training.

Great program builders are likely to be deft politicians and great administrators. Ken Heilman built an enduring behavioral neurology program at UF, but he does not have a political bone in his body, and he hates the bureaucratic demands of administration. The behavioral neurology program prospered principally because of the enthusiasm he generated in faculty and, more significantly, residents and students in various disciplines. He had an immediate impact on neurology residents, who theretofore had practically no instruction in behavioral neurology. R.T.W., who began his neurology residency on July 1, 1970, the same day that Ken joined the faculty, recalls one of his first encounters with this new attending physician:

> An early memory was calling him on a Saturday morning about a patient on the VA service, even though he was not the attending physician. To my surprise, he drove in to see the patient with me. As I would come to learn and even expect, Dr. Heilman made the experience enjoyable; he used the opportunity to teach. His enthusiasm was uplifting and the lessons learned enduring. There was something about Dr. Heilman's teaching and enthusiasm that quickly aroused my interest in behavioral neurology. The way he could explain aphasia, neglect, apraxia, and other disorders could turn what previously had been just another unfortunate patient with a stroke into a magnificent mind opening learning experience. He suggested that I might enjoy reading Dr. Geschwind's classic 1965 articles in *Brain*, "Disconnection Syndromes in Animals and Man." These articles were fascinating, and I enjoyed discussing them with Dr. Heilman. He, in his classic Socratic method, encouraged me to sometimes see patients as "experiments of nature," and to think about ways that these patients could help us understand how the brain functions.

It was also evident to graduate students in psychology and speech pathology that behavioral neurology was a wide-open field that leant itself to research, and that Ken Heilman could be an effective and enthusiastic mentor. Ken soon organized a weekly research meeting, and welcomed faculty from other disciplines: psychiatry, psychology, speech pathology, and experimental psychology, for starters. The interactions were mutually beneficial. Paul Satz, a neuropsychologist, was an active participant, and Ken learned much from Paul about experimental techniques and statistical analysis.

Later in his residency, R.T.W. decided that we needed a primate lab in which to test hypotheses about unilateral neglect. He described proposing this to Ken:

I thought it would be a great idea to utilize non-human primates to do behavioral research. It seemed to me that if we could design appropriate experiments, then make specific lesions, that we might be able to expand our knowledge beyond "experiments of nature." It would not be possible to describe how aghast Kenny was at the thought of working with "monkeys." He told me that if I really wanted to do it that I could, but never expect to see him at the primate colony. It was with that understanding that we moved forward. Kenny and I would spend untold hours thinking about a study, lesion localization, and how to measure the effects of specific lesions. It would often get humorous since we both have right-left confusion, which extended even to the diagrams we would sketch on his blackboard. With his encouragement, these experiments thrived and did add to our knowledge of higher cortical function. Even though he may never have seen one of the experimental subjects except on videotape, none of the ideas or experiments could have happened without his wisdom and encouragement.

R.T.W. continued his primate research after residency, having joined the faculty. By 1974, four years after Ken had arrived in Gainesville, R.T.W. had been on the faculty for one year. There was a well-run primate lab with a technician who treated the animals like pets, and there were several graduate students participating with Ken in human research. At that time, Fred Vroom, a fine clinical neurologist and the institution's sole electromyographer, left the university, leaving only four full-time faculty members in the department: the Chief, B.J. Wilder (the epileptologist), R.T.W., and Ken. Even though two of the four were behavioral neurologists, the Chief was so pleased with Ken's progress that he allowed him to travel to New Hampshire to persuade E.V. to move down from Dartmouth. He had to agree to do EMGs, and thus became a rare breed: a neurologist with expertise in both neuromuscular disease and cognitive neurology. Despite its size, neurology was profitable, and Mel was able to obtain departmental status in 1974. Mel remained chair of neurology until 2000. When he stepped down, he was the longest-serving head of neurology in the country. He had kept the department small and focused: in 2000 the department had only 11 full-time neurologists: five behavioral neurologists, four epileptologists, one electromyographer and the Chief.

In 1975, we decided at Ken's suggestion to advertise to a national audience for a continuing education course. We had enough faculty members at UF in psychology, speech and neurology to give most of the lectures, but Arthur Benton agreed to come from Iowa as a special guest. Because it was as much neuropsychology as neurology, we called it a Course in Behavioral Neurology and Neuropsychology. It was a great success, and under the sponsorship of the Florida Society of Neurology, it has been held annually ever since (the 35th Annual Course was presented in 2009). Most participants in all specialties were appreciative of the multidisciplinary nature of the course; but there were occasional persons who felt that we should not be attempting to venture outside the confines of our own profession. But we have always felt that reaching across disciplines was healthy and productive. Ken later sought Arthur Benton's advice about developing a text, and it was with Arthur's encouragement and help (he contributed two chapters) that the first edition of *Clinical Neuropsychology* was conceived in 1977 and published in 1979 (Heilman and Watson, 1979).

Ken decided to add a fellowship in 1977. Tom Van den Abell, Dawn Bowers (both psychologists) and Leslie Rothi, a speech pathologist, were early fellows. Subsequently, the fellowship attracted neurologists, psychologists, speech pathologists, and even one anthropologist. Many have contributed to this book. Ken could have had fellows earn their keep by seeing patients, but he wanted them to be learning and doing research. As the fellowship evolved, Ken got State support to run a memory disorder clinic each Wednesday afternoon. A psychiatrist and a social psychologist were also on its staff. One to three fellows (Ken was able to get research funding so that fellows could stay for two or more years) would see up to four patients each afternoon. Ken carefully examined each patient, and had a knack for finding new areas of interest. Many patients became case reports. When E.V. became Chair in 2000, he was under tremendous pressure from the administration to improve the department's clinical efficiency. Ken was a good friend, but resisted all entreaties that he improve clinic throughput. In retrospect, he was right. The memory disorder clinic was a true academic exercise that benefitted both patients and science.

Looking back, the 1970s seem almost idyllic. We were young and enthusiastic. Although each of us had clinical responsibilities— three or four months a year on the wards, which is nearly double our current schedule—clinical work paid well, and was much less intense than today and there seemed always to be time to talk over new ideas and plan new research projects. Research was also simpler. The tools we used were easily comprehensible. Anatomic imaging was in its infancy; there was no functional imaging. Physiological studies were still largely non-digital. There were also fewer bureaucratic impediments to research: no institutional review boards, no institutional animal care and use committees. So there was little delay between the conception and the execution of many of our research projects. When R.T.W. came up with an idea to disentangle attentional and intentional aspects of neglect, it took a while, with their combined right-left disorientation, to realize that it really made sense. It was really simple: you gave the monkey a tactile stimulus on one side of the body and trained it to respond with the opposite hand. The monkey lab was up and running, so Barbara Haws, our great lab technician, was soon training the monkeys. When Ken came up with the idea that some apraxics may have lost the concepts of correct praxic movements, while others may still have the concepts, but could not execute them, he and E.V. took 8mm movies under the live oak trees in the medical school parking lot of each of us making correct and incorrect movements, to create a test of praxis comprehension. To test grammatical comprehension, we drew stick-figure pictures illustrating reversible sentences.

Over the years, of the three of us, Ken has changed the least. While R.T.W. was becoming a national figure in medical education, and E.V. was assuming more clinical and administrative responsibilities, Ken has remained focused on behavioral neurology research, teaching, and mentoring a long and increasingly illustrious line of residents and fellows. At 70, he is as energetic and productive as he was in his 30s. The only difference is that now, every couple of years, Ken publishes a monograph. When E.V. and Kenny were on call together at Boston City Hospital, Ken would regale E.V. with stories of his early schooling—like his taking a bathroom break in the middle of an achievement test, that resulted in his being grouped with the slower learners in his class—his experiences in Turkey, how he dealt with bullies, and the like, but sometimes he would just sit and write. E.V. recalled that Ken told him he was writing a novel; but it turns out he was writing notes on his experiences in internship. He just recently published a book of them (Heilman, 2009). He has published a fascinating monograph on creativity (Heilman, 2005), and he is currently working on additional monographs.

Ken's behavioral neurology program has also stayed faithful to its original conception to study brain-behavior relationships. As an example, in the 1980s, an engineer who was working on a prototype magnetoencephalogram suggested that we might want to use this technique to study behavior. It was attractive, because magnetoencephlography offered a window on physiological events not restricted to the surface of the brain, like conventional electroencephalography. Ken resisted the temptation, reasoning that it would be largely a distraction, with more time spent in validating the technique than learning about the brain. Similarly, although interested in dementia, and skilled in its diagnosis and management, he did not gravitate toward disease-oriented research or clinical trials, even when funding sources favored this kind of research. But he encouraged two of his former fellows (now both professors of neurology), Leslie Gonzalez-Rothi and Steve Nadeau, to branch into neurorehabilitation research, and he is happy to use validated new techniques to further his research.

Kenny Heilman is a person of many interests, but he lives to be creative, to understand how the brain works. R.T.W. often told him that nothing seemed to excite him more than a good idea. Nothing seemed to give him as much pleasure as a paper being published showing fruition of that idea. Kenny and I have laughed about what I might say if I delivered his eulogy, particularly that I'm sure he would walk up to God and whisper in his ear, "Okay God, you can tell me now, how does the brain work?"

Dr. Heilman is one of the greatest teachers we have ever known. He has that rare ability, one he shared with Dr. Geschwind, of being able to teach anyone, and feeling that any interested person should receive his complete attention. Interestingly, he needs to teach using nothing but a blackboard or a flip chart. Somehow slides distract his stream of thinking. R.T.W. recalls the first of his talks that he attended at an Academy of Neurology meeting: Kenny was using slides, but they seemed to break his train of thought. R.T.W. suggested that he not use slides, and he never or rarely used slides (note that this should be "slides", not "slide")in subsequent presentations. Just last year, Kenny gave a talk to first year medical students without using slides. Students loved it: "Awesome! A lecture without PowerPoint!"

Kenny is usually a terrific speaker, but he can get inarticulate, particularly when describing mundane details. He once gave a talk on neglect of non-touch, a difficult concept, and during his talk he compounded the difficulty by getting right and left confused. R.T.W. was sitting behind three women during his talk and at the conclusion of his talk; Kenny asked if there were any questions. One of the women turned to another and whispered, "Can you repeat the entire talk?" Kenny was later told about this, and found it hilarious. R.T.W. comments, "His teaching ability is so amazing that whenever my wife, Carolyn, and Kenny's wife, Patricia, went to a meeting where Kenny was giving a talk, both wives would attend the talk. My wife, who has no background in neurology, would sit enthralled and talk excitedly about his talk later in the day. When my daughter, Mary, had a chance to spend time in clinic with Dr. Heilman as a fourth year medical student, she later wrote me an email letting me know that Dr. Heilman was the "greatest" teacher she had ever seen. Even though I agreed with her, I admit to being a little offended since I had tried many times to teach her myself."

There are very few people in one's life that are so special. Special because of the kind of person they are, their love of family, tradition, creativity, and joy in helping others learn. We have had the good fortune of knowing many fine and productive people both within academics and in other arenas. There is no one as special as Dr. Kenneth Martin Heilman. He stands alone as a thinker, innovator, teacher, and friend.

*Dr. Edward Valenstine died on March 8, 2013 after a long battle with cancer. Dr. Heilman and I continue to profoundly miss Ed. As I edit this last chapter that Ed and I worked on together it brings back so many memories of Ed as a friend, colleague and exemplary person. In some way this final book chapter that Ed and I wrote has special meaning.

References

Heilman, K. M. (2005). *Creativity and the Brain.* New York: Psychology Press.
Heilman, K. M. (2009). *Postgraduate Year One: Lessons in Caring.* New York: Oxford University Press.
Heilman, K. M., Pandya, D. N., & Geshchwind, N. (1970). Trimodal inattention following parietal ablations. *Transactions of the American Neurological Association, 95,* 259–261.
Heilman, K. M., & Valenstein, E. (1979) (Eds.). *Clinical Neuropsychology.* New York: Oxford University Press.
Vilensky, J. A., Gilman, S., & Sinish, P. R. (2004). Denny-Brown, Boston City Hospital, and the history of American neurology. *Perspectives in Biology and Medicine, 47,* 505–518.

INDEX